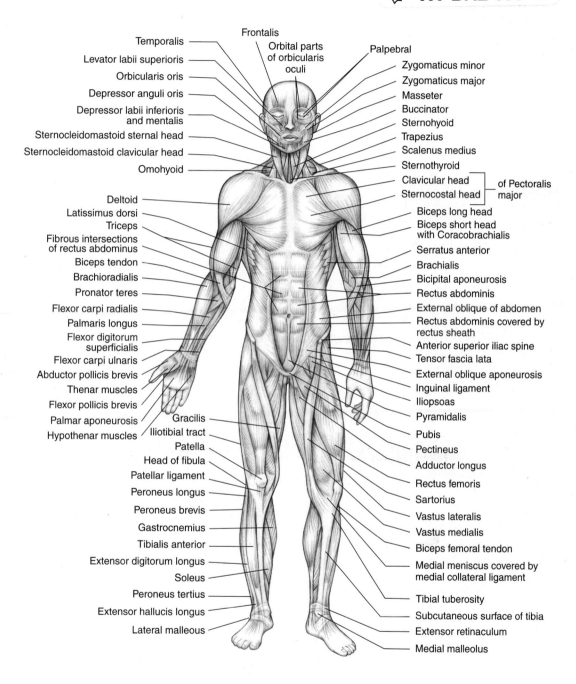

Frontalis
Temporalis
Orbital parts of orbicularis oculi
Palpebral
Levator labii superioris
Zygomaticus minor
Orbicularis oris
Zygomaticus major
Depressor anguli oris
Masseter
Depressor labii inferioris and mentalis
Buccinator
Sternohyoid
Sternocleidomastoid sternal head
Trapezius
Sternocleidomastoid clavicular head
Scalenus medius
Omohyoid
Sternothyroid
Clavicular head
Sternocostal head
of Pectoralis major
Deltoid
Latissimus dorsi
Biceps long head
Triceps
Biceps short head with Coracobrachialis
Fibrous intersections of rectus abdominus
Serratus anterior
Biceps tendon
Brachialis
Brachioradialis
Bicipital aponeurosis
Pronator teres
Rectus abdominis
Flexor carpi radialis
External oblique of abdomen
Palmaris longus
Rectus abdominis covered by rectus sheath
Flexor digitorum superficialis
Anterior superior iliac spine
Flexor carpi ulnaris
Tensor fascia lata
Abductor pollicis brevis
External oblique aponeurosis
Thenar muscles
Inguinal ligament
Flexor pollicis brevis
Iliopsoas
Palmar aponeurosis
Gracilis
Pyramidalis
Hypothenar muscles
Iliotibial tract
Pubis
Patella
Pectineus
Head of fibula
Adductor longus
Patellar ligament
Rectus femoris
Peroneus longus
Sartorius
Peroneus brevis
Vastus lateralis
Gastrocnemius
Vastus medialis
Tibialis anterior
Biceps femoral tendon
Extensor digitorum longus
Medial meniscus covered by medial collateral ligament
Soleus
Peroneus tertius
Tibial tuberosity
Extensor hallucis longus
Subcutaneous surface of tibia
Lateral malleous
Extensor retinaculum
Medial malleolus

TAPPAN'S
HANDBOOK *of*
HEALING
MASSAGE
TECHNIQUES

Classic, Holistic, and Emerging Methods

Third Edition

Frances M. Tappan, PT, EdD
Former Associate Dean
School of Allied Health Professions
University of Connecticut
Storrs, Connecticut

Patricia J. Benjamin, PhD
Academic Dean
Chicago School of Massage Therapy
Chicago, Illinois
Former Director of Education
Connecticut Center for Massage Therapy, Inc.
Newington, Connecticut

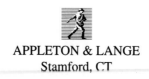

APPLETON & LANGE
Stamford, CT

Copyright © 1998 by Appleton & Lange
A Simon & Schuster Company
Copyright © 1988 by Appleton & Lange
Copyright © 1980 through 1987 by Reston Publishing Company, Inc.
"Shiatsu: An Overview," Chapter 17, Copyright © 1986 by Pauline E. Sasaki

02/ 10 9 8 7 6 5

Prentice Hall International (UK) Limited, London
Prentice Hall of Australia Pty. Limited, *Sydney*
Prentice Hall Canada, Inc., *Toronto*
Prentice Hall Hispanoamericana, S.A., *Mexico*
Prentice Hall of India Private Limited, *New Delhi*
Prentice Hall of Japan, Inc., *Tokyo*
Simon & Schuster Asia Pte. Ltd., *Singapore*
Editora Prentice Hall do Brasil Ltda., *Rio de Janeiro*
Prentice Hall, *Upper Saddle River, New Jersey*

Library of Congress Cataloging–in–Publication Data

Tappan, Frances M.
    Tappan's handbook of healing massage techniques : classic, holistic, and emerging methods / Frances M. Tappan, Patricia Benjamin. — 3rd ed.
        p.   cm.
    Rev. ed. of: Healing massage techniques. 2nd ed. c 1988.
    Includes bibliographical references and index.
    ISBN 0–8385–3676–X (pbk : alk. paper)
    1. Massage therapy.   2. Acupressure.   I. Benjamin, Patricia J., 1947–   .II. Tappan, Frances M. Healing massage techniques.
III. Title.
    [DNLM: 1. Massage—methods.   WB 537 T174h 1998]
RM721.T2178   1998
615.8′22—dc21
DNLM/DLC
for Library of Congress   97-30651

Acquisitions Editor: Kimberly Davies
Production Editor: Jeanmarie M. Roche
Art Coordinator: Eve Siegel
Designer: Mary Skudlarek

ISBN 0-8385-3676-X

9 780838 536766   90000

Contents

PART VI   SUPPLEMENTAL LEARNING MATERIALS

Contributors

Gary Bernard
Director and Head Instructor
Amma Institute
San Francisco, California

Pauline E. Sasaki
Certified Practitioner and Instructor
American Oriental Bodywork Therapy Association
Teacher of Zen Shiatsu throughout the United States and Europe
Norwalk, Connecticut

Beverly Shoenberger, RPT
Expressive Arts Therapist
Co-Founder, Connecticut Center for Massage Therapy
Newington, Connecticut

Iona Marsaa Teeguarden, MA, MFCC
Author of *Acupressure Way of Health: Jin Shin Do®* and
A Complete Guide to Acupressure—Jin Shin Do®
Director, Jin Shin Do® Foundation for Bodymind Acupressure™
Watsonville, California

Jasmine Ellen Wolf, BA
Authorized Instructor of Jin Shin Do® Foundation
Nationally Certified in Therapeutic Massage and Bodywork
Teacher of Jin Shin Do® throughout New England
Coventry, Connecticut

Preface

The third edition of *Healing Massage Techniques* is a culmination of 50 years of Dr. Frances Tappan's dedication to the study and teaching of hands-on healing. "Tappan's Handbook" has been added to the title to acknowledge Dr. Tappan's work in developing the text over the years and in setting its basic structure, tone, and philosophical direction. Her vision of having descriptions of massage techniques from around the world accessible to students of the healing arts has made this the standard massage training text.

Dr. Tappan began her life-long study of massage in the 1940s with research into the techniques used in physical therapy in the United States. The results of her initial research are found in Appendix A. Created in 1948, this chart compares the systems of massage used in the developing profession of physical therapy as reflected in the work of Albert Hoffa, Mary McMillan, and James Mennell. The chart was published in 1961 in Dr. Tappan's first book, *Massage Techniques: A Case Method Approach*.

Dr. Tappan continued her study of massage techniques studying Bindegewebsmassage in Germany at the Elizabeth Dicke School in Uberlingen. She also traveled to Taiwan in 1975 to learn about acupuncture and how finger pressure on acupuncture points could be incorporated into massage sessions to enhance healing. The subtitle of the first edition of *Healing Massage Techniques* published in 1980 reflects an expanding awareness of massage worldwide—*A Study of Eastern and Western Methods*.

The current subtitle, *Classic, Holistic, and Emerging Methods*, was adopted for the second edition in 1988. This subtitle identifies the broad scope of the book as well as Dr. Tappan's basic philosophical position, which may be summed up as follows: value the traditional, look worldwide, include the whole person, and seek new insights and methods. Dr. Tappan was in the forefront of recognizing what are now called alternative, complementary, and integrative approaches to healing.

The third edition is a continuation of Dr. Tappan's work into the 21st century, and I feel privileged to be part of this latest update. The text has been reorganized, important concepts clarified, sections expanded, and techniques added. The inside covers represent two major world views of the human body; one from the Western perspective showing muscular structure, and the other from the Eastern perspective showing energy meridians. These illustrations may also serve as useful references.

Part I, General Information, contains background material that serves as a professional foundation and sets the stage for the remainder of the book. Important concepts are defined in Chapter 1. A discussion of the wellness and treatment perspectives begins to develop the context for the uses of massage described later. Travis' Illness/Wellness Continuum is particularly useful in helping us get beyond the dichotomy of wellness versus treatment to see these two perspectives as forming a whole view of healing. It is reminiscent of the yin/yang symbol from Taoist philosophy usually depicted with one white side and one black side, but with a dot of white in the black and a black dot in the white. In every treatment application, there is also a wellness intent and many wellness applications involve some treatment of specific conditions.

The history of massage is told in Chapter 2 from the context of it being an ancient and global practice. The use of massage for health and healing long predates current professions, and its history from this fuller perspective is testament to its universality. Massage belongs to no one profession but is the province of the many different practitioners who value it as a means to promote well-being.

The efficacy of massage, although unquestionable in many ways, continues to be studied using scientific methods. Especially as practitioners from mainstream medicine in the United States consider integrating more touch in general, and specific hands-on techniques into their work, massage will be studied in this way. All practitioners can benefit from the knowledge about massage gained through science. Chapters 3 and 25 review some of the most important research being done about the effects and uses of massage.

The performance of massage techniques by health practitioners requires some basic knowledge and skills to help both giver and receiver benefit optimally from the experience and avoid harm. Since the most basic aspect of massage is touch, an understanding of what touch means to both giver and receiver is an essential professional foundation. Although information on these topics is sprinkled throughout the text, Chapters 4 and 5 specifically address contraindications, endangerment sites, and general principles for giving massage.

Part II is devoted entirely to classic Western massage. Chapters 6 and 7 look at classic massage techniques and joint movements that form the basis of most of the therapeutic applications of massage found in physiotherapy, in natural healing, and for health and fitness. Classic texts from the 19th and early 20th centuries, as well as more current authorities, have been used to develop an authentic description of these useful and enduring techniques. Chapters 8 and 9 describe applications of classic massage both in a full-body routine and in more detailed massage to different parts of the body. A unique aspect of Chapter 9 is a consideration of each body part from a holistic perspective, exploring the meaning that each part might have to the individual and the implications for the massage practitioner.

Part III looks at five different well-respected forms of contemporary massage and bodywork. Each chapter provides an overview of the form and describes its basic techniques. The approaches presented are very different from each other and represent the wide variety of bodywork forms that have been developed for various effects. For example, the main focus of polarity therapy is energy balancing; myofascial techniques separate, soften, and lengthen fascia; trigger point therapy relieves trigger points in myofascial tissues; light massage techniques enhance the movement of lymph; and foot reflexology stimulates areas in different parts of the body.

Four different Asian bodywork traditions are explored in Part IV. Each form is based on traditional Chinese medicine and meridian theory and focuses on normalizing the movement of energy or chi (ki) through the body. Finger pressure to acupuncture points traces its history to ancient China, while amma continues this tradition in Japanese-style massage. More modern forms include shiatsu from Japan, and Jin Shin Do® from the United States. These forms are examples of evolving approaches to the ancient Chinese healing arts.

Part V addresses the practical aspects of massage in its applications for different populations. The common applications presented include massage for athletes and fitness participants, for pregnant woman, for infants and children, in the workplace, for mental and emotional well-being, for healthy aging, for the terminally ill and dying, and in medical settings. The book ends with an essay on the "art of healing touch," which highlights Dr. Tappan's personal insights and message for practitioners of the art of massage. In the end it becomes clear that the techniques themselves are only part of the equation and that intention, communication, and caring are equally important in any formula for true health and healing.

Rounding out the content of the book is reference material including a bibliography, glossary, a list of organizations and publications (Appendix B) and a list of states which license massage therapists (Appendix C). The sample performance evaluations forms presented in Appendix D provide teachers of massage with simple instruments for giving feedback to students. Appendix E contains a short form and a long form for taking health histories in order to plan safe and effective massage sessions.

It is our hope that those of you who read and study from this book not only value the basic information presented, but also sense the wonder and potential of hands-on healing for the simplest of intentions—to help individual human beings in their quest for good health and well-being.

Patricia J. Benjamin, PhD

Acknowledgments

It would be humanly impossible to give adequate acknowledgment to all who have contributed to the writing and updating of this book. Many of those involved in writing the first two editions continue to deserve our thanks. These include Lucille Daniels, whose vision assisted Dr. Tappan in writing her master's thesis, which became the foundation for this project; the School of Physical Therapy at the University of Connecticut, especially Vera Kasaka; Dorothy McLaughlin, who traveled with Dr. Tappan to Taiwan to study acupuncture; Joseph Yao, Donald Courtial, and Dorothy McLaughlin for their assistance with descriptions of acupuncture points; and Steve Kitts and Beverly Shoenberger for their consultations in preparing the previous edition.

We are also indebted to those involved in this most recent update. So many people contributed in so many ways. We would especially like to thank Victoria Carmona for her thoughtful critiques, computer expertise, help with photographs, and miscellaneous odd jobs. We are also grateful to Angelus Infinity for her general support throughout the project. Various members of the faculty and staff of the Connecticut Center for Message Therapy helped review drafts of the text, and special thanks go to Eric Mosher and Alicia Davis. Thanks also go to Sage Defronzo for manuscript preparation. Several people helped with photographs from which illustrations were made. Great appreciation goes to Ruth Chapman, Lorraine Davis, Rick Haesche, Caroline Harrison, Bridget Healy, John Julian, Marie Mips, Robin Roth, Lee Stang, James Thompson, and Deby Van Ohlen.

A project like this a culmination of a lifetime of study and experience. Therefore, we would be remiss not to express gratitude to all of those with whom we have studied and worked and to the many patients and clients who have taught us so much. Thanks also to those in various professions who have kept the flame burning and continue to value and practice healing massage in their work.

The many people at Appleton & Lange who contributed to the success of this project also deserve recognition, especially Kim Davies, our editor, for her encouragement and understanding through the last stages of the project.

I

General Information

1

Introduction

Touch and movement have been used since ancient times to enhance well-being and to heal. Today healing massage techniques are used in several different health professions, including therapeutic massage and bodywork, physical therapy, athletic training, nursing, chiropractic, osteopathy, and naturopathy. Massage is used somewhat differently in these professions according to their scope of practice and theoretical perspectives, but they share a common bond, that is, the massage techniques themselves. The heart of this book is the description of techniques and of how massage techniques are applied to enhance the well-being of the recipient.

The information in this chapter will help define the context for the presentation of healing massage techniques that follow. Key concepts from the title of the text, the general terminology used, the wellness and treatment models, and the uses of massage are discussed to help set the stage for the remainder of the book.

■ KEY CONCEPTS

The title of this book, *Healing Massage Techniques: Classic, Holistic, and Emerging Methods,* describes the scope of the text. The meaning of each word in the title is explored in the following paragraphs.

To *heal* means to make healthy, whole, or sound; restore to health; or free from ailment. The word *healing* is used in this text to mean enhancing health and well-being, as well as the process of regaining health or optimal functioning after an injury, disease, or other debilitating condition. In the holistic context, it means to make whole or restore integrity.

Massage is the intentional and systematic manipulation of the soft tissues of the body to enhance health and healing. Joint movements and stretching are commonly performed as part of massage. The primary characteristics of massage are touch and movement.

The description of what the practitioner actually does is the *technique*. Massage techniques may be generally described in terms such as sliding, percussing, compressing, broadening, kneading, frictioning, vibrating, stretching, and holding. Although massage may be applied using electrical and mechanical devices, this text focuses on the age-old art of using the hands to perform massage techniques.

The broader concept of the term *technique* also includes the intent. Onlookers can see how the practitioner and receiver move during an application of technique, but the intent can only be inferred. The choice of technique is determined by what practitioners hope to accomplish according to their theoretical perspective. The intent might be to enhance a biophysical process such as relaxation or circulation, or to balance energy, or to evoke a positive emotional state. It might also be expressed in a more functional way, such as to recover from an athletic competition, to improve posture, or to diminish pain.

Massage techniques that have endured the test of time and remain in use today are called *classic*. Classic also suggests simplicity, style, excellence, and enduring value. In this sense, the ancient systems of bodywork from China and India are classic. Classic Western massage refers to those techniques used traditionally in Europe and the United States since the late nineteenth century, when the word *massage* itself came into general use. Part II of this book is devoted entirely to classic Western massage because of its simplicity, adaptability, and continued usefulness as a system of healing massage techniques.

Holistic massage refers to those approaches that take into account the wholeness of human beings, that is, body, mind, and emotions. The spiritual, often included in the concept of holistic, means different things to different people. In the holistic paradigm, massage is applied to the physical body, yet it affects all other aspects of the whole person. Although the word *holistic* is relatively new in the health profession, the concept is of ancient origin.

This book also addresses *emerging methods* of massage, that is, those that have come into the mainstream in the past few decades. Emerging methods may have been developed within one of the established health professions, or from alternative practitioners, and sometimes from creative individuals who may not be in a recognized health profession. The late twentieth century has seen an explosion of interest in various forms of massage as people have rediscovered their many benefits for promoting optimal health and healing. The terms *classic, holistic,* and *emerging* are not mutually exclusive, but refer to different ways of thinking about massage techniques. Many of the classic systems are holistic, as are many of the emerging methods.

■ GENERAL TERMINOLOGY

The general terminology used in the different health professions varies slightly. Some health professionals will say they have clients, while others use the term patients. Some call themselves therapists, while others refer to themselves as technicians or practitioners. Some refer to what they do as treatments or procedures, while others use the term sessions. Massage is described variously as a modality, massage therapy, bodywork, physiotherapy, and manual therapy.

In this text, we will use a universal terminology to be more inclusive. The one who performs massage will be called the *giver* or *practitioner,* while the one receiving massage will be called the *receiver* or *recipient.* The word *practitioner* specifically refers to someone trained in massage techniques who uses massage in the practice of his/her profession. *Session* will refer to the period of time in which massage is performed. The term *treatment* will be reserved for descriptions of medical applications.

■ THE WELLNESS AND TREATMENT MODELS

The wellness and treatment models are concepts that add clarity to defining *intention* in performing massage and to describing *scope of practice.* The models are also useful for framing theoretical and historical discussions of healing massage techniques.

The association of these two models has ancient origins in Greek mythology. Aesclepius, son of Apollo and the first physician, had two daughters named Hygeia and Panacea. Hygeia is the goddess of health, and Panacea the goddess of cures. Ancient Greeks went to Aesclepian temples for healing of various ills, and a form of massage is thought to have been given there. The memory of the Greek goddesses is still with us in the terms *hygiene* and *panacea.* In the late nineteenth and early twentieth centuries, the word *hygiene* referred generally to those practices that promote health. Today, the common understanding of the word *hygiene* is largely confined to practices of cleanliness. *Panacea* has come to mean a cure-all, or remedy for all ills.

The Wellness Model. Massage is often included along with good nutrition, adequate exercise, bathing, proper rest, sunshine, fresh air, and good cheer in prescriptions for good health. This is true across time and in many different cultures. For example, these health practices were found in some form in ancient China and India, medieval Europe, natural healing in late nineteenth-century Western society, and physical culture in early twentieth-century United States. *Wellness* is a reincarnation of this idea in the late twentieth century.

Wellness refers to a condition of optimal physical, emotional, intellectual, spiritual, social, and vocational well-being. Therapeutic massage and bodywork can promote well-being in these dimensions in a number of ways. The components of wellness and a healthy lifestyle are explained in practical terms by Seiger, Vanderpool, and Barnes (1995, pp. 5–6).

- **Physical** well-being involves being physically fit; eating nutritiously; being free from chemical dependency and other harmful behaviors; being aware of early signs of illness; getting adequate sleep and rest; preventing accidents.

- **Emotional** well-being involves balance in emotions; expressing emotions appropriately and comfortably; showing respect and affection for others; coping successfully with stress and personal problems; seeking counsel when needed.
- **Intellectual** well-being includes clear thinking and problem solving; processing information; questioning and evaluating; learning from life experiences; being flexible, creative, and open to new ideas.
- **Spiritual** well-being is whatever brings meaning and purpose in your life; knowing your purpose in life and being more comfortable expressing love, joy, peace, and fulfillment; feeling connected to your inner self, significant others, and the universe; having hope after setbacks; appreciating nature.
- **Social** well-being means having satisfying relationships and interacting well with others; having a network of family, friends, and others who can help you in time of need; establishing a sense of belonging within your community.
- **Vocational** well-being includes school and job satisfaction; working in harmony with others to accomplish something worthwhile.

The wellness model is also a holistic model in that it views people in light of their "wholeness," within themselves and in the world. It goes beyond the idea of the absence and prevention of disease (a medical perspective), to one of achieving a vibrant, meaningful life. It emphasizes personal responsibility and, in its broadest sense, aims to improve individual, organizational, and community well-being.

The contemporary wellness movement was pioneered by John Travis, MD, in the 1970s. He founded the Wellness Resource Center in 1975 and conducts seminars to educate the general public and health professionals about the concept of wellness. His illness/wellness continuum, shown in Figure 1–1, is a well-recognized diagram used to show the relationship between the wellness and treatment models (Travis & Callander, 1990).

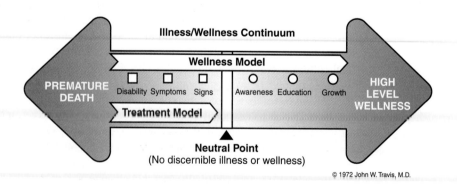

FIGURE 1–1. The wellness model. *(Reprinted with permission,* Wellness Workbook, *Travis & Ryan, Ten Speed Press, Berkeley, CA. ©1981, 1988, John W. Travis, MD)*

Travis's wellness model includes the treatment model, but goes beyond disability and the signs and symptoms of disease in a movement toward awareness, education, and growth, that is, toward high-level functioning. Using the wellness model, the massage practitioner may specifically address conditions found during the course of a session, but the overall intent remains to promote optimal health beyond the alleviation of specific symptoms. From the time of birth to old age, massage supports nature in the process of moving toward and maintaining high-level wellness.

Practitioners in professions that can be broadly defined as *wellness* or *health-related professions* tend to work with people who come to them for help in achieving a greater state of well-being. There may or may not be any medically significant condition present. Medical providers will sometimes refer people to practitioners working in the wellness model as an adjunct to medical therapies. That has given rise to the term *complementary* for approaches that fall outside of standard medical practice.

Many practitioners working within the wellness model do not diagnose or treat specific illnesses or injuries and may not do so unless their professional licenses permit it. Massage therapists in most states are prohibited from diagnosis and treatment by law, although some states allow limited treatment by referral from a physician.

Practitioners performing massage within the wellness model tend to think of themselves as working with people, and not solely with medical conditions. Their intent is to use massage with its health-enhancing effects in such a way as to benefit the person in whatever way possible. In the wellness model, it makes more sense to talk about massage as having *benefits* for people with certain diseases or injuries, rather than it being *indicated* for a specific condition, which is a treatment model concept.

The Treatment Model. Practitioners in the medical or health care professions usually have patients who present themselves with some symptoms of disease or injury, and they use massage to help treat or cure the condition. They may assess or diagnose the condition or accept referral from a primary health care provider who diagnoses and then refers the patient. In the treatment or medical model, the key concept is to diagnose and treat the condition. When the condition subsides, the goal is accomplished and the treatment is discontinued. In the wellness model developed by Travis, this is the *neutral point.*

In the treatment model, massage is considered a *modality,* or method of treating the presenting condition. In this sense, it is in the same category of modalities such as ice packs, hot packs, ultrasound, or whirlpool baths. For example, massage is one of the modalities used in the practice of physical therapy.

In the treatment model, the term *indication* is used to mean that when a specific condition is present, then massage is indicated or advised to alleviate the condition. For example, light effleurage is indicated to induce relaxation, deep transverse friction is indicated to create a strong mobile scar, and tapotement on the back is indicated in treatment of respiratory congestion. Recent studies confirm that massage is indicated to help premature infants gain weight and to reduce anxiety in adolescents hospitalized for psychiatric care. Chapters 3 and 25 explore many of the situations for which massage is indicated and review some of the pertinent research.

Practitioners in professions that can be broadly defined as *medical* or *health care* work with people who come to them for relief of specific diagnosed diseases or injury rehabilitation. Physical therapists, athletic trainers, nurses, physiatrists, chiropractors, and osteopaths often incorporate massage and bodywork into their treatments. Depending on the profession, it may be called manual therapy, physiotherapy, or simply a modality.

Relationship Between the Models. The treatment model is at one end of the continuum of the wellness model, and is, therefore, part of the wellness model. Practitioners working primarily in the wellness model may in fact "treat" or address certain conditions within their scope of practice. It is also possible that a practitioner in a health care profession working traditionally in the treatment model may address the general well-being of their patient. In real life, the distinctions may not be as clear as in theory, but generally speaking, certain professions and certain practitioners tend to approach their clients or patients with either a wellness or a treatment intent.

■ USES OF MASSAGE

Massage has many uses according to the Western scientific viewpoint. It may be used to affect specific body structures, for example, in relaxing specific muscles, increasing range of motion at a joint, or freeing the fascia. It may be used to affect more general body processes such as general relaxation, lymph flow, or growth and development in infants. It may be used to affect emotional states such as in reducing anxiety. It may increase body awareness and foster structural and functional integration. Or it may simply provide an avenue of connection between practitioner and receiver in which caring and compassion are communicated.

In Asian cultures, which view health and disease from the paradigm of Chinese medicine, massage is used to enhance the flow of energy called *chi.* In Ayurvedic medicine from India, massage may be used to balance energy centers called *chakras.* Practitioners often integrate theories and techniques from different cultures and develop more eclectic practices of massage.

Recipients seek massage for a variety of reasons. Many who feel stressed out seek relaxation. Some seek relief from pain or sore and stiff muscles. Athletes may use massage as part of a training program. Some use massage as a complement to medical treatment, chiropractic, or psychotherapy. Infants and children are massaged to enhance growth and development. People in midlife may use massage to slow the effects of aging. The elderly seek massage to improve body function and to receive caring touch. Healing massage techniques are found in all cultures of the world today and are mentioned throughout recorded history. In Chapter 2 we will take a closer look at the history of massage to help us understand its universality and how it came to be the way it is in the United States today.

■ SUMMARY

Massage is the systematic manipulation of soft tissues of the body to enhance health and healing. Joint movements and stretching are often performed as part of a massage session. The heart of this text is the description of massage techniques and how they are applied. The term *technique* includes how the movements are performed and the intent of the practitioner. The term *healing* is used both in a wellness sense (ie, to maintain optimum well-being) and in a treatment sense (ie, to regain health after injury or illness).

Classic massage techniques are those that have endured the test of time because of their simplicity and effectiveness, for example, classic Western massage as developed in Europe and the United States in the nineteenth century. *Holistic* massage takes into account the wholeness of human beings, that is, body, mind, emotions, and spirit. *Emerging* methods are those that have come into the mainstream in the past few decades. These concepts are not mutually exclusive.

The terminology used in the text will be inclusive, except when speaking of a particular profession. The one who performs the massage will be called the *giver* or *practitioner,* while the one receiving massage will be called the *receiver* or *recipient.* The term *session* will describe the time period in which massage is performed, and the term *treatment* will be reserved for strictly medical applications.

The intent of giving massage can be understood using the wellness and treatment models. In the illness/wellness continuum developed by John Travis, MD, the treatment model includes the half of the continuum that addresses signs, symptoms, and disability to avert premature death. The treatment model is that part of a comprehensive wellness model that brings a person to a neutral point. The complete wellness model continues toward awareness, education, and growth to reach high-level wellness. Generally speaking, certain professions and certain practitioners tend to approach their clients or patients with either a wellness or a treatment intent.

From the wellness perspective, massage is used to achieve high-level well-being in a number of areas. From the medical or treatment perspective, massage helps in the healing of a diseased or injured person or body part. In the wellness model, it makes more sense to talk about massage as having benefits for people with certain diseases or injuries, rather than it being indicated for a specific condition, which is a treatment model concept. Practitioners use massage for a variety of reasons such as to affect specific body structures, general body processes, and emotional states; or to increase body awareness, foster structural and functional integration, communicate compassion, or balance energy. People seek massage for many different reasons such as relaxation, relief from pain, conditioning, to slow the effects of aging, or to receive caring touch.

▪ REFERENCES

Robbins, G., Powers, D., & Burgess, S. (1994). *A wellness way of life.* 2nd edition. Madison, WI: Brown & Benchmark.

Seiger, L., Vanderpool, K., & Barnes, D. (1995). *Fitness and wellness strategies.* Madison, WI: Brown & Benchmark.

Travis, J. W., & Callander, M. G. (1990). *Wellness for helping professionals.* Mill Valley, CA: Wellness Associates Publications.

History of Massage

The history of massage is both ancient and global. The practice goes back to before recorded history and is found in some form in every known culture in the world. Different cultures have developed their own unique forms of massage and body-work, and these practices have been transformed when peoples come in contact with each other and share information. Travel, war, trade, international study, and modern forms of communication have all facilitated the exchange of ideas and the evolution of the practice of massage on a global scale. The United States is one place where the ancient and modern practices of many cultures have come together and formed a vibrant multi-ethnic mix. The eclectic nature of massage therapy in the United States today, and the many forms of massage available here, is a testa-ment to the United States as a center of global commerce.

In this chapter we will present some interesting facts about the uses of massage at various times and in a variety of places. We will also outline some of the major forces that have shaped the work in the United States in the latter twentieth century. The aim is to give practitioners a sense of the vast heritage of which they are a part.

To organize the historical picture somewhat, different forms of massage will be described as falling into three different spheres of practice: wellness (including health and fitness), healing (including medical applications), and sports. These three categories overlap somewhat but are useful in thinking about how techniques and systems were used and handed down through the ages. Some of these forms may be both historical *and* contemporary to the extent that they continue to be performed in their traditional ways.

As is the custom in many history texts, we will use the more universal designa-tion of dates. The abbreviation "B.C.E." will be used to denote "before the common era," often referred to as "B.C." "C.E." is used to mean "in the common era," referred to as A.D. in the Roman calendar.

■ NATIVE AND FOLK CULTURES

In cultures without written records, historical evidence of health practices like massage is difficult to find. The knowledge and skills were handed down in families and in communities through the generations from person to person, and many of these oral traditions have been lost. However, we can learn some things from explorers who first came in contact with indigenous peoples of the world and who described their daily lives in written records. In addition, some ancient forms are still performed by groups who continue to practice their honored traditions. Massage in the South Sea Islands before their contact with Western civilization and the curanderas of the southwest United States are examples of native and folk traditions for which we have some information.

South Sea Islands. Descriptions from nineteenth-century European and American travelogs offer glimpses of massage as practiced in the native cultures of the South Sea Islands. It was reported that the Maoris of New Zealand called their version of massage *romi-romi,* and the natives of Tonga Island performed *toogi-toogi* for relief of sleeplessness and fatigue. "Melee denotes rubbing with the palm, and fota kneading with the thumb and fingers" (Kellogg, 1923, p. 12). In 1874 Nordhoff described a wellness massage called *lomi-lomi* performed by the natives of the Sandwich Islands (Hawaii):

> To be lomi-lomied you lie down upon a mat, or undress for the night, if you prefer. The less clothing you have on the more perfectly the operation can be performed. To you thereupon comes a stout native with soft fleshy hands, but a strong grip, and beginning with your head and working down slowly over the whole body, seizes and squeezes with indefatigable patience, until in half an hour, whereas you were weary and worn out, you find yourself fresh, all soreness and weariness absolutely and entirely gone, and mind and body soothed to a healthful and refreshing sleep.
>
> (Murrell, 1890, p. 10)

The Maori of New Zealand are reported to have had a tradition of treating club feet in infants with massage. In his study of the genetics of club feet, Beals tells of the practice of continuous massage of the club feet by the older women of the family, which he said had surprisingly good results. It was a practice passed down from generation to generation, which has virtually disappeared today with the advent of European medicine in New Zealand (Beals, 1978).

Curanderas. Today in the Southwestern United States, Hispanic healers called *curanderas* continue a folk healing tradition from Spain and Mexico embellished by native American remedies. Its roots may be traced to the Moors of eighth-century

Spain, then to the Spaniards who came to the Americas in the fifteenth century, and also to native Americans, particularly the Aztecs of ancient Mexico (Torres).

Curanderas are women healers called upon when a family's chief caregiver needs assistance. *Curanderas totals* practice all the various healing specialties including herbs, midwifery, massage, and spiritual techniques. *Curanderas totals* have a strong spiritual dimension to their methods and are described as using "ritualism and symbolism in their art and are able to move in and out of dimensions not bound to earth." It is believed that *curanderas* inherit their power to heal, although some families with no heritage of healing may be given the *don,* translated as "gift," or more loosely as the "heart" (Perrone, Stockel, & Krueger, 1989, p. 90).

Sobardoras are *curanderas* who specialize in massage and may also use herbal remedies in their work. They perform soft tissue manipulations and "bonesetting" types of joint manipulations. *Sobardoras* learn their art by apprenticeship.

■ ANCIENT CIVILIZATIONS

Written and pictoral records from the ancient civilizations of Sumer, China and Japan, India, Greece, and Rome contain descriptions of massage and exercise. Many of the forms of massage and bodywork practiced today trace their roots to these ancient practices.

Sumer. A clay tablet from Sumer dating from 2100 B.C.E. describes a remedy that uses an herbal mixture and "rubbing" and "frictions."

> *Pass through a sieve and then knead together turtle shells, naga-si plant, salt, and mustard. Then wash the diseased part with beer of good quality and hot water, and rub with the mixture. Then friction and rub again with oil, and put on a poultice of pounded pine.*
>
> *(Time-Life Books, 1987, p. 41).*

China and Japan. Since Chapters 15–18 each begin with a history of bodywork based in Chinese medicine, in this chapter, we will simply mention some of the highlights. Please consult Chapters 15–18 for more detailed information.

The Yellow Emperor's Classic of Internal Medicine, believed to have been written over 2500 years ago, is often cited as the first book on Chinese medicine. It became the foundation for traditional medicine practiced in Asian countries of China, Japan, and Korea (Monte, 1993, p. 20). Essential concepts in Chinese medicine include yin and yang, life energy called *qi* or *chi,* which moves in patterns defined by energy channels, and the five element (fire, wood, water, metal, earth) theory. Ancient health practices and therapies from China include *acupuncture* with needles, *acupressure* using finger pressure on acupunture points, a form of massage called *tuina,* and forms of exercise called *chi kung* and *tai chi.*

Anma, or *amma,* is a form of Japanese massage that was brought from China via the Korean peninsula in the sixth century B.C.E. At that time, the Japanese assimilated the Chinese medical philosophies that came to them as *kampo* ("the Chinese way"), and amma became an accepted Japanese healing practice. See Chapter 16 for a more detailed history of amma.

Shiatsu is a modern form of Japanese bodywork developed in the 1940s by Torujiro Namikoshi. Shiatsu incorporates many of the ideas from Western science with traditional Japanese amma. Shiatsu was introduced into the United States in the 1950s by Torujiro's son, Toru Namikoshi. See Chapters 15 and 17 for more detailed information about the history of shiatsu.

India. Ayur-Veda, "knowledge of long life" and the traditional medicine of India, is said to have been given to a Hindu seer by the god Indra. The Ayurvedic system goes back to at least fifth century B.C.E. and is based on the Vedas, the ancient philosophical and spiritual writings of India (Monte, 1993, p. 30).

Ayurvedic health practices include guidelines for vegetarian eating, forms of cleansing, movements and postures (hatha yoga), breathing exercises, meditation, and massage. Essential concepts in Ayurvedic theory include a life force called *prana,* energy centers called *chakras,* the five great elements (earth, water, fire, air, ether), and the three *doshas (vata, pita, kapha).* The ancient wisdom of Ayurveda continues to be practiced today and has been popularized in the West in the writings of Deepok Chopra (Chopra, 1991).

The recent revival of infant massage in the United States has been patterned in part on the ancient practice of baby massage in India. Leboyer's popular book, *Loving Hands: The Traditional Indian Art of Baby Massage* (1982), shows Shantala, an Indian woman, massaging her baby as she learned from her mother, who learned from her mother, and so on back in time.

Greece. In ancient Greece, the uses of massage for wellness, healing, and sports were well advanced. Hippocrates (450–377 B.C.E.) wrote of the utility of friction after sprains and reduced dislocations and recommended abdominal kneading and chest clapping (Kleen, 1921, p. 2). Aristotle (384–322 B.C.E.), a Greek philosopher and tutor of Alexander the Great, is said to have recommended rubbing with oil and water as a remedy against weariness. Alexander the Great (356–323 B.C.E.), who ruled a vast empire from Egypt to India, reportedly had a personal *triptai* (massage specialist) named Athenophanes, "whose business it was to rub the great emperor and to prepare his bath" (Kleen, 1921, p. 2).

The gymnasia in ancient Athens and Sparta were centers run by the State for free men and youths, which contained facilities for exercises, frictions, and baths. The exercises included wrestling, boxing, running, jumping, throwing the quoit and spear, and some ball games. Massage with oil was used to prepare the young men before their exercises and to refresh them after their exercises and after their baths (Johnson, 1866, pp. 15–16).

A description of massage performed in the Greek gymnasia is offered by Galen (c. 130–200 C.E.), a respected Roman physician who early in his career was physician to the gladiators. Galen's writings preserve knowledge of the Greek traditions and contain valuable descriptions of how massage was performed in those times. Galen describes the effects of massage before exercises (*tripsis paraskeuastike*) and after exercises (*apotherapeia*):

Rubbing which prepares for gymnastic exercises, and that which follows the same, is subservient to the exercises. The former heats and moderately opens the pores, and liquifies the excretions retained in the flesh, and softens the solid parts, and this is termed preparatory or paraskeuastic *rubbing. But the other is termed after-administering (*apotherapeutic*); and as it is applied with a larger amount of oil, it at the same time moistens by means of the grease, and softens the solid parts, and carries off what is contained in the pores.*

(Johnson, 1866, pp. 19–20)

Rome. The Roman Empire dates from approximately 27 B.C.E. to 476 C.E. At the height of its power, the Roman Empire extended from present-day Turkey and Asia Minor in the east to the British Isles in the west and included the territories of southern Europe and northern Africa. The Romans adopted much of Greek culture and spread it throughout their empire.

Aulus Cornelius Celsus (25 B.C.E.–50 C.E.), a Roman physician, is credited with compiling a text called *De Medicina,* a series of eight books covering all of the medical knowledge of his time. In the text, he describes the use of exercises, frictions, inunctions (ie, applying oil or ointment), rubbing, brushing, ligatures, and dry cupping to prevent and treat certain diseases. Active movements prescribed include walking, running, swimming, riding on horseback, and playing at ball (Georgii, 1880, p. 3).

The Romans borrowed many of the features of the Greek gymnasia to create the Roman Baths. The ruins of a famous Roman Bath may still be toured in the former Roman city of Aquae Sulis, now the city of Bath, England. Also at this site is a temple to the Roman goddess of wisdom, Minerva. The Aquae Sulis baths were in operation from approximately 60 to 410 C.E. The baths themselves consisted of a space for undressing (*apodyterium*), an exercise court, a warm room (*tepidarium*), a type of steamroom (*caldarium*), and a cold pool (*frigidarium*). At Aquae Sulis, there was also a great swimming pool and immersion baths where one could sit up to the neck in hot curative waters. Both men and women came to these baths.

The Roman writer Seneca (4 B.C.E.–65 C.E.) left a vivid description of the noise of the Roman bath above which he was trying to study. The passage included complaints about the noise of people exercising and the following passage about massage:

Or perhaps I notice some lazy fellow, content with a cheap rub-down, and hear the crack of the pummelling hand on his shoulder varying in sound according as the hand is laid on flat or hollow.

(Cunliffe, 1978, p. 16)

After the fall of the Roman Empire in 476 C.E., the idea of the Roman bath was preserved in Turkey and brought back into Western civilization as the Turkish Bath during the Renaissance. In Turkey it was customary for women, as well as men, to go to the baths as part of their health regimen. The Turkish Bath became very popular in the big cities of Europe and the United States in the nineteenth century.

After partaking of the various forms of hot and cold waters at the *hammam* or Turkish Baths, a patron would receive a rather rigorous form of bodywork. The following is a description of a bodywork session given at the *hammam* in Constantinople in the mid-nineteenth century:

> *The tellack (two, if the operation is properly performed) kneels at your side, and bending over, grips and presses your chest, arms, legs, passing from part to part like a bird shifting its place on a perch. He brings his whole weight on you with a jerk; follows the line of muscle with an anatomical thumb . . . draws the open hand strongly over the surface, particularly round the shoulder, turning you half up in doing so . . . You are now turned on your face; and . . . he works his elbow round the edges of your shoulder-blades, and with the heel, hard, the ankle of the neck . . . You are then raised for a moment to a sitting posture, and a contortion given to the small of the back with the knee, and a jerk to the neck by the two hands holding the temples.*
>
> (*Johnson, 1866, pp. 29–30*)

Turkish Baths can still be found in some of the major cities of the world. I think that it is also important to note that the tradition of the Greek gymnasia, the Roman Baths, and the Turkish Baths is still with us in the form of the modern health club. The basic format of exercise space, swimming pool, showers, steamroom, sauna, whirlpool, and massage room continue this ancient tradition.

■ MIDDLE AGES AND RENAISSANCE EUROPE

The Middle Ages in Europe extended roughly from the sixth to the fourteenth centuries. This is often considered a period of darkness for Europe when much of the classical culture of the Greeks and Romans disappeared. The classical writings about the medical use of friction and rubbing were destroyed and not brought back to Europe until the Renaissance in the fourteenth to seventeenth centuries. These writings were preserved by the Arabic peoples in Turkey and the Near East. Some of the information concerning rubbing and frictions was also preserved at this time in the folk healing traditions in Europe.

The Middle Ages was not all darkness, however. A book translated from Arabic into Latin in the eleventh century, called the *Tacuinum Sanitatis,* expounded on the six things that are necessary for everyone in the daily preservation of health. These were listed as the treatment of air, right use of foods and drink, correct use of movements and rest, proper sleep, correct use of elimination and retention of humors, and the regulating of the person by moderating joy, anger, fear, and distress. It notes that "the secret of the preservation of health, in fact, will be in the proper balance of all these elements, since it is the disturbance of this balance that causes illnesses" (Arano, 1976, p. 6).

The *Tacuinum Sanitatis* is evidence of the rich knowledge about healthy living that was known in the Middle Ages and of an early holistic philosophy of health and disease in Europe. It contains the seeds of the philosophy and practices of natural health and healing, which were in full swing by the late nineteenth century.

This is one of the major traditions of which healing massage techniques are a significant part.

It should be noted that the Arabic physician Avicenna (980–1037 C.E.) wrote about massage in his famed medical texts. Avicenna said "the object of massage is to disperse the effete matters formed in the muscles and not expelled by exercise. It causes the effete matter to disperse and so remove fatigue" (Wood & Becker, 1981).

The classical writings of the Greeks and Romans were reintroduced into Europe during the Renaissance in the fourteenth to seventeenth centuries. This included writings about the use of frictions and rubbing in the treatment of disease and injuries. This no doubt renewed interest in massage as a medical treatment in the great learning centers of Europe in France, England, Germany, Russia, and Sweden.

One of the founders of modern surgery, Ambrose Pare (1517–1590) of France, wrote about the use of frictions for joint stiffness and wound healing. Pare described different types of frictions simply as gentle, medium, and vigorous.

▪ CLASSIC WESTERN MASSAGE

Two figures loom large in the history of massage in the nineteenth and early twentieth centuries: Pehr Henrik Ling of Sweden and Johann Georg Mezger of Amsterdam. Their pupils have taken their systems of active and passive movements, combined and expanded upon them, and spread them throughout the world. Classic western massage is a synthesis of techniques developed by these two men.

Per Henrik Ling. Ling (1776–1839) was a fencing master, poet, playwright, and educator. He believed that movements of the body had the power to protect, educate, express, and heal. Ling developed four different systems of movement (ie, military, educational, aesthetic, and medical) that are described in his treatise *The General Principles of Gymnastics,* published one year after his death in 1840. In the late nineteenth and early twentieth centuries, Ling's educational gymnastics were taught in the public schools of the United States as Swedish gymnastics, and his system of medical gymnastics was known popularly as the Swedish movement cure. The movement cure consisted of passive and active movements used to treat chronic disease conditions.

Ling is eulogized as having put medical gymnastics on scientific ground. However, a reading of his treatise in the original Swedish reveals the more metaphorical thinking of a poet. He believed that human beings are made up of mechanical, chemical, and dynamic forces. The mechanical force is roughly equivalent to movements of the muscles, and the chemical force has to do with processes like digestion, elimination, and the secretions of glands. The dynamic force is an interesting mix of mental, emotional, and spiritual aspects. Balance in these three forces is necessary to maintain health, while imbalance results in disease. The mechanical force, the realm of passive and active movements, is sometimes used to reestablish balance and, therefore, health, in the human organism (Roth, 1851, pp. 25–32).

Ling's medical gymnastics included both active and passive movements. In his *Notations to the General Principles,* Ling identified the passive movements with descriptive terms like shaking, hacking, pressing, stroking, pinching and squeezing, kneading, clapping, vibrations, and rolling (eg, passive range of motion). He instructed that oil may be used to decrease skin friction, but that "this hinders the manipulation of the inner abdominal organs" (Ling, 1840).

The types of diseases treated by medical gymnastics in the nineteenth century included a variety of ailments such as congestion of the head, humming in the ears, asthma, emphysema, gastritis, constipation, incontinence, and hernia. Nervous conditions such as epilepsy, neuralgic pain, and paralysis were also treated. Explorations into the treatment of mental diseases by movements were also conducted (Roth, 1851).

Ling believed that practitioners of his work need a thorough grounding in anatomy and physiology. However, in the *Means or Vehicles of Gymnastics,* he cautioned his pupils against a mechanistic view of the human body with these words:

> *May anatomy—that holy genesis, which reveals the great work of the Creator to the eye of man, and teaches him at one and the same time how small and yet how great he is—be the gymnast's most treasured fundamental principle; but let him contemplate these forms—not as if they were lifeless ones—but . . . as though they were living, not as constituting an inert mass, but the instrument of the soul, animated with the latter throughout.*
>
> *(Ling, 1840c).*

Ling established the Royal Institute of Gymnastics in Stockholm in 1813 to teach his systems of gymnastics. His pupils took educational and medical gymnastics to major cities all over the world, and by the late nineteenth century, people interested in natural health and healing were going to the Royal Institute to learn Ling's systems as further developed by those who carried on his work.

Ling's major legacy to the practice of massage lies in his belief that active and passive movements skillfully applied can help maintain and restore health and balance in the human organism. His broad view of human beings has persisted, and his work was part of the evolution of the modern concepts of holistic health and wellness. The exercises of Ling's educational gymnastics were the forerunners of modern forms of calisthenics and physical fitness. The Swedish movement cure, and systems like it, have been combined with other methods of natural healing to form an alternative or complement to allopathic medicine. In addition, the Swedish movements were carried on in the early practice of physical therapy.

Johann Mezger. Mezger (1838–1909), a physician in Amsterdam, also believed that passive movements had the power to heal. Although he never published a detailed description of his work, his pupils von Mosengeil and Helleday did write articles about Mezger's massage. Mezger categorized the methods of soft tissue manipulation into four broad technique categories using the French terms *effleurage* (stroking), *petrissage* (kneading), *friction* (rubbing), and *tapotement* (tapping).

The popularity of Mezger's work was instrumental in reviving the interest in massage in medical settings (Nissen, 1920, pp. 7–8). The general categories of movements he defined have proved very useful and form the basis of classic Western massage. Vibration was added later as a fifth category as it gained popularity in the late nineteenth century.

Swedish Movement Cure in the United States. Ling's medical gymnastics, or movement cure as it was known in English-speaking countries, was well established in England and in the United States by the late nineteenth century. Dr. M. Roth studied at the Royal Institute and wrote the first book in English on Ling's system in 1851, *The Prevention and Cure of Many Chronic Diseases by Movements.* Figure 2–1 shows two drawings from Roth's book. One drawing depicts superficial friction being performed for respiratory congestion, and the other shows passive rotation of the foot used to increase circulation in the lower limbs to affect circulation in the head and chest. Note that the patient (recipient) and the operator (practitioner) are in various positions to best facilitate the movements being performed. The convention of lying on a table during the entire session was a later development adopted after the introduction of Mezger's massage.

The Swedish movement cure was first brought to the United States in 1854 by Dr. George Taylor of New York. Other prominent names in the early history of the movement cure in the United States are Hartvig Nissen in Washington, D.C. (1889),

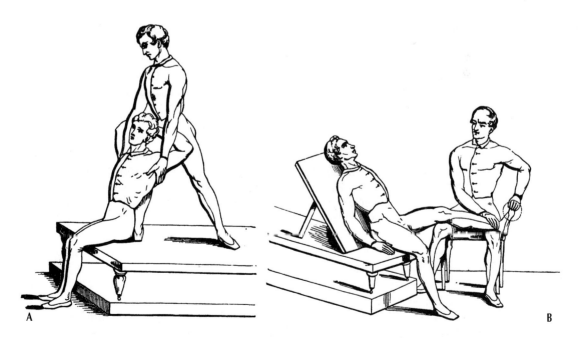

A   B

FIGURE 2–1. Drawings from Dr. Roth's book, *The Prevention and Cure of Many Chronic Diseases by Movements,* published in 1851. **A.** Superficial friction on the sides of the chest for respiratory congestion. **B.** Passive rotation of the foot to increase circulation.

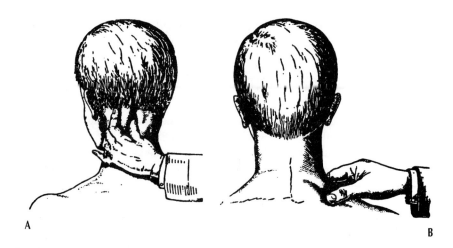

A   B

FIGURE 2–2. Drawings of kneading the neck muscles from Ostrom's book, *Massage and the Original Swedish Movements,* published in 1905. **A.** Kneading the posterior neck muscles. **B.** Kneading the upper trapezius.

Baron Nils Posse in Boston (1894), Kurre Ostrom in Philadelphia (1905), and Axel Grafstrom in New York (1904).

In the latter nineteenth and early twentieth centuries, Mezger's massage was adopted by practitioners of the Swedish movement cure, and you begin to see the two terms used together. For example, they are both used in the title of Ostrom's book, *Massage and the Original Swedish Movements* (1905). Figure 2–2 shows drawings of kneading of the neck muscles from Ostrom's book.

■ EARLY TO MID-TWENTIETH CENTURY

Various forms of soft tissue manipulation and passive movements continued to be developed in the United States into the twentieth century as methods for promoting health and healing. The mainstream form continued to be massage and the Swedish movements, which were used in the spheres of medical treatment, natural health and healing, and sports and fitness.

Massage in Regular Medicine. The use of massage in regular medicine (as opposed to folk remedies, natural healing, and other "alternative" practices) can be found in the medical literature of Europe and the United States dating from the 1700s. It was generally called *frictions, rubbing, or medical rubbing.* In 1866 Walter Johnson wrote a history of medical massage with the lengthy title, *The Anatripic Art: A history of the art termed anatripsis by Hypocrates, tripsis by Galen, friction by Celsus, manipulation by Beveridge, and medical rubbing in ordinary language, from the earliest times to the present day.*

Marie Marcellin Lucas-Championnière (circa 1880) claimed that in fractures, the soft tissue union as well as the bony union should be considered from the start. Sir William Bennett of England was impressed with Lucas-Championnière's idea and started a revolutionary treatment with the use of massage at St. George's Hospital in circa 1899. Albert J. Hoffa published his book, *Technik der Massage,* in Germany in 1900. This book is still a good basic text on massage, giving clear descriptions of how to execute the stokes and advocating the procedures that underlie all modern techniques. The book by Max Bohm, *Massage: Its Principles and Techniques,* written in 1913, includes interpretations of Hoffa's techniques. In 1902, Douglas Graham published *A Treatise on Massage, Its History, Mode of Application and Effects.* This text finally aroused the interest of the medical profession in the United States in massage and its therapeutic effects.

Sir Robert Jones, a leading orthopedic surgeon in England, was an enthusiast of the Lucas-Championnière treatment of fractures. Jones was to have an influence on two of the great figures of physical therapy in the United States. Mary McMillan was associated with Jones's clinic at Southern Hospital in Liverpool, England, from 1911 to 1915, and James B. Mennell worked with Jones at the Special Military Surgical Hospital, Shepherd's Bush, England. Mennell (1880–1957) wrote his text, *Physical Treatment by Movement, Manipulation and Massage,* in 1917 during World War I. Mennell's text was a compilation of the manual therapeutics that he saw in various European countries, and he considered it to be a rationale of massage treatment. He endeavored to show the importance of care and gentleness in giving massage. Mennell was a medical officer and lecturer of massage at the Training School of St. Thomas' Hospital in London, England, from 1912 to 1935. He was very influential in shaping the practice of physical therapy in its early years.

During World War I, E. G. Bracket and Joel Goldthwait became interested in the reconstruction (ie, rehabilitation) work that was being done among the Allied nations. They initiated the Reconstruction Department of the United States Army in 1918. The department consisted of physiotherapy, occupational therapy, and curative workshop divisions. Short intensive courses were arranged in recognized schools of physical education throughout the country to train women to perform physiotherapy, including massage, on wounded soldiers (McMillan, 1925, p. 10).

In his book, *A Practice of Physiotherapy* (1926), C. M. Sampson, MD, describes the types of modalities used in the developing field of physiotherapy, including massage. Figure 2–3 is a photograph of a corner of the general massage section of an army hospital. It shows four operators, as practitioners were then called, working with soldiers who are seated in chairs, and lying or sitting on tables. Massage was applied to the injured site to assist in rehabilitation.

Mary McMillan, who later figured prominently in the development of the profession of physical therapy, received her special training in London at the National Hospital for Nervous Diseases, at St. Bartholomew's Hospital, and at St. George's Hospital with William Bennett. At the Southern Hospital in Liverpool, McMillan was in charge of massage and therapeutic exercises at Greenbank Cripples' Home. She came to the United States as Director of Massage and Medical Gymnastics at Children's Hospital in Portland, Maine. She later served as chief aide at Walter

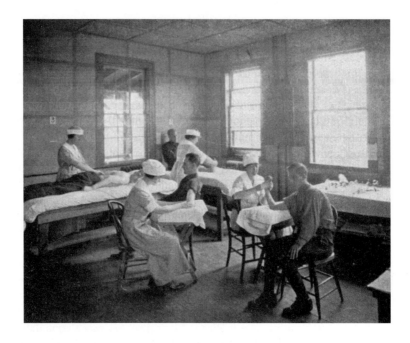

FIGURE 2–3. Photograph of a corner of the general massage section of an army hospital from Sampson's book, *A Practice of Physiotherapy,* published in 1926.

Reed Hospital and instructor of special war emergency course at the Reed College Clinic for training reconstruction aides in physiotherapy during World War I. McMillan was director of physiotherapy at Harvard Medical School while she was writing her book, *Massage and Therapeutic Exercise,* from 1921 to 1925.

Physical therapists trained for rehabilitation work during and after World Wars I and II continued to expand the field of physical therapy for treating a number of orthopedic conditions. They were called upon in the 1940–50s to treat victims of the polio epidemic of that time. But as Gertrude Beard noted, the amount of massage being prescribed by physicians in the United States declined in the decades following World War II. She speculates that this was due to the fact that massage is time-consuming, sometimes strenuous, demands real skill, and the basis for prescribing it is largely empiric rather than scientific (Beard, 1964, p. 1).

Natural Health and Healing. Massage and the Swedish movements were also practiced by proponents of natural healing. These practitioners used various natural remedies to treat different ailments and generally rejected the allopathic methods of drugs and surgery. The philosophy of natural healing includes the belief that humans are created with innate healing powers that can be facilitated by various natural methods such as rest, sunshine, heat and cold applied by water (hydrotherapy), exercise, massage, proper nutrition, laughter, and herbal remedies. Natural healing in the late nineteenth and early twentieth centuries also included magnetic healing, a form of energy work (Bilz, 1898).

The Battle Creek Sanitarium in Battle Creek, Michigan, run by John Harvey Kellogg (1852–1943), was a natural healing resort of the early twentieth century. Kellogg advocated a host of natural health practices he called "biologic living" including vegetarianism, physical exercise, sunshine, fresh air, colonic irrigation, various forms of bathing, and massage. There was no alcohol, no coffee, no tea, and no smoking. Kellogg and his brother invented the first cold cereal and started the breakfast cereal industry (Armstrong & Armstrong, 1991, pp. 107–111). Kellogg's book, *The Art of Massage,* was first published in 1895.

C. W. Post (1854–1914), of Post brand cereal fame, opened a competing sanitarium on the outskirts of Battle Creek called La Vita Inn. Post featured what he called "mental healing." In 1895 in a self-published book called *I Am Well,* Post offers this advice, which sounds much like relaxation techniques used today:

> *Seek an easy position where you will not be disturbed. Relax every muscle, close your eyes and go into silence where mind is plastic to the breathings of Spirit, where God talks to son.*
>
> *(Armstrong & Armstrong, 1991, p. 111)*

Bernarr Macfadden (1868–1955) was a popular proponent of natural health, which he called *physical culture.* In the early 1900s, he opened a string of physical culture resorts in the East and Midwest. His *Physical Culture* magazine was launched in 1898 and was popular well into the 1930s. Macfadden's Physical Culture Training School in Chicago graduated "doctors" of hydropathy, kinesitherapy, and physcultopathy. His health regimen consisted of proper breathing, relaxation, diet, fasting, bathing, singing, exercise, and massage. He was considered a huckster by some, but was successful in bringing the tradition of natural health to the general public. (Armstrong & Armstrong, 1991, pp. 203–213).

Swedish Massage. The heyday of Swedish massage was from about 1920 to 1950. During this time, the genre called Swedish massage came to include massage, Swedish movements, various forms of hydrotherapy, heat lamps, diathermy, and colonic irrigation. The focus was on health. "Reducing massage" was popular in the 1930–40s, since massage was believed at that time to be a beauty aid that helped reduce fat on the thighs and waistline.

Practitioners were trained in private vocational schools called "colleges" such as the College of Swedish Massage in Chicago. A typical women's class in "scientific massage technique" in the 1940s is shown in Figure 2–4. At this time, women and men were separated, and there was very little cross-gender legitimate massage outside of medical facilities (Benjamin, 1993). Graduates of these colleges of Swedish massage often opened their own establishments called massage parlors or health centers. Women worked in upscale beauty parlors such as Helena Rubenstein and Elizabeth Arden. Sometimes exercise classes were offered along with Swedish massage services. Graduates of colleges of Swedish massage could also find jobs in the YMCA, private health clubs, resorts, hospitals, and with professional sports

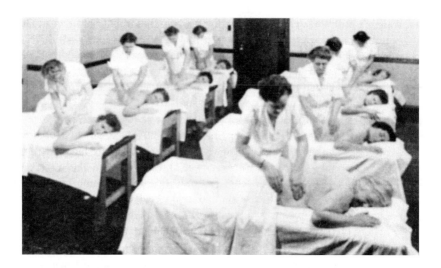

FIGURE 2–4. Photograph of a women's class in "scientific massage techniques" from a catalog of the College of Swedish Massage in Chicago, circa 1940s.

teams. Many practitioners of Swedish massage were proponents of the tradition of natural healing and worked with alternative medical practitioners, especially chiropractors and naturopaths.

Sports. Massage has been part of the sports and fitness scene since ancient Greek times. The rubdown was a well-established practice by athletes in the United States and England in the late nineteenth century. It consisted of superficial skin friction with the hand, a brush, a coarse towel, or a horsehair glove. It was said that "Oxford athletes are never allowed to do cross country running without first rubbing their legs with horsehair gloves or with hands" (Pollard, 1902, p. 21).

H. Joseph Fay wrote about the use of massage in sports in 1916. In his book, *Scientific Massage for Athletes,* he describes massage as being used for ridding the muscles of wastes, which bring about fatigue and stiffness, and to produce additional growth of bone and muscle. He says that the practical trainer "works the meat, or muscle, between the hide and the bone so that it's in its highest state for exercise" (Fay, 1916, p. 20).

Massage performed by trainers was a familiar sight at college and amateur athletic events in the first part of the twentieth century. Albert Baumgartner, a former trainer at the State University of Iowa, wrote *Massage in Athletics* in 1947. He describes massage as being used in preparation for a workout or competition, during rest periods between activities, for reconditioning or recuperation to revitalize the body, and in the treatment of minor injuries. Baumgartner also recognized the psychologic benefits of massage to the athlete.

By the 1950s, massage had largely disappeared from the American sports scene. The profession of athletic training was growing, and trainers specialized in the prevention and treatment of athletic injuries using many of the methods of physical therapy. As physical therapy decreased its use of massage in the 1950s, so did athletic training.

In the 1970s, the tradition of massage for athletes was revived within the growing profession of massage therapy. Impressed by the success of European athletes who used massage in their training regimens, athletes in the United States began seeking massage to enhance performance and to complement other restorative methods. The American Massage Therapy Association launched its National Sports Massage Team and certification program in 1985 (Benjamin & Lamp, 1996, p. 3). Sports massage was included as part of the official medical team at the centennial Olympics in Atlanta in 1996.

Fitness. Just as the ancient Greek gymnasia were not solely for elite athletes, YMCAs and health clubs offer various physical fitness activities for the general population. The YMCA tradition of exercise and massage was well established by 1915 when R. Tait McKenzie described the workouts at the "Y" as consisting of a mixture of Swedish gymnastics, German gymnastics, and games, ending with a bath and a rubdown (McKenzie, 1915, p. 70). By 1953 the health services at the YMCA offered massage and related services for general wellness. The scope of services offered was described by Frierwood:

> *The technician uses massage, baths (shower, steam, electricity cabinet), ultraviolet irradiation (artificial and natural sunlight), infrared (heat), instruction in relaxation and in some cases directed exercise. The adult members secure a relief from tensions, gain a sense of well-being, give attention to the personal fitness and develop habits designed to build and maintain optimum health and physical efficiency throughout the lifespan. (1953, p. 21)*

▪ LATER TWENTIETH-CENTURY UNITED STATES

In the 1950s, the practice of massage went into a period of decline. The term *massage parlor* was being used as a cover for prostitution, ruining the image of legitimate practitioners. Other modalities were taking precedence in physical therapy, and the therapeutic value of massage was being questioned. In the sports arena, trainers were specializing in injuries and the tradition of massage as a training aid was largely forgotten. It was a time of social conservatism, and the undressing and touching that happen in a massage session were uncomfortable for many of the general public. Most private massage schools closed down.

The Human Potential Movement. Two things happened in the 1960s to help revive the practice of massage: the counterculture and the human potential movement. Young people in the 1960s rejected the conservative, conformist, "untouchable" values of the 1950s, and began a search for a deeper meaning in life. These were the post–World War II baby-boomers reaching young adulthood at mid-century.

At the same time, a group of accomplished professionals started meeting at the Esalen Institute in Big Sur, California, to search for the limits of human potential. In the seminars at the Esalen Institute, people explored their feelings in encounter groups and delved into meditation, various spiritual practices, physical practices from Asia such as tai chi, and various forms of massage and bodywork. TV, movies, and popular magazines such as *Look* and *Life* brought knowledge of the Esalen experience to the American public. Americans were breaking out of the confines of the 1950s and exploring their potential in new ways (Leonard, 1988).

A form of massage was developed at the Esalen Institute that was to dramatically affect the field of massage therapy. This form of massage was not about technique, although it was loosely based on a simple form of classic Western massage. It was about making connection with the inner self, and with each other. It was not about professional massage at first, but about friends connecting with friends on a deep level. It is explained by George Downing in his *Massage Book* (1972):

> The core of massage lies in its unique way of communicating without words . . . When receiving a good massage a person usually falls into a mental-physical state difficult to describe. It is like entering a special room until now locked and hidden away; a room the very existence of which is likely to be familiar only to those who practice some form of daily meditation . . . Trust, empathy and respect, to say nothing of a sheer sense of mutual physical existence, for this moment can be expressed with a fullness never matched by words. (p. 1)

Many of those who embraced the ideals of the counterculture and the human potential movement tried Esalen-style massage as part of that experience. Others searching for drugless spiritual or mystical experiences studied Eastern philosophy and cultures. Many joined ashrams where they learned health practices of India, which include vegetarianism, meditation, yoga, and massage. Some studied Taoism, and tried health practices from China and Japan including acupuncture, tai chi, *chi kung, tuina,* and shiatsu. China had opened its doors to Western trade in 1972.

Many of the values, as well as the practices, of the tradition of natural health and healing from earlier in the century were revived in the 1970s. Some of those who learned massage in ashrams, growth centers, or out of books wanted to try making a living doing massage professionally. Many still hold onto the values of the counterculture and resist efforts to "professionalize" the field of massage. Others join professional associations and are active in legislative efforts for the profession of massage therapy.

The opening up to massage that happened in the 1960–70s had a tremendous impact on the emerging profession of massage therapy. There was a significant growth in the number of practitioners and potential receivers of massage. The number of massage and bodywork training programs increased dramatically, and there was an infusion of youthful energy, spirit, and hope. The concept of holistic health and healing were revived and expanded. There was an openness to new ideas and diversity, and an expansion of thinking beyond Western science and medicine. The values of caring, heart, and connection became defining qualities of the work (Benjamin, 1996).

Continued Recognition of Healing Massage. The cultural revival of the 1960–70s has impacted health professions other than massage therapy. The wellness movement took hold in the 1970s within the traditional fields of health, physical education, and recreation. It was undoubtedly influenced by the human potential movement. The concept of wellness was developed by people like John Travis, MD, who developed the wellness model mentioned in Chapter 1 (see Figure 1–1).

Methods that "touch" patients in a human way are being reexamined for their therapeutic value. For example, the American Nurses Association has recognized massage therapy as an official nursing subspecialty; and Therapeutic Touch, a form of energy work, has become a well-researched and respected practice among nurses.

Research is now being performed on the benefits of massage in medical fields such as psychiatric care, pediatrics, gynecology, hospice care, as well as in physical therapy. The Touch Research Institute at the University of Miami was created in 1991 by the school of medicine. It is the first center in the world devoted to basic and applied research in the use of touch in human health and development (Collinge, 1996, p. 290). Chapters 3 and 25 review some of this research.

The Office of Alternative Medicine (OAM) was also established in 1991 to explore "unconventional medical practices," and to recommend further research on the subject. *Alternative Medicine: Expanding Medical Horizons: A Report to the National Institutes of Health on Alternative Medical Systems and Practices in the United States* (1994) was published to summarize their findings to date. The 372 page book contains descriptions of many alternative practices including hypnosis, homeopathic medicine, herbal medicine, Ayurveda, various manual healing methods including massage therapy, and many more. The NIH has subsequently awarded several Exploratory Grants from its Office of Alternative Medicine, which includes research projects on manual healing methods.

In January 1993, a special article appeared in the *New England Journal of Medicine* called "Unconventional Medicine in the United States." It was a report of a national survey that looked at the prevalence of the use of what was called "unconventional medicine," which included therapies such as chiropractic, acupuncture, relaxation techniques, herbal remedies, energy healing, hypnosis, spiritual healing, and massage therapy. Massage ranked third in alternative therapies used by the general public, with only relaxation techniques and chiropractic reported more frequently. The article concluded that the frequency of use of unconventional therapy in the United States is much higher than previously reported (Eisenberg et al, 1993, pp. 246–252).

It is interesting that massage was considered to be "unconventional medicine" even with its long tradition within regular medicine. Perhaps it is considered by some to be "alternative" because it is also found in the traditions of natural healing and sports, and in the human potential movement, and because practitioners of massage are often not in the standard health care professions. In any case, people are turning to healing massage techniques to improve their health and healing in record numbers as we approach the twenty-first century.

■ SUMMARY

The history of massage is both ancient and global. It is used for health and healing in native and folk cultures all over the world. In the writings of the ancient civilizations of Sumer, China, India, Greece, and Rome we find descriptions of highly developed forms of massage. During the Middle Ages in Europe, classical Greco-Roman culture was preserved by the Arabic peoples in Turkey and the Near East and brought back to Europe during the Renaissance. The Turkish Bath, which included a form of massage, was an evolution of the Greek gymnasia and Roman Baths. Today's health clubs with their workout facilities, swimming pools, steamrooms, whirlpools, and massage rooms are part of this legacy.

Two men were very influential in the development of today's classic Western massage: Pehr Henrich Ling (1776–1839) and Johann Mezger (1838–1909). Ling developed a system of active and passive movements to treat medical conditions, which was commonly called the Swedish Movement Cure in nineteenth-century United States. Johann Mezger popularized the use of the familiar French terms to describe four broad categories of massage: *effleurage, petrissage, tapotement, frictions.* In the twentieth century, the work of Ling and Mezger was further developed by their pupils and found its way into regular medicine, as well as in the alternative field of natural health and healing. Swedish massage, a popular genre of classic Western massage, included massage, Swedish movements, various forms of hydrotherapy, heat lamps, diathermy, and colonic irrigation. Swedish massage was offered at places such as health clubs, the YMCA, resorts, and private clinics. Its heyday was between the 1920s and 1940s.

Massage went through a period of decline in the United States in the 1950s. It was being used as a cover for prostitution, and its popularity as a health practice for the general public waned in the conservative climate of that decade. Massage was also losing credibility as a therapeutic modality within the medical professions at that time.

Massage was revived as a valuable health and healing method beginning in the late 1960s. The counterculture and the human potential movement helped bring to light the benefits of massage as a holistic health practice. Since that time, massage therapy has been recognized as an important part of the alternative or complementary healing movement. It is increasingly used by a public interested in natural means toward health and fitness.

■ REFERENCES

Alternative Medicine: Expanding Medical Horizons: A Report to the National Institutes of Health on Alternative Medicine Systems and Practices in the United States. (1994). Available from the Office of Alternative Medicine, National Institutes of Health, 6120 Executive Blvd. #450, Rockville, MD 20892-9904.

Arano, L. C. (1976). *The medieval health handbook: Tacuinum sanitatis.* New York: George Braziller.

Armstrong, D., & Armstrong, E. M. (1991). *The great American medicine show: Being an illustrated history of hucksters, healers, health evangelists, and heroes from Plymouth Rock to the present.* New York: Prentice-Hall.

Baumgartner, A. J. (1947). *Massage in athletics.* Minneapolis, MN: Burgess.

Beals, K. R. (1978). Clubfoot in the Maori: A genetic study of 50 kindreds. *New Zealand Medical Journal, 88,* 144–146.

Beard, G., & Wood, E. C. (1964). *Massage principles and techniques.* Philadelphia: W. B. Saunders.

Benjamin, P. J. (1993). Massage therapy in the 1940's and the College of Swedish Massage in Chicago. *Massage Therapy Journal, 32*(4), 56–62.

Benjamin, P. J. (1996). The California revival: Massage therapy in the 1970–80's. Presentation at the AMTA National Education Conference in Los Angeles, CA, June 1996.

Benjamin, P. J., & Lamp, S. P. (1996). *Understanding sports massage.* Champaign, IL: Human Kinetics.

Bilz, F. E. (1898). *The natural method of healing: A new and complete guide to health.* Translated from the latest German edition. Leipiz: F. E. Bilz.

Bohm, M. (1913). *Massage: Its principles and techniques.* Translated by Elizabeth Gould. Philadelphia: Lippincott.

Chopra, D. (1991). *Perfect health: The complete mind/body guide.* New York: Harmony Books.

Collinge, W. (1996). *The American Holistic Health Association complete guide to alternative medicine.* New York: Warner Books.

Cunliffe, B. (1978). *The Roman baths: A guide to the baths and Roman museum.* City of Bath: Bath Archeological Trust.

Downing, G. (1972). *The massage book.* New York: Random House.

Eisenberg, D. M., Kessler, R. C., Foster, C., Norlock, F. E., Calkins, D. R., & Delblanco, T. L. (1993). Unconventional medicine in the United States. *New England Journal of Medicine, 328*(4), 246–252.

Fay, H. J. (1916). *Scientific massage for athletes.* London: Ewart, Seymour & Co.

Frierwood, H. T. (1953). The place of the health service in the total YMCA program. *Journal of Physical Education, 21.*

Georgii, A. (1880). *Kinetic jottings.* London: Henry Renshaw.

Grafstrom, A. (1904). *A text-book of mechano-therapy (massage and medical gymnastics), prepared for the use of medical students, trained nurses, and medical gymnasts.* Philadelphia: W. B. Saunders.

Graham, D. (1902). *A treatise on massage, its history, mode of application and effects.* Philadelphia: Lippincott.

Hoffa, A. (1978). *Technik der massage* (13th ed). Stuttgart, Germany: Ferdinand Enke. Translated for Fran Tappan by Ruth Friedlander.

Johnson, W. (1866). *The anatriptic art.* London: Simpkin, Marshall & Co.

Kellogg, J. H. (1923). *The art of massage.* Battle Creek, MI: Modern Medicine Publishing Co.

Kleen, E. A. (1921). *Massage and medical gymnastics.* New York: William Wood & Company.

Leboyer, F. (1982). *Loving hands: The traditional art of baby massage.* New York: Alfred A. Knopf.

Leonard, G. (1988). *Walking on the edge of the world: A memoir of the sixties and beyond.* Boston: Houghton Mifflin.

Ling, P. H. (1840a). The general principles of gymnastics. In *The collected works of P. H. Ling.* (1866). Stockholm, Sweden. Translated by Lars Agren and Patricia J. Benjamin. Unpublished.

Ling, P. H. (1840b). Notations to the general principles. In *The collected works of P. H. Ling.* (1866). Stockholm, Sweden. Translated by Lars Agren and Patricia J. Benjamin and published in *Massage Therapy Journal,* Winter 1987.

Ling (1840c). The means or vehicle of gymnastics. Translated by R. J. Cyriax. In *American Physical Education Review, 19*(4), April 1914.

McKenzie, R. T. (1915). *Exercise in education and medicine,* 2nd ed. Philadelphia: W. B. Saunders.

McMillan, M. (1925). *Massage and therapeutic exercise,* 2nd ed. Philadelphia: W. B. Saunders.

Mennell, J. B. (1945). *Physical treatment,* 5th ed. Philadelphia: Blakiston.

Monte, T., & the Editors of East West Natural Health. (1993). *World medicine: The East West guide to healing your body.* New York: Putnam.

Murrell, W. (1890). *Massotherapeutics or massage as a mode of treatment.* Philadelphia: Blakiston

Nissen, H. (1889). *A manual of instruction for giving Swedish movement and massage treatment.* Philadelphia: F. A. Davis.

Nissen, H. (1920). *Practical massage and corrective exercises with applied anatomy.* Philadelphia: F. A. Davis.

Ostrom, K. W. (1905). *Massage and the original Swedish movements.* Philadelphia: Blakiston.

Perrone, B., Stockel, H. H., & Krueger, V. (1989). *Medicine women, curanderas, and women doctors.* Norman, OK: University of Oklahoma Press.

Pollard, D. W. (1902). Massage in training. An unpublished thesis, International Young Men's Christian Association Training School, Springfield, MA.

Posse, N. (1895). *The special kinesiology of educational gymnastics.* Boston: Lothrop, Lee & Shepard.

Roth, M. (1851). *The prevention and cure of many chronic diseases by movements.* London: John Churchill.

Sampson, C. W. (1926). *A practice of physiotherapy.* St. Louis: C. V. Mosby.

Time-Life Books. (1987). *The age of god-kings: Timeframe 3000–1500 B.C.* Alexandria, VA: Time-Life Books.

Torres. (no date). *The folk healer: The Mexican-American tradition of curanderismo.* Kingsville, TX: Nieves Press.

Wood, E. C., & Becker, P. D. (1981). *Beard's massage,* 3rd ed. Philadelphia: W. B. Saunders.

Effects, Benefits, and Indications

Massage is valued for its ability to enhance general health and well-being and for its specific therapeutic effects. Through the years, many theories have been proposed for how massage works its healing wonders. In this chapter we will explore some of those theories and review the research that has been done to confirm its therapeutic value.

■ TERMINOLOGY

The terms *effects*, *benefits*, and *indications* will be used to discuss the values of massage. The *effects of massage* refer to the basic physiologic and psychologic changes that occur to the recipient during a massage session. Depending on the situation, these effects may be either beneficial or harmful to a recipient. Chapter 4 discusses how to avoid harm to the receiver when giving massage.

Benefits are experienced by receivers when the effects of massage support their general health and well-being or their healing process. It is in this sense that someone with a medical condition may benefit from massage even though the intent is not to treat a specific condition.

Massage is said to be *indicated* when it is used in the treatment model to have a specific effect on a particular medical condition. The success of the use of massage as a treatment is determined by how much it contributes directly and measurably to the alleviation of that condition.

▪ THE EFFECTS OF MASSAGE

The focus of this section will be on the changes produced in the body, mind, and emotions of the recipient during massage. Practitioners in various professions use massage to accomplish the goals of their sessions or treatments with these effects in mind.

The literature will often refer in general to the "effects of massage," but it must be noted that different techniques of soft tissue manipulation and joint movement have different effects. For example, a light sliding effleurage usually has a relaxing effect. Tapotement has a stimulating effect if received for a short time and may have a sedating effect if received for a longer period of time. Practitioners choose specific techniques to obtain specific effects and need to know what those are for effective application. Whenever possible, we will be specific about which techniques tend to produce which effects. Table 3–1 summarizes the effects of massage mentioned in this chapter.

The discussion of the effects of massage in this chapter will be kept primarily to those effects that have practical applications in the wellness and treatment models. Technical discussions of the mechanisms involved and of activity at the cellular and molecular levels will be kept to a minimum and mentioned only if they shed light on more practical considerations.

Physical Effects of Massage

The major physical effects of massage are related to its effects on the skin and its ability to elicit the relaxation response, improve blood circulation, affect immune system function, assist metabolic balance in muscle tissue, promote muscle relaxation, maintain connective tissue pliability and mobility, increase joint mobility and flexibility, and reduce pain. Touch, an essential characteristic of massage, is also linked to proper growth and development of infants.

Effects on the Skin. The skin is the primary point of contact between the giver and receiver of massage. One of the major effects of pressure to the skin is stimulation of the sensory receptors found here. This stimulation may have additional effects such as general relaxation, body awareness, and pain reduction.

The skin helps remove excretory products, and its pores must be kept open to maintain health. Exfoliating, by scraping or frictioning off, the outermost layer of dead skin cells is an old health and beauty practice. In unusual situations, for example, if a broken arm has been in a cast for weeks, the buildup of dead cells may be extreme. If there are layers of dead cells inhibiting the normal functions of skin, they can be removed by first bathing, showering, or sitting in a whirlpool, followed by massage or another exfoliation process.

Besides helping to remove dead skin cells, the friction of massage creates heat, which promotes perspiration and increases sebaceous excretions. The skin also caries out a certain amount of respiration (exchanging carbon dioxide and oxygen), which can be assisted by the action of massage.

SUMMARY OF THE POTENTIAL EFFECTS OF MASSAGE ON THE BODY–MIND[a]

TABLE
3–1

Physical Effects

Integumentary system	Stimulate sensory receptors in skin
	Increase superficial circulation
	Remove dead skin
	Add moisture with oil or lotion
	Increase sebaceous gland excretions
Connective tissue (fascia)	Improve pliability of fascia
	Separate tissues
Circulatory system	Increase local circulation
	Enhance venous return
	Reduce blood pressure and heart rate with regular relaxation massage
Muscular system	"Milk" metabolic wastes into venous and lymph flow
	Relax muscles (general and specific)
	Relieve myofascial trigger points
Skeletal system	Increased joint mobility and flexibility
Nervous system	Stimulate parasympathetic nervous system (relaxation)
	Reduce pain (neural-gating mechanism)
	Increase body awareness
Endocrine system	Release of endorphins (also involves nervous system)
Immune system	Increase lymphatic flow
	Improve immune function via stress reduction
Digestive system	Movement of contents of the large intestines
	Better digestion with relaxation

Mental and Emotional Effects

Mental	Increased mental clarity
Emotional	Reduced anxiety
	General feelings of well-being
	Release of unexpressed emotions

[a]These effects do not occur during every massage session. The massage techniques used and the qualities of movement (eg, rhythm, pacing, pressure, direction, duration) help determine which effects are likely to occur. The physical, mental, and emotional condition of recipients and their openness to massage also might have impact on which effects occur.

Oil or lotion applied to the skin during massage may also be beneficial in dry climates, on aging skin, and on certain dry skin conditions. Moisture may be added with topical substances worked into the skin during massage.

Where nerve injury is present, sensory nerve endings may be hypersensitive. In these cases, massage may not bring sedation, but may only increase the pain of the recipient and would be contraindicated. Sometimes skillful practitioners can lower the pain threshold by altering their approach. For example, firm contact may be tolerated better than superficial contact.

The condition of the skin following extreme injury is often abnormal. Parts that have been in a cast will have layers of dead skin under which tender, new skin has developed. In cases where the skin has been burned, massage would not be advisable until adequate scar tissue has formed. In these cases, a physician would indicate when massage may be applied safely.

Relaxation Response. Soothing massage is commonly recognized as an effective relaxation technique. It is one of several stress-management methods known to trigger the relaxation response. Others are meditation, autogenic training and imagery, progressive relaxation, abdominal breathing, hatha yoga, biofeedback, and flotation tanks (Robbins, Powers, & Burgess, 1994, pp. 191–196).

Relaxing back massage is especially effective for stress management. It is used by practitioners in a variety of settings including general wellness massage and with patients in the medical environment (Bauer & Dracup, 1987; Fakouri & Jones, 1987; Fraser & Ken, 1993). Back massage for relaxation is described in Chapter 9.

The relaxation response is a physiologic phenomenon activated by the parasympathetic nervous system. Inducing the relaxation response counters the damaging effects of a chronic stress response by bringing balance to the systems. Specific health benefits of the relaxation response cited by Robbins, Powers, and Burgess (1994, pp. 191–192) include:

- Decreased oxygen consumption and metabolic rate, thus less strain on the bodies energy resources
- Increased intensity and frequency of alpha brain waves associated with deep relaxation
- Reduced blood lactates, blood substances associated with anxiety
- Significantly decreased blood pressure in hypertensive individuals
- Reduced heart rate and slower respiration
- Decreased muscle tension
- Increased blood flow to arms and legs
- Decreased anxiety, fears, and phobias, and increased positive mental health
- Improved quality of sleep

During the relaxation response, a person feels totally relaxed and is in a pleasant semi-awake state of consciousness. General full-body massage consisting predominantly of effleurage and petrissage, with fewer specific techniques that cause discomfort, is most likely to evoke the relaxation response. The qualities of such a session could be described as light, smooth, and flowing. The relaxing effects of this type of session may be enhanced with certain types of music, soft lighting, warm room temperatures, and little talk.

Blood Circulation. Massage can affect both general and local blood circulation. Several studies have shown that capillary vessel dilation and increased blood flow in an area occur with massage. Even light pressure is shown to have an effect (Wood & Becker, 1981, pp. 25–26).

Superficial skin friction improves local circulation in the skin and underlying connective tissue. The heat and redness produced is evidence of increased local circulation. The mechanical action of deep effleurage on the extremities enhances venous flow. The resulting decreased venous pressure provides a favorable situation for increased arterial circulation. This direct mechanical effect includes mainly the more superficial veins.

Whenever possible, gravity should be considered to assist, rather than inhibit, the flow of blood within the veins. The valves within the veins prevent any back-flow of blood once it has moved forward. That is the reason for the dictum in classic Western massage that deep effleurage should always be "toward the heart," or moving distal to proximal on the limbs. The valves in the veins could be damaged if the blood were to flow too hard backward against them.

The mechanical action of kneading and other forms of petrissage also assist in venous return, much the same way muscle contraction does during exercise. Compression of the tissues increases local circulation as blood in the capillaries is moved along toward the larger veins.

Deep stroking and kneading specifically have been known to increase blood volume in an area, and the increased flow is thought to last for some time after massage. For example, Bell (1964) reported that after a 10-minute massage of the calf, blood flow to the area doubled, an effect that lasted 40 minutes. This effect has beneficial implications for bringing nutrients to an area, as well as removing metabolic waste products.

Venostasis is a condition in which the normal flow of blood through a vein is slowed or halted. Muscular inactivity can bring about venostasis, particularly in the dependent limbs where gravity inhibits normal venous return. Other causes for venostasis may be varicose veins, thrombosis, or pressure on the vessels by edema within the surrounding tissues.

Massage should obviously not be given if there is a possibility of spreading inflammation or dislodging a thrombus, or if the obstruction is such that the mechanical assistance of massage could not improve the venous flow. Massage given first to the proximal aspects of an injured limb will ensure that these circulatory pathways are open enough to carry the venous flow along toward the heart.

As mentioned above, one of the long-term effects of eliciting the relaxation response regularly and learning to control stress is decreased blood pressure in hypertensive individuals. This saves wear and tear on the circulatory system and improves circulation overall.

Immune System Function. Massage affects immune system function by improving lymphatic flow and by reducing the negative effects of stress. The first effect is a direct result of massage, while the latter is indirect, but no less important.

LYMPHATIC FLOW. Lymph is a viscous fluid that moves slowly through the lymphatic vessels. These vessels are, for the most part, noncontractile. The movement of lymph through the capillaries, ducts, and nodes of the lymphatic system depends on outside sources such as the contraction of muscles, action of the diaphragm, and pressure generated by filtration of fluid from the capillaries. The lymphatics have a lower pressure and slower flow than venous flow.

Lack of mobility due to a sedentary lifestyle, confinement to bed or a wheelchair, pain, or paralysis seriously interferes with lymph drainage. Most massage techniques, especially effleurage and petrissage, will mechanically assist general lymphatic flow. Special lymphatic massage techniques have been developed to maximize the effects of moving lymph through superficial capillaries. Lymphatic massage has been described as involving a light, smooth pumping action, as well as scooping, rotary, and stationary circles applied along the lymph pathways (Knaster, 1996, pp. 167–169). Lymphatic massage is described in more detail in Chapter 13.

STRESS REDUCTION. To the extent that massage helps reduce the effects of chronic stress and pain, it can be linked to improved immune system function. The hormonal and nervous system responses to stress are known to have harmful effects if continued over a long period of time. Immune system disorders caused by chronic stress include frequent infections, autoimmune disease, and possibly, cancer (Corwin, 1996, 233–238).

A study appeared in 1995 in *Lancet*, a British medical journal, that showed that wounds healed more slowing in people suffering from chronic stress. Researchers found that the stressed group had lower levels of interleukin-1 beta, an immune system substance known to play a role in wound repair (Greene, 1996, p.16).

Massage designed to help elicit the relaxation response, as described above, can assist in bringing the body back to balance and thus improve immune system function. Massage can be an important part of a stress-reduction program, along with other health practices such as proper nutrition, exercise, and rest.

Digestion. To the extent that massage helps reduce stress, it can be thought of as improving digestion. Chronic stress is known to disrupt the normal digestive process, leaving people with indigestion and possibly stomach and intestinal ulcers.

Abdominal massage is also used to enhance movement of the contents of the large intestine. See Chapter 9 for a description of abdominal massage. Massage has been used for decades to aid movement of the bowels in people suffering from constipation.

Metabolic Balance in Muscle Tone. Metabolically, the muscles maintain a chemical balance through normal activity. As the muscles contract, they rid themselves of metabolic waste products by "milking" these toxins into the lymphatic and venous flow. Muscles additionally assist lymphatic and venous flow toward the heart through mechanical pressure that pushes the fluids through vessels where valves prevent a backflow. Thus, these metabolic by-products are carried away. As the muscles relax, fresh blood flows into them, bringing necessary nutrients to the area. This balancing action may be disturbed through overactivity or underactivity.

Overactivity disturbs the balance by not allowing sufficient relaxation time for the inflow of nutritive products. At the same time, due to exertion, metabolic waste products are formed faster than they can be eliminated. Thus the muscle becomes loaded with irritant acids and may experience oxygen deficiency or ischemia.

Underactivity also disturbs the balance by not providing the "milking" effect to assist venous and lymphatic return. Hence, the irritant products that accumulate in the muscle tissue are not carried away as they should be, and the muscle becomes more or less "stagnant." When partial or total muscular inactivity occurs, massage can mechanically assist the "milking" process. However, it cannot totally replace the action of normal muscular activity.

Following strenuous physical activity, metabolic waste products can be hastened back into the venous return by massage. The stiffness and soreness that often follow such strenuous activity can be lessened or prevented by massage immediately following the activity. This is a primary consideration in post-event and recovery sports massage (Benjamin & Lamp, 1996). This also has implications for patients performing strengthening exercises during rehabilitation.

Muscle Relaxation. Massage is often used to help return hypertonic muscles to a relaxed state. There are several ways that muscle relaxation may be effected. Reduction of general muscle tension may be due in part to the effects of the relaxation response as mentioned above. There may also be a conscious letting go of muscle tension by the higher brain centers as the recipient assumes a passive state during a massage session.

General muscle relaxation may also be traced to increased sensory stimulation that accompanies the application of massage techniques. Yates (1990) reasons that massage causes a massive increase in the sensory input to the spinal cord, which results in readjustments in reflex pathways, which leads to spontaneous renormalization of imbalances of tonic activity between individual muscles and muscle groups. Residual muscle tension left over from past activity or emotional stress is released as the system rebalances itself (pp. 11–12). Thus, muscular relaxation may result from the general application of a variety of basic massage techniques such as effleurage, petrissage, friction, tapotement, and vibration.

More technical methods may be used to relax specific muscles. For example, the reflex effect of muscle spindles may be used to reduce tonicity in individual muscles. In a technique called muscle approximation, the attachments of the muscle are slowly and forcibly drawn together, or approximated. This decreases the stretch of the muscle spindle, thus decreasing gamma firing and reducing muscle tone. The approximation is held until the muscle fibers relax (Rattray 1994, pp. 44–45).

Stimulation of the sensory receptors in the muscluotendinous junction is believed to reflexly reduce alpha neuron firing, thus reducing muscle tone. This reflex action may be induced using the origin and insertion technique. This technique is used when direct work on the muscle belly is too painful. Cross-fiber and with-fiber techniques are performed on the attachments of the targeted muscle in small segments until the tissue releases; eventually overall muscle tone is reduced (Rattray, 1994, pp. 43–44). Muscular relaxation is one of the basic effects of massage. Other specific methods for inducing muscular relaxation will be mentioned throughout the text.

Connective Tissue Pliability and Mobility. Connective tissue is the most pervasive tissue in the body. It is found in ligaments, tendons, and fascia. Fascia is the connective tissue that surrounds all muscles, bones, and organs and helps to give them shape. Fascia literally holds the body together and can be thought of as continuous sheets of supportive tissue that envelop the entire body and its parts.

In healthy bodies the connective tissue is pliable and moves freely. With chronic stress, chronic immobility, trauma, or disease, connective tissue may become thickened or rigid or may stick to other tissues, forming adhesions. This causes restrictions in movement and impairs the ability of the affected tissues to conduct exchanges of nutrients and cellular wastes.

Massage can help restore connective tissue pliability and improve tissue function. Connective tissue has a property called *thixotropy*, that is, it becomes more fluid and pliable when it is stirred up, and more solid when it is immobile. The pressing, stretching, and other movements of massage raise the temperature and the energy level of the tissue slightly and creates a "greater degree of sol (fluidity) in organic systems that are already there but are behaving sluggishly" (Juhan, 1987, pp. 69–70).

Certain massage techniques can also help break adhesions formed when connective tissues stick to each other or to other tissues. The simple mechanical actions of lifting, broadening, and applying a shearing force across the parallel organization of fibers helps separate tissues. Kneading, deep transverse friction, broadening techniques, and myofascial techniques are very effective for separating and "unsticking" tissues that are adhering.

In addition to promoting healthy connective tissue function, massage helps prevent some tissue abnormalities and dysfunction. For example, massage techniques such as kneading and deep friction have been found to help prevent the formation of abnormal collagenous connective tissue called *fibrosis* (Yates, 1990). Deep transverse friction is used in rehabilitation to help the body form strong mobile scar tissue during the remodeling phase of soft tissue healing. Deep friction helps break interfibrillary adhesions by forcibly broadening the tissues. This in turn helps produce more parallel fiber arrangement and fewer transverse connections in the tissue that inhibit movement (Cyriax & Cyriax, 1993). Subcutaneous scar tissue may at times be loosened by careful and persistent friction; however, it remains to be seen whether deeper scarring in connective tissue can be relieved once it is formed.

Increased Joint Mobility and Flexibility. Tense muscles, scarring in muscle and connective tissues, adhesions, trigger points, and general connective tissue thickening and rigidity may all restrict movement at joints. Massage and passive joint movements can be used effectively to help maintain joint mobility and normal range of motion by addressing any abnormal conditions found in the soft tissues surrounding the joint.

A cooperative study by sport physical therapists and a massage therapist found that massage can significantly increase range of motion in the hamstrings (Crosman, Chateauvert, & Weisburg, 1985). Increased flexibility lasted for at least seven days after the massage. The massage techniques used in the study were light and deep effleurage, stretching effleurage, petrissage (kneading), and friction (deep circular and deep transverse).

Pain. Pain is defined in *Taber's* as "a sensation in which a person experiences discomfort, distress, or suffering due to irritation of or stimulation of sensory nerves, esp. pain sensors" (Thomas, 1985). Pain reduction is one of the benefits of massage that follows from its ability to elicit the relaxation response, relieve muscle tension, and improve circulation.

Massage may be used effectively to reduce pain caused by conditions that respond well to soft tissue manipulation such as hypertonic muscles, ischemia, and myofascial trigger points. Muscle relaxation and improved local circulation can help relieve pain associated with tense muscles and the accompanying ischemia. Massage may also be used to help interrupt a pain–spasm–pain cycle induced by hypertonic muscles by the use of specific techniques such as approximation as described above (Kresge, 1983; Rattray, 1994; Yates, 1990).

It is also thought that massage may reduce pain by activating the neural-gating mechanism in the spinal cord through increase in sensory stimulation. The theory is that by activating fast, large fibers that carry tactile information, transmission from slower, smaller pain-transmitting fibers is blocked. The perception of pain may be reduced for minutes or hours through the additional sensory input created by massage techniques. Activation of the neural-gating mechanism has been suggested as an explanation for the temporary analgesia associated with deep friction massage in the treatment of tendinous and ligamentous injuries (Yates, 1990). Research by de Bruijn (1984) noted that the high degree of analgesia resulting from deep transverse friction is preceded by painful irritation of the affected tissues. De Bruijn concluded that friction massage was a promising treatment for soft tissue injuries since the eventual pain-reduction effect allowed the patient to use the affected tissue for better healing.

Myofascial trigger points (TP) are known to cause pain at the site of the TP, as well as at satellite trigger points, and in muscles that lie within the reference zone of the TP. Massage (ischemic compression and muscle stripping) and stretching are therapies used in deactivating trigger points (Travell & Simons, 1983, 1992). See Chpater 12 for further discussion of trigger points and their relief.

There is some evidence that massage induces the release of neurochemicals called endorphins and enkephalins. These substances modulate pain-impulse transmission in the central nervous system and induce relaxation and feelings of general well-being. The mechanism involved in not clearly understood and may be a combination of psychologic, as well as physical, reactions to massage. More research is needed for a fuller understanding (Yates, 1990).

Growth and Development

Touch has been found to be essential for the proper growth and development of infants and children. Holding, cuddling, rocking, and stroking are all necessary for infants to thrive. There is also evidence that adequate pleasurable tactile experience in early life can influence the development of personality traits such as calmness, gentleness, and nonaggressiveness (Brown, 1984, pp. 41–120; Juhan, 1987, pp. 43–55; Montagu, 1978, pp. 76–157).

The importance of stimulation to the skin for proper growth and development cannot be overestimated. The skin develops from the same primitive cells as the brain and is a prime sensory organ. Stimulation of the tactile nerve endings in the skin provides information about the outside world and helps the brain organize its circuitry for proper development. This is also true for movement and information received through the kinesthetic sense. Thus "the use of touch and sensation to modify our experience of peripheral conditions exerts an active influence upon the organization of reflexes and body image deep within the central nervous system" (Juhan, 1987, p. 40).

As infants learn about the world around them through touch and movement, they also learn about themselves and their own bodies. Juhan expresses this idea, "by rubbing up against the world, I define myself to myself" (Juhan, 1987, p. 34).

Massage is an excellent way to provide systematic and regular touching to growing infants. The massage of infants has been practiced widely in places such as India, and is increasing in use in the United States.

Mental and Emotional Effects

The effects of massage on the mind and emotions are less well understood than the physical effects, although they are related to the physical effects in many ways, and vice versa. The mental and emotional effects include increased mental clarity, reduced anxiety, and feelings of general well-being. A phenomenon called *emotional release*, which is an interesting interface of body, mind, and emotions, may also occur during massage.

Mental Clarity. Two studies performed at the Touch Research Institute in Miami, and reported in *Massage* magazine in July/August 1996, suggest that massage may help improve mental clarity. In one study, 15-minute massage sessions were given to hospital personnel over a five-week period during their lunch hour. People reported feeling more relaxed, in better moods, and more alert after receiving massage. Similarly, students who received massage during finals week reported being more relaxed and less anxious and said that they remembered information better after an 8-minute massage session.

In a job stress study conducted in 1993, subjects received a 20-minute massage in a chair twice weekly for a month. They reported less fatigue and demonstrated greater clarity of thought, improved cognitive skills, and lower anxiety levels. EEG, alpha, beta, and theta waves were also altered in ways consistent with enhanced alertness (Field, Fox, Pickens, Ironsong, & Scafidi, 1993).

Massage is used with athletes in pre-event situations to help spark the alertness necessary for competition. For pre-event readiness sports massage sessions are 15–20 minutes in duration, have an upbeat tempo, and use techniques to increase circulation and joint mobility. Tapotement is frequently employed for stimulation (Benjamin & Lamp, 1996, pp. 67–68).

In each of the cases mentioned above, the massage sessions were relatively short, that is, between 8 and 20 minutes. It is likely that increased mental alertness is related to increased circulation to the brain and sensory stimulation, as well as mental clarity possible with a calm mind.

Reduced Anxiety. The studies mentioned above, which showed an increase in mental alertness with massage, also reported a reduction in anxiety level. This would be an expected result of the relaxation response and action of the parasympathetic nervous system. It may also be related to the release of endorphins thought to occur during some forms of massage (Kaard & Tostinbo, 1989).

Feelings of General Well-Being. Stated in positive terms, massage is shown to increase feelings of general well-being. This most likely involves the same mechanisms as anxiety reduction, that is, relaxation response and release of endorphins. Tactile pleasure associated with relaxation massage and simple caring touch may also contribute to feelings of well-being.

It is interesting to note that prolonged exposure to pain and other stressors has been shown to deplete the stores of endorphins, leading to an increased perception of pain and dispair. To the extent that massage helps to manage pain and stress, and to release endorphins, it may seem to contribute to a positive outlook.

Emotional Release. A phenomenon called *emotional release* sometimes occurs during a massage session. Unexpressed emotions that are held in the receiver's body may come to the surface in various forms such as weeping or feelings of anger or fear. It is possible that during deep relaxation, a person's natural psychologic defenses are lowered, allowing them to feel or express emotions held inside.

Releasing trapped emotions may be an important step in a physical or psychologic healing process. Although this is a process familiar to many massage practitioners, relatively little is known about the mechanisms involved. Clyde Ford, DC, talks about this phenomenon in his books, *Where Healing Waters Meet: Touching Mind & Emotion Through the Body* (1989) and *Compassionate Touch: The Role of Human Touch in Healing and Recovery* (1993).

A Holistic View

Theoretically dividing the human organism into body, mind, and emotions is a useful exercise for discussing the effects of massage. Perhaps it is a product of Western thought and science to think of human beings as divided in this way. However, it should always be remembered that we live as whole persons and that these effects interact with each other in complex ways to produce an overall effect that may be greater than the sum of its parts. The specialties of Western medicine are just beginning to explore the interconnections in these aspects of persons.

Practitioners experience the interconnectedness of human beings in many ways. For example, a practitioner may be focused on some physical aspect such as relaxing hypertonic muscles, and the recipient's experience might also have an emotional component such as painful memories of an accident that caused trauma to the area. A psychotherapist may witness the physical effects of stress, such as tension headaches, in their clients. Awareness of how the body, mind, and emotions interact will help practitioners better serve their clients or patients.

How Effects Are Produced

Several mechanisms have been identified to explain how the effects of massage and bodywork techniques are produced. Some of these theories are recognized within the Western biomedical model, while others are on the cutting edge of alternative

and body–mind studies. The mechanisms presented here include mechanical, physiologic, reflex, body–mind, and energetic. Table 3–2 outlines the mechanisms used to explain the effects of massage. Some effects may be produced by more than one mechanism.

Mechanical Effects. Mechanical effects are the result of physical forces such as compression, stretching, shearing, broadening, and vibration of body tissues. These effects occur on the more gross level of physical structure. Examples of mechanical effects include increased superficial skin circulation using superficial warming friction; enhanced venous return using deep effleurage; elongation of muscles using stretching; improved lymph flow using lymphatic drainage techniques; and breaking adhesions with deep transverse friction.

Physiologic Effects. Physiologic effects refer to organic processes of the body. These may involve biochemical processes at the cellular level, but may also occur at the tissue and organ system levels. Examples of physiologic effects include the various results of the relaxation response produced by activating the parasympathetic nervous system; decrease in anxiety by facilitating the release of endorphins; and proper development and growth in infants assisted by the tacile stimulation that occurs during massage.

Reflex Effects. Sir James MacKenzie (1923) defines the reflex process as "that vital process which is concerned in the reception of a stimulus by one organ or tissue and its conduction to another organ, which on receiving a stimulation produces the effects" (p. 47). In massage, the hands stimulate the sensory receptors of the skin and subcutaneous tissues, causing reflex effects. The stimuli pass along the afferent

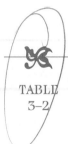

MECHANISMS TO EXPLAIN THE EFFECTS OF MASSAGE

TABLE 3–2

Mechanical effects	The result of physical forces such as compression, stretching, shearing, broadening, and vibration of tissues. Occurs on the gross level of physical structure.
	Examples: venous return, lymph flow, breaking adhesions
Physiologic effects	Organic processes of the body on cellular, tissue, or organ system levels.
	Examples: activation of parasympathetic nervous system; release of endorphins
Reflex effects	The result of pressure or movement in one part of the body having an effect in another part.
	Examples: capillary vasodilation or constriction, pain reduction, reflexology
Body–mind effects	The result of the interplay of body, mind, and emotions in health and disease processes.
	Examples: relaxation response, anxiety reduction
Energetic effects	The result of balancing or improving the flow of energy within and around the body.
	Examples: improving flow of *chi* (energy) by pressing traditional acupuncture points (see Chapter 15).

fibers of the peripheral nervous system to the spinal cord. From there, it is conceivable that these stimuli may disperse through the central and autonomic nervous systems, producing various effects in any zone supplied from the same segment of the spinal cord.

Some of these reflex effects are capillary vasodilation or constriction, relaxation or stimulation of voluntary muscle contraction, and gooseflesh. In addition, there is possible sedation or stimulation of sensory reception with accompanying reduction or increase in pain. In some cases the reflex effects may be unpleasant, causing nausea, vomiting, and depression of the heart's action with resulting pallor and sweating.

Reflex effects may also refer to the phenomenon of pressing one part of the body and having an effect on an entirely different part of the body. For example, in zone therapy, the theoretical basis for reflexology, pressing on certain spots on the body such as on the ears, hands, or feet is thought to have a normalizing effect on corresponding organs and structures in other parts of the body. Chapter 14 explains more about reflexology.

Body–Mind Effects. Body–mind effects acknowledge the interplay of body, mind, and emotions in health and disease. This concept has a long tradition in natural healing, in most native cultures, and in healing traditions of China and India. Western medical science is beginning to confirm demonstrable links between our physical bodies and our mental and emotional states. The new science of psychoneuroimmunology has grown out of these studies.

The body–mind connection can be easily seen in the relaxation response, a physiologic process involving the parasympathetic nervous system. The relaxation response can be elicited by practices such as meditation, which quiets the mind, or by the tactile stimulation of massage. Other examples of body–mind effects of massage include reduction in anxiety and release of emotions held in the body.

Energetic Effects. Massage and bodywork have been described as balancing, or improving the flow, of energy. What this energy is, and how it relates to the body are yet to be determined in terms of Western science. However, there are ancient traditions of massage and bodywork, primarily from China and India, based in concepts of energy flow. Therapeutic touch, a form of energy work adopted by many nurses, addresses the energy field of the recipient (Claire, 1995, pp. 251–268).

There are many theories about how energy flows in and around the body, and practitioners and receivers alike report "feeling" energy. Energy work is currently outside of the understanding and general acceptance of Western biomedicine, but it has persisted over time and is found to be useful by many people.

■ BENEFITS OF MASSAGE FOR EVERYONE

When the effects of massage support general health and well-being or the ongoing healing process, there are *benefits* by definition. A general wellness or health massage aims to normalize body tissues and to optimize function. Everyone can benefit from the health-promoting effects of wellness massage.

The main intention in a wellness massage is to promote general and muscular relaxation and to enhance circulation of fluids, digestion, and elimination. The effects of general relaxation alone have impact on many physiologic and psychologic aspects of health and well-being. Massage also provides healthy touch, which is a basic human need.

■ BENEFITS FOR SPECIAL POPULATIONS

The effects of massage may be especially beneficial for people in certain situations. Such benefits are not intended in the sense of the treatment model, but are the natural effects of a general wellness massage tailored for a unique individual. For example, pregnant women who tend to have back and leg strain may find special benefit in the effects of massage related to muscle relaxation and improved circulation. Infants benefit from the extra tactile stimulation provided by regular massage for their normal growth and development. Chapter 20 discusses massage for mother and child. The elderly may find massage beneficial for mitigating the normal effects of the aging process and providing healthy caring touch. Massage for healthy aging is discussed in Chapter 23.

Some practitioners are going to workplaces and providing wellness massage for people who sit at desks or similar workstations all day. Massage chairs are commonly used in this environment. The special chairs offer a convenient delivery model and give access to the upper body, which is more stressed in office workers. Workplace wellness massage is described more fully in Chapter 21.

For centuries, athletes have benefited from massage as part of their training regimen. The intent of sports massage is to help athletes stay in top condition during strenuous training, prepare for competition, recover after competition, and recover from injury. See Chapter 19 for more information about sports massage.

People going through stressful life situations may benefit from the relaxing effects of massage. Massage may be used by those in psychotherapy treatment to help reduce anxiety as they process emotional issues. Massage for mental and emotional wellness is described in Chapter 22.

People with life-threatening illnesses, those in hospices, and their caregivers may benefit from the psychologic benefits of massage. Even those for whom treatment of a condition is not an option may improve the quality of their lives with massage, as explained in Chapter 24.

■ INDICATIONS: MASSAGE AS TREATMENT

Practitioners in several health care professions use massage and related bodywork forms to treat specific medical conditions. Physical therapists, nurses, respiratory therapists, chiropractors, and osteopaths have all used massage for certain treatment effects. Chapter 25 is devoted to looking at the research related to the use of massage in the medical environment.

■ SUMMARY

Massage is valued for its ability to enhance general health and well-being and for its specific therapeutic effects. The terms *effects*, *benefits*, and *indications* are used in this text to discuss the values of massage. *Effects of massage* refers to the basic physiologic and psychologic changes that occur in the recipient as a result of massage. *Benefits* are experienced by receivers when the effects of massage support their general wellness or their healing process. Massage is said to be *indicated* when it is used in the treatment model to have a specific effect on a particular medical condition.

It is difficult to generalize about the effects of massage, since the actual effects depend on the specific techniques used, as well as the condition and reaction of the receiver. However, massage has the potential to produce a number of physical, mental, and emotional effects. The physical effects of massage may include healthy skin, general relaxation, improved blood circulation, enhanced immune system function, metabolic balance in the muscles, muscle relaxation, connective tissue pliability, increased joint mobility and flexibility, reduction of pain, and optimal growth and development. The mental and emotional effects may include increased mental clarity, reduced anxiety, feelings of general well-being, and emotional release.

Mechanisms that may be used to explain the effects of massage include mechanical or physical forces, physiologic processes, reflex effects, body–mind effects, and energetic effects. In some cases, more than one of these mechanisms may be involved in producing a specific effect of massage.

Massage has benefits for everyone to the extent that it supports general health and well-being and enhances a person's healing process. It has special benefits for certain populations such as pregnant women, elders, athletes, and those who work in offices. The relaxation effects of massage benefit those in psychotherapy, those in hospitals, and people with life-threatening illnesses. Chapter 25 is devoted to exploring the use of massage in medical settings.

■ REFERENCES

no author. 1996. Massage helps lower stress of working, taking final exams. In *Massage, 62* (July/August), 148.

Bauer, W. C., & Dracup, K. A. (1987). Physiological effects of back massage in patients with acute myocardial infarction. *Focus on Critical Care, 14*(6), 42–46.

Bell, A. J. (1964). Massage and the physiotherapist. *Physiotherapy, 50*, 406–408.

Benjamin, P. J., & Lamp, S. P. (1996). *Understanding sports massage.* Champaign, IL: Human Kinetics.

Brown, C. C., ed. (1984). *The many facets of touch.* Johnson & Johnson Baby Products Company.

de Bruijn, R. (1984). Deep transverse friction: Its analgesic effect. *International Journal of Sports Medicine, 5*(suppl), 35–36.

Claire, T. (1995). *Bodywork: What type of massage to get, and how to make the most of it.* New York: William Morrow.

Corwin, E. J. (1996). *Handbook of pathophysiology.* Philadelphia: Lippincott.

Crosman, L. J., Chateauvert, S. R., & Weisburg, J. (1985). The effects of massage to the hamstring muscle group on range of motion. *Massage Journal,* 59–62.

Cyriax, J. H., & Cyriax, P. J. (1993). *Illustrated manual of orthopedic medicine,* 2nd ed. Boston: Butterworth & Heinemann.

Fakouri, C., & Jones, P. (1987). Relaxation Rx: Slow stroke back rub. *Journal of Gerontological Nursing, 13*(2), 32–35.

Field, T. M., Fox, N., Pickens, J., Ironsong, G., & Scafidi, F. (1993). Job stress survey. Unpublished manuscript. Touch Research Institute, University of Miami School of Medicine. Reported in *Touchpoints: Touch Research Abstracts, 1*(1).

Ford, C. W. (1989). *Where healing waters meet: Touching mind & emotion through the body.* Barrytown, NY: Station Hill Press.

Ford, C. W. (1993). *Compassionate touch: The role of human touch in healing and recovery.* New York: A Fireside/Parkside book.

Fraser, J., & Kerr, J. R. (1993). Psychophysiological effects of back massage on elderly institutionalized patients. *Journal of Advanced Nursing, 18,* 238–245.

Greene, E. (1996). Study links stress reduction with faster healing. *Massage Therapy Journal, 35*(1), 16.

Juhan, D. (1987). *Job's body: A handbook for bodywork.* Barrytown, NY: Station Hill Press.

Kaard, B., & Tostinbo, O. (1989). Increase of plasma beta endorphins in a connective tissue massage. *General Pharmacology, 20*(4), 487–489.

Knaster, M. (1996). *Discovering the body's wisdom.* New York: Bantam.

Kresge, C. A. (1983). Massage and sports. In O. Appenzeller & R. Atkinson (eds.) *Sports medicine: Fitness, training, injuries* (pp. 367–380). Baltimore: Urban & Schwarzenberg.

MacKenzie, J. (1923) *Angina pectoris.* London: Henry Frowde and Hodder and Stoughton.

Montagu, A. (1978). *Touching: The human significance of the skin,* 2nd ed. New York: Harper & Row.

Rattray, F. S. (1994). *Massage therapy: An approach to treatments.* Toronto, Ontario: Massage Therapy Texts and MA Verick Consultants.

Robbins, G., Powers, D., & Burgess, S. (1994). *A wellness way of life,* 2nd ed. Madison, WI: Brown & Benchmark.

Thomas, C. L. (ed.). (1985). *Taber's cyclopedic medical dictionary.* Philadelphia: F. A. Davis.

Travell, J. G., & Simons, D. G. (1983). *Myofascial pain and dysfunction: The trigger point manual.* Baltimore: Williams & Wilkins.

Travell, J. G., & Simons, D. G. (1992). *Myofascial pain and dysfunction: The lower extremities.* Vol. 2. Baltimore: Williams & Wilkins.

Wood, E. C., & Becker, P. D., (1981). *Beard's massage,* 3rd ed. Philadelphia: W. B. Saunders.

Yates, J. (1990). *A physicians guide to therapeutic massage: Its physiologic effects and their application to treatment.* Massage Therapists Association of British Columbia, Vancouver, B.C., Canada.

Endangerment Sites, Contraindications, and Cautions

One of most basic rules of giving therapeutic massage is to *do no harm.* In this chapter we will present some guidelines for helping you make decisions about what to do and what to avoid to protect the health and safety of your clients and patients. Endangerment sites, contraindications, and cautions are all important considerations for practitioners.

The great variety of massage forms used today complicates the issue somewhat. These forms vary from deep tissue structural massage of the physical body to light work affecting the energy within and around the physical body. An endangerment site or a contraindication in one form of bodywork may be perfectly safe for a different form.

This chapter will focus on endangerment sites, contraindications, and cautions that are important when giving classic Western massage and forms that use similar techniques. This includes all techniques applied to the physical body that involve pressing, stroking, frictions, kneading, tapping, and vibrating. Chapters devoted to other types of massage, bodywork, or techniques that affect energy will contain information about contraindications and cautions for that particular type.

The practitioner's knowledge of Western anatomy and physiology is essential to ensure the safety of the person receiving massage and bodywork. It is particularly important to know the location of major nerves and blood vessels, glands, and visceral organs. Endangerment sites, contraindications, and cautions will be discussed in this chapter in terms of Western science and concepts of pathology.

ENDANGERMENT SITES

Endangerment sites are areas of the body where delicate structures are less protected and, therefore, may be more easily damaged when receiving massage. Caution is required when performing massage in or around endangerment sites. The following paragraphs identify common endangerment sites for classic Western massage and similar massage techniques and discuss cautions that should be taken when working in those areas. Figure 4–1 shows the general location of these endangerment sites on the anterior and posterior body.

Neck Area. The anterior neck is the triangular area on the front of the neck defined by the sternocleidomastoid (SCM) and includes the sternal notch, which is the depression found just superior to the sternoclavicular joint. Delicate structures located in the anterior neck region are the carotid artery, jugular vein, vagus nerve, larynx, and thyroid gland. Deep pressure on any of these structures could be dangerous.

Pressure within the anterior triangle of the neck, including the depression formed by the sternal notch, should be avoided entirely in most forms of massage. There are some advanced techniques that address cervical muscles from the anterior neck, but these should be performed only by experienced therapists with special training. The gentle superficial stroking during lymphatic drainage and noncontact forms of energy work are possible exceptions to the no-touch rule.

Great care should be taken when performing neck massage on the elderly due to the likelihood of atherosclerosis and potential further damage to major blood vessels in the area. Only light pressure should be used on the neck, if massage is applied to the neck at all.

Axillary Area. Delicate circulatory and nervous structures are relatively exposed in the axillary or armpit area. These include the brachial artery, axillary artery and vein, cephalic vein, and the nerve complex of the brachial plexus. Deep pressure in this area should be approached with caution.

Elbow Area. There are two places in the elbow area that require caution. One is the space just medial to the olecranon process where the ulnar nerve is relatively exposed. This is the "funny bone" area that causes sharp pain when hit.

The second area is the anterior surface, or fold, of the elbow. This area is similar to the popliteal fossa found posterior to the knee as described later on. Vulnerable structures found in this area include the brachial vein and artery, median cubital vein, and median nerve. These structures are all close to the surface and unprotected by muscle. Moderate broad pressure may be applied to the area, but deep specific pressure should be restricted to the surrounding muscles.

Umbilicus Area. The umbilicus is a sensitive area superficial to the descending aorta and abdominal aorta. Avoid direct heavy pressure to the umbilicus.

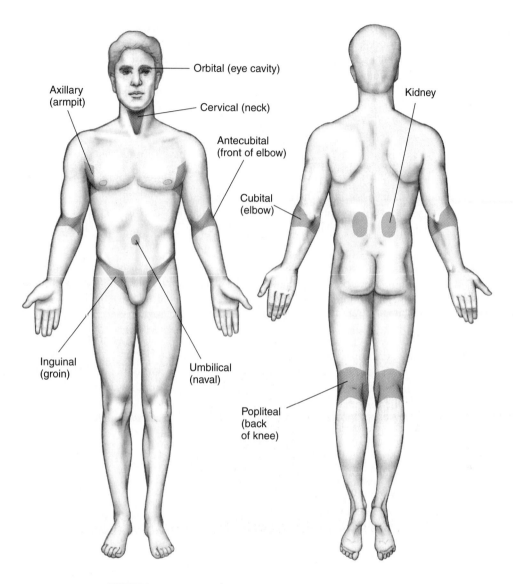

FIGURE 4–1. Important endangerment sites, anterior and posterior body.

Kidney Area. The kidneys are located on either side of the spine generally at the level between the 3rd lumbar and 12th thoracic vertebrae. They are positioned behind the parietal peritoneum and against the deep muscles of the back. Superficial or deep stroking and pressing techniques may be applied carefully to the muscles of the back located in the kidney area. However, only very light pressure should be used when performing percussion techniques over this area.

Inguinal Area (Groin). The inguinal or groin area is located roughly where the thigh and the trunk meet on the anterior side of the body. The femoral nerve and major blood vessels to the lower extremities cross there, for example, femoral artery, great saphenous and femoral veins. When the thigh is flexed, a depression is created in the area exposing the more delicate structures. Great care should be taken when applying deep pressure into this area, for example, when reaching for the iliopsoas. This should be attempted only by experienced practitioners.

Popliteal Fossa. The muscles of the posterior lower extremity cross the knee laterally and medially, leaving the center space relatively unprotected. This is the popliteal fossa area. The popliteal artery and vein and the tibial nerve are located there. Avoid any pressure over this area, and follow the muscles around the area when massaging them.

Eyes. Great care should be taken when working on the face around the eyes. Be careful not to slip and hit the eyeball by accident. Only the very lightest pressure is used when stroking the eyelid.

Major Veins in Extremities. Major veins in the extremities are being included under endangerment sites because structural damage can occur to the valves within the veins if deep effleurage is applied improperly. Always apply deep flushing effleurage to the arms and legs from distal to proximal, that is, toward the heart, and with the flow that opens the valves.

■ GENERAL PRINCIPLES FOR SAFETY AROUND ENDANGERMENT SITES

Here are some general principles to keep in mind to protect the receiver's body from structural damage during massage. Remember, your first responsibility is to do no harm.

1. Always adjust the pressure you use to match the part of the body, the condition of the tissues, and the person you are working on. Any part of the body can be damaged if too much pressure is used for the person receiving.
2. Avoid heavy pressure anyplace where nerve, blood, or lymph vessels and structures are close to the surface or relatively unprotected by muscle or bone.
3. Be careful around joints where delicate structures are less protected by skeletal muscle.
4. If you feel a pulse, it means that you are on a major artery. Move to a different place immediately.
5. If the receiver feels searing, burning, shooting, electrical sensations, "pins and needles," or numbness, you may be pressing on a nerve. Move to a different place immediately.

6. Any abnormal structure is a potential endangerment site. Get information about structural abnormalities, and proceed with caution when you are sure it is safe to do so.
7. Always work with awareness, and when in doubt, do not take a chance that might lead to injury.

■ CONTRAINDICATIONS AND CAUTIONS

Contraindications are conditions or situations that make the receiving of massage inadvisable because of the harm it might do. *Regional* or *local contraindications* refer to a specific area of the body and *general contraindications* refer to the whole person. In the treatment model, a contraindication is "any symptom or circumstance indicating the inappropriateness of a form of treatment otherwise advisable" (Thomas, 1985).

Practitioners should be alert to possible contraindications for every recipient. A health history taken at the initial visit will provide information about previous conditions or situations to be aware of and current health status. Practitioners should check in with recipients periodically to see if their health status has changed in significant ways, particularly related to a known condition that is a contraindication or for which special cautions apply.

Knowledge of normal anatomy and physiology, as well as the nature of common pathologies, is important for the wellness practitioner. Such knowledge may help prevent a well-meaning practitioner from causing harm to a client and increase the possibility of benefit. Practitioners operating from the treatment model need to be especially well versed in the pathologies with which they are working.

There are some general principles that can be used to help determine if harm could be done by performing massage. An understanding of these principles is far more important than memorizing a long list of specific pathologies.

1. *Do not perform massage when the recipient (general circumstances):*
   • Feels physically ill or nauseated
   • Is in severe pain
   • Has a fever
   • Has been seriously injured recently (local contraindications)

2. *Do not touch areas of the skin where there is a pathologic condition that is contagious or that may be worsened or spread by applying pressure or rubbing.* For example:
   • Rashes
   • Boils
   • Open wounds
   • Athlete's foot (tinea pedis)
   • Herpes simplex (eg, cold sores)
   • Impetigo. A skin infection usually caused by staph or strep.

3. *Do not perform soft tissue manipulation or massage when there is a pathologic condition that might be spread through the lymph or circulatory systems.* For example:
   - Lymphangitis. Inflammation of the lymphatic vessels [blood poisoning].
   - Malignant melanoma. A cancerous mole or tumor that metastasizes or spreads easily through the bloodstream or lymph.
   - Swollen glands. The glands are attempting to filter out bacteria and other pathogens, and draining them may cause an infection to spread.

4. *Do not perform soft tissue manipulation or massage near or over any area where there is bleeding.* For example:
   - Ecchymosis. A bruise; avoid pressure to immediate area.
   - Whiplash or other acute trauma. Any situation in which there is tearing of tissue and where there may be bleeding into the tissue during the first 24 to 48 hours after the trauma; avoid massage in area.

5. *Do not perform soft tissue manipulation or massage in the presence of acute inflammation.* For example:
   - Acute febrile conditions. Elevated body temperature for which infection is suspected (fever), avoid massage entirely.
   - Appendicitis. Massage will spread inflammation throughout abdomen; avoid massage entirely.
   - Rheumatoid arthritis. Avoid massage over acutely inflamed joints.
   - Locally inflamed tissues. Signs are redness, heat, swelling; avoid the surrounding area.

6. *Research the condition carefully, including getting a physician's recommendation, when working with recipients with circulatory system disorders.* For example:
   - Cardiac arrhythmias or carotid bruit. Avoid lateral and anterior neck.
   - Phlebitis or thrombophlebitis. Avoid site of disease completely, usually the legs.
   - Severe atherosclerosis. Massage only with the physician's permission, and then only very superficially.
   - Severe varicose veins. Tissues easily damaged and tendency to clotting; avoid massage of the area.

7. *Be especially careful in areas of abnormal sensation.* For example:
   - Decreased sensation. May be due to stroke, diabetes, medication (eg, muscle relaxants); recipient cannot give accurate feedback on pressure and may have abnormal vasomotor response to the massage; use extreme care in amount of pressure.
   - Hyperesthesia. Increased sensitivity to touch; massage only to recipient's tolerance or comfort.

8. *Understand the physician's recommendations and the relevant anatomy and physiology in cases where there is a loss of integrity in an area.* For example:

- Over recent surgery. Only those specifically trained to work with recent scar tissue should attempt this work.
- Artificial joint replacements. Check recommended restrictions in range of motion in replaced joints.
- Chronic sacroiliac joint subluxation. Avoid unilateral deep pressure over one ilium.
- Severe rheumatoid arthritis. Affects joints and joint capsule; use extreme caution even when not acute. Avoid passive stretch into neck flexion in all cases of rheumatoid arthritis in the neck.

9. *Edema, or accumulation of fluid in the interstitial spaces, may be either an indication or contraindication for massage depending on the circumstances.* Acute edema resulting from trauma, edema resulting from inflammation due to bacterial or viral infection, pitted edema indicating tissue fragility, lymphatic obstruction due to parasites, and edema due to deep vein thrombosis are all contraindications for massage (Rattray, 1994, pp. 119–125). If edema is significant, consult the recipient's health care provider for further instructions.

10. *Take care to follow physician's recommendations regarding hygiene when working with recipients with compromised immune systems.* For example:
    - Following organ transplant. Immune system suppressed with medication.
    - AIDS (acquired immune deficiency syndrome)
    - Chronic fatigue syndrome

11. *Understand the pathogenesis of any symptom of disease. Once the origin of a symptom is understood, select appropriate techniques and positioning to best support the health of the recipient.*

12. *Medication that a client or patient is taking may require avoidance of massage or adjustment to the session. Some medications require more caution than others. Check with the health care provider who prescribed the medication if in doubt.* The types of medications that require caution include, but are not limited to: those that alter sensation (eg, numbing); affect the blood and circulation (eg, prevent clotting, regulate blood sugar level); or alter mood (eg, depressants, antidepressants). Persons under the influence of alcohol or recreational drugs should not receive massage. These drugs alter sensation, affect mood, and in many cases, reduce good judgment.

Conditions That Require Caution

There are certain circumstances for which caution is advised while giving massage. The following are some examples of simple cautions.

- Low blood pressure. Someone with low blood pressure may be more susceptible to fainting after receiving massage either on a table or on a massage chair. Be sure that such a recipient gets up slowly.

- Osteoporosis. For someone with diagnosed osteoporosis, someone whom you suspect to have the disease, or those in a high-risk category (eg, small, sedentary postmenopausal women; frail elderly; or someone with hyper-kyphosis ["dowager's hump"]), deep pressure and vigorous joint movements should be avoided. If the condition is advanced, the receiver's health care provider should be contacted for further instructions.
- Contact lenses. If someone is wearing contact lenses, take special care when working around the eyes to avoid pressure on the lenses and to avoid dis-lodging or moving the lenses. If using a face cradle when the recipient is prone, make sure that no pressure is put on the recipient's eyes. Taking the contact lenses out during massage is preferable.
- Psoriasis. Psoriasis is an example of a skin condition that may be helped or hurt by the type of topical substance used during massage. Some massage oils or lotions may irritate the affected areas. Check with recipient for sub-stances to avoid, and be alert to skin reactions during the session.

The Person, Not the Pathology

In the wellness model, practitioners work with people with pathologies, and not only on the pathologies themselves. In fact, practitioners often find themselves working around pathologies.

Massage may be a valuable adjunct to regular medical care, as it reintroduces the element of touch and stress reduction, in addition to other physical benefits it might have. In the hands of a skilled practitioner, the touch may vary from very light to very deep and may actually be involved in the treatment of a condition. However, even in the hands of a child, massage given with love and sensitivity can be very supportive and helpful. Simple massage techniques that give comfort and support to a person in need can be learned by friends and family.

Most of the contraindications and cautions mentioned above are based on com-mon sense. If the giver of massage is motivated by sincere concern, is gentle in giv-ing, and is receptive and responsive to feedback from the recipient, the experience will most likely be a healthy one for both people.

■ RESOURCES

Practitioners' own professional libraries should include the resources needed to do research on conditions and pathologies commonly encountered in their practices. Less common pathologies may be researched at a local library or a library at a school of medicine.

A basic professional library for massage practitioners should include a good anatomy and physiology text, an atlas of human anatomy, a general pathology text, and a medical dictionary (eg, *Taber's Cyclopedic Medical Dictionary; Mosby's Pocket Dictionary*). Practitioners specializing in certain populations should have ap-plicable references for basic information. There are books available on massage with specific populations (eg, pregnant women, children, elderly). A reference book for common medications and their effects and side effects might also be useful.

One of the best resources for information may be the recipient himself or herself. Recipients are often very knowledgeable about their own pathologies, especially if they have lived with a chronic condition for some time. The recipient's health care providers may also serve as valuable resources when there is any doubt as to the safety of someone receiving massage.

■ SUMMARY

One of the most basic rules of giving therapeutic massage is to *do no harm.* Practitioners should be aware of *endangerment sites* on the body where damage may easily be done and should follow the guidelines for safe performance of massage.

Endangerment sites are found in the following areas of the body: anterior neck, axillary or armpit, elbow, umbilicus, kidney, inguinal triangle (groin), popliteal fossa (behind the knee), eyes, major blood vessels. Some general principles for safety around endangerment sites include using appropriate pressure in applying techniques, avoiding heavy pressure where delicate structures are close to the surface and unprotected, being careful around joints, avoiding pressure over major arteries and nerves, and proceeding with caution around any abnormal structures. When in doubt, do not take a chance that could lead to injury.

Contraindications are conditions or situations that make receiving massage inadvisable. *Regional* or *local contraindications* refer to a specific area of the body, and *general contraindications* refer to the whole person. Massage should be avoided in all circumstances where its application would worsen an existing condition, spread an infection, cause bleeding, or damage already weakened structures. Caution should be used when giving massage to people on medication, especially drugs that alter sensation, affect blood and circulation, or alter mood.

Most contraindications are based on common sense and knowledge about abnormal conditions and pathologies. Every massage practitioner should have a basic professional library containing resource materials for researching the conditions that their clients or patients present. Information from the recipient himself or herself is also valuable, but when in doubt consult the person's primary health care provider for direction.

■ REFERENCES

Anderson, K. N., & Anderson, L. E. (1990). *Mosby's pocket dictionary of medicine, nursing, & allied health.* St. Louis: C. V. Mosby.

Rattray, F. S. (1994). *Massage therapy: An approach to treatments.* Toronto, Ontario: Massage Therapy Texts and MAVerick Consultants.

Thomas, C. L., ed. (1985). *Taber's cyclopedic medical dictionary.* Philadelphia: F. A. Davis.

General Principles for Giving Massage

These general principles are guidelines for providing safe, effective massage and bodywork. They take into consideration the interpersonal nature of the work, the physical environment, the comfort and safety of the recipient, and the performance of the massage itself. These guidelines hold true no matter what the specific form, approach, or style of massage you practice.

■ THE PROFESSIONAL RELATIONSHIP

Professional Demeanor

The professional appearance and behavior of the practitioner are important in putting the receiver of massage at ease. They should inspire confidence and a sense of safety. They also help establish appropriate professional boundaries between practitioner and receiver, which is especially important in a relationship based primarily on touch.

Clothing should be neat, clean, modest, and comfortable, allowing freedom of movement. Avoid clothing that may be sexually suggestive such as tight pants, short shorts, and shirts that expose the chest. Jewelry should be minimal and should not touch the receiver at any time.

The practitioner should be free from offensive body odors. This includes odors from the body and clothes and strong perfumes and colognes. Some practitioners bathe or change shirts during the day to stay fresh. After a spicy meal, or just a long day, you may want to consider a breath freshener. Smokers should be particularly aware to eliminate odors on their clothes, hands, and breath.

Language used by the practitioner also sets the tone of the professional relationship. Practitioners should speak in a way that can be clearly understood, avoiding unduly technical and scientific language and jargon. Practitioners should speak to the understanding and educational level of the receiver. However, care should be taken in referring to the body, and sexually suggestive words and expressions avoided.

The physical contact inherent in massage establishes a close relationship between practitioner and receiver. This relationship should be understanding and sympathetic, but never personal.

Touching Another Person

The primary mode of personal interaction during massage is touch. It is essential that the practitioner be knowledgeable about the psychosocial implications of touch, as well as its physical nature. Practitioners giving massage need to be skilled in touch.

Touch is more basic than technique. To touch means "to come into contact with." In massage that contact happens primarily on a physical and energetic level and is achieved primarily through the hands of the practitioner. From the holistic perspective, you touch the whole person, and what may seem to be only physical touch often has profound effects on the mind, emotions, and spirit of the receiver.

Touch can communicate care and compassion, confidence, calmness, focus, and skillfulness. It can also convey anxiety, apprehension, anger, distractedness, disinterestedness, and unsureness. Practitioners should always be aware of their state of being, because whatever it is, it will be communicated through touch to a sensitive receiver. Prepare yourself to give massage by being aware of your intention to be caring and compassionate, and by becoming calm and focused.

It is also important that the practitioner be clear about the difference between friendly, caring, and even affectionate touch and sexual touch. Sexual touch is never appropriate in a professional setting.

Comfort levels with touch vary for a number of reasons. People from different cultural backgrounds will have different experiences with and attitudes toward touch. For example, studies have shown that people from Great Britain and northern Europe experience touch less in social interaction than those from some Mediterranean countries such as Spain, Italy, and Greece (Montagu, 1978).

Many men and women have been the victims of physical and sexual abuse. Many more have endured the traumatic stress of natural disaster, war, or other disturbing events. These people need special care regarding touch. The practitioner should be aware of each receiver's reaction to touch, and ensure that he or she feels safe and comfortable.

It is possible that the receiver of massage may interpret your touch in a way that was not intended. He or she may project his or her own issues regarding touch onto you. Your touch may be perceived as abusive or sexual when you had no such intention. When that happens, clear verbal communication is essential to clear up any misperceptions.

A unique feature of touch is that when you touch another person, you are touched yourself. When you are giving touch, you are also receiving touch. This is one reason why giving massage can be such a rewarding experience. However, this can also be a source of caution. For example, a practitioner who comes in contact with someone who is experiencing grief, anger, anxiety, or extreme stress can pick up some of the disturbing affects of these emotions. There are self-care techniques that you can practice to limit the degree to which you pick up the negative "vibes" of the people you touch during a session, while remaining a source of care and compassion.

Gender Issues

Because of the use of touch and the interpersonal nature of massage, there are certain gender issues to be aware of. These may be peculiar to a particular culture or person's cultural background and the professional setting, and may differ with the specific gender mix. The following comments are made with the late twentieth-century culture of the United States in mind. Appropriate professional demeanor, knowledge, and skill regarding touch and good verbal communication skills will help make the following issues less troublesome. This is true regardless of the gender of the practitioner and the receiver.

Legitimate cross-gender massage, except in a strictly medical setting, was not generally practiced until the latter twentieth century. Women worked with women, and men worked with men at places like the YMCA, health clubs, spas and salons, and resorts. Athletic massage was given to male athletes by male trainers. As American society changed in the 1970s, cross-gender massage became more common.

In cross-gender situations, practitioners need to be especially clear about the nonsexual nature of their work and establish clear professional boundaries. Verbal intervention should be immediate if a misunderstanding of intention seems evident. Sexualizing the professional relationship by either party is unacceptable, and if allowed by the practitioner, is unethical.

A receiver's homophobia or aversion to homosexual orientation may present problems in a same-gender situation, whether the practitioner is homosexual or not. This is generally not a problem for women receiving from women practitioners, but is a frequent issue for men receiving massage from men. Because men in our culture seem to equate touch with sexual touch, any touch by another person may have sexual overtones for them. Male practitioners need to be mindful of this cultural dilemma and behave so that the receiver is comfortable. This poses special problems when nurturing and compassion are called for. Male practitioners need to meet those needs of the receiver in a socially acceptable manner.

Male practitioners working with women recipients have special considerations. Most cases of sexual harassment and abuse are committed by men to women. Chances are high that some of the women recipients of massage have such histories. It is also possible that the women may not identify this past experience as a problem in the present. Men must approach all women as possible survivors of abuse and must be aware of and especially sensitive to their need for clear boundaries.

Permission to Touch

When a person agrees to receive massage from a practitioner, there is an inherent permission to touch. However, when the touch occurs in certain areas, especially those which can be sexually sensitive, there should be an additional permission to touch that specific area for therapeutic purposes. This is true for areas like the upper or inner thigh, the lower abdomen, and around breast tissue in women.

In cases where the recipient has suffered physical or sexual abuse, there may be additional sensitive areas. For example, if a man was physically abused by a parent with beatings on the back of the legs and buttocks, these may be emotionally sensitive areas to be considerate of and receive permission to work on. You may not know beforehand about these situations, so it is wise to be aware of the recipient's reactions to touch throughout the session. If you sense that the recipient is uncomfortable physically or emotionally with your touch, it is best to ask permission to continue.

Talking and Feedback

Whether, and how much, talking occurs during a massage session depends on the purpose of the session and the needs of the receiver. The practitioner should be aware of the amount and nature of verbal interaction taking place, and structure the session in the best interests of the receiver.

When relaxation is a primary goal, talking should be kept to a minimum. Silence allows receivers to sink further into a relaxed state and be quietly with themselves. They are more likely to be receptive to the relaxing effects of music playing and to the "letting go" that happens during relaxation. A soft voice should be used for necessary communications.

People who are nervous about receiving massage, especially for the first time, may need more verbal interaction. The practitioner may want to give more direction, describe what he or she is doing, and ask for frequent feedback to help put the person at ease.

Certain types of techniques require frequent feedback on pain level for the safety of the recipient, and for information on the effectiveness of techniques. For example, the receiver may give feedback to help pinpoint the precise location of trigger points, or to determine how much to stretch a muscle safely. Feedback can take different forms. A receiver whose face winces in pain, or whose muscles tighten up, or who gives a deep sigh is offering feedback on his or her state of being. The practitioner should be aware of this nonverbal feedback and use it during the flow of the session.

Sometimes a recipient will experience what is called an "emotional release." It is known that our bodies store suppressed emotions, and these may be released in a massage session as a person is touched, or as the recipient relaxes and lets down emotional defenses. This may be as simple as a sigh or crying. Practitioners not trained in psychotherapy should not attempt to delve into the meaning of such a release of emotions, but should simply be present and supportive.

Practitioners can also give useful feedback to recipients. For example, they may call the receiver's attention to a muscular holding pattern or mention when a formerly tense muscle relaxes. In this way, a person can become more aware of his or her own body.

Talking may also be of a more social nature. This should be kept to a minimum in most cases during a session. An exception may be an elderly person who has little other social contact and wants to talk, or a person who has recently experienced something upsetting and needs to talk about it. Careful judgment is needed in instances like these. Professional boundaries should never be violated. Practitioners should avoid talking to receivers about their own lives and troubles. A good rule of thumb is to follow the lead of the receiver by listening and responding only to the receiver's questions or comments. This helps you determine whether the interaction is coming from your own or the receiver's needs. You should not get your needs met at the expense of the professional relationship. Practitioners should be especially mindful of their scope of practice and not delve into psychotherapy unless properly trained. It may be useful to keep a referral list for receivers who ask for help finding a psychotherapist.

Practitioners should develop skill in recognizing and establishing the amount and nature of verbal interaction that is best in a given situation. Since the primary mode of communication in massage is touch, usually less talk is better.

Confidentiality

In a professional relationship, there is an implicit trust that the practitioner will keep information about the receiver confidential. This includes information found on a health history form; information told to the practitioner during a session, or before or after a session; and observations about a client related to physical, mental, or emotional condition. It is a matter of respecting the privacy of the receiver.

There are exceptions to the general rule of confidentiality; for example, talking to another health professional about a receiver's condition in order to serve him or her better. A practitioner receiving professional supervision may discuss a case with a supervisor. The degree of strictness of confidentiality varies with the setting. For example, in a medical setting or cooperating with psychotherapists in treating their patients, the strictest measure of confidentiality applies. There may be legal restrictions also.

In places like a health club or salon or spa, the degree of confidentiality required is less strict and is governed more by ethics and respect for the receiver than by law. It is considered unethical to gossip about a receiver or to give information about him or her without permission.

■ THE PHYSICAL ENVIRONMENT

Massage Tables and Chairs

Massage tables are specially designed for the needs of the massage practitioner. A massage table should be adjustable in height and have a removable, adjustable face cradle. Tables vary in length, width, and type of covering over the padding (eg, soft

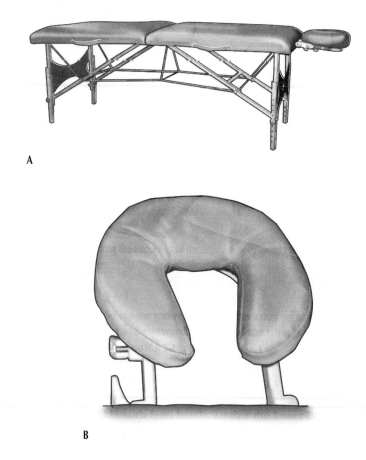

A

B

FIGURE 5–1. **A.** Typical adjustable massage table. **B.** Face cradle.

or hard vinyl). A typical portable massage table and a face cradle are shown in Figure 5–1.

The type of table you choose depends on the type of work you do, and under what circumstances. For example, if you work in a clinic, you may want a stationary table. If you carry your table from place to place, you will want a lightweight portable table. If you do sports massage, you may want a narrow table. Some shiatsu practitioners get up on the table for better leverage, and so a wider table is more practical. Your table is an important investment. To see a variety of tables, you may want to visit a massage supplies showroom or a massage therapy trade show or convention.

The massage chair is specially designed to provide maximum comfort while receiving massage in a seated position while fully clothed. Chairs usually have a seat, knee rests, arm rest, chest cushion, and face cradle. There should be adjustments for the chest cushion and the face cradle. A typical massage chair is shown in

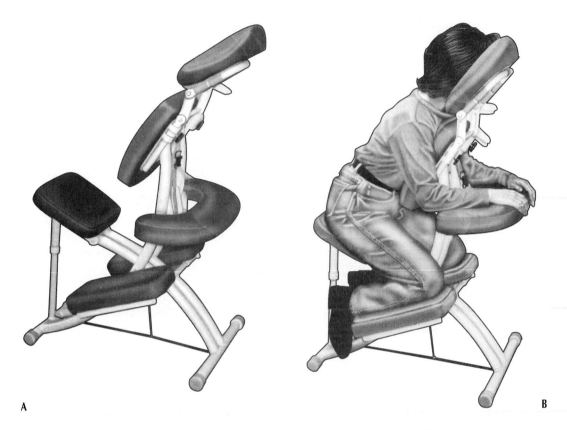

A

B

FIGURE 5–2. **A.** Special adjustable massage chair. **B.** Recipient supported in special massage chair; head in face cradle, arms and legs on supports, chest leaning into pad.

Figure 5–2. This type of massage chair is a recent innovation from the 1980s, and chairs are continually undergoing improvement in design.

Whenever possible, practitioners should use equipment specially designed for massage. However, sometimes practitioners have to improvise in less than ideal situations. For example, massage may be given to people in wheelchairs, to the bedridden elderly or ill, to workers at their desks, or even at poolside at a swim meet. In these circumstances, care should be taken to ensure the safety and comfort of the receiver while providing for good body mechanics for the practitioner.

The General Environment

Massage is given in a variety of locations. It is found in private office settings, chiropractic clinics, health clubs, spas or salons, training rooms, medical clinics and hospitals, nursing homes, hospices, and other places. On-site massage in special massage chairs is given in commercial businesses and other public places. Whatever the location, there are certain factors in the environment that will help make the session more successful. Important factors to consider include the room temperature, air quality, lighting, sound, dressing arrangements, and overall cleanliness and neatness.

The room temperature should be warm enough so that the receiver is comfortable. When the receiver is partially or fully unclothed under a drape, a comfortable room temperature is usually around 75°F. Receivers often get cold during massage as they relax. Ways to help keep them warm include an electric mattress pad underneath the bottom sheet, a heat lamp overhead, or an electric or other blanket on top. Turning up the heat in the room is a less desirable solution, because the practitioner may then get overheated while working.

Air quality should be fresh and pleasant, and rooms well ventilated. This may be a challenge in some places where strong odors are present, or in buildings where smoking is allowed. Also consider allergens such as pollen and animal hair. Electric air cleaners may be used, and in the summer, air conditioners can help keep air fresh. However, when using an air conditioner, be mindful of the warmth of the room.

Lighting is an important consideration. Soft and indirect lighting are more restful than harsh and direct lighting. Overhead lighting may shine in the receiver's eyes when he or she is supine on a table, as will the sun if doing massage in an outdoor setting such as at a spa or at an athletic event. In places where overhead lighting cannot be controlled, you may provide the receiver with a light shield for the eyes when he or she is supine.

Sound can help create a peaceful and healing environment, or a stimulating one. Music elicits certain emotions and is often used to create a particular effect. In general, popular and vocal music should be avoided if the intent is to relax. Use of popular music may also confuse the professional relationship, since it is normally heard in social situations. Numerous CDs and tapes are available with music specifically designed for relaxation, and some specifically for massage. Sometimes it is desirable to have a background of more stimulating music; for example, when the receiver must go back to work immediately, or for an athlete receiving massage just before an event. Music that is stimulating, while not stressful or frenetic, is appropriate in these situations. The receiver's taste in music should be taken into consideration and a variety of choices made available.

For some people, silence, or a fish tank bubbling in the background, is most restful. Fish tanks are known to have a relaxing effect on people in the room. There are also machines that produce "white noise" to mask annoying outside noises.

Dressing arrangements should be convenient and provide a private space for receivers to disrobe and get onto the table. If there is only one table in a room, then the practitioner may simply leave the room while the recipient is disrobing. In a situation where there is more than one table in the room, such as in a training room or clinic, gowns may be provided for the receivers to use when walking from the dressing area to the massage table. Robes are often provided for this purpose at spas.

It is generally considered a breach of professional boundaries for recipients to be seen naked as they are preparing for massage. Exceptions are in cases where the person receiving massage needs assistance dressing, such as with the elderly or disabled. Even in these cases, care should be taken to preserve the modesty of the recipient as much as possible.

Overall cleanliness and neatness of the space where massage is given should be maintained. Not only does this provide a sanitary environment for the recipient, it helps create a calm, peaceful, and cheerful atmosphere. Oil bottles should be neatly arranged and wiped clean, and clean linens neatly stacked or stored away. Used sheets and towels should be placed in a closed container and kept out of sight. Floors should be cleaned, carpets vacuumed frequently, and furniture dusted.

There may be local health department regulations concerning sanitation in places where massage is provided. These may include the materials used on the floor, how sheets and towels are stored, and how floors should be cleaned.

Topical Substances

Many forms of massage and bodywork use some kind of topical substance to enhance their effects or to minimize skin friction during the application of techniques. These may be classified as liniments, oils, lotions, or combinations of these.

A liniment is a liquid or semiliquid preparation for rubbing on or applying to the skin for therapeutic purposes. Liniments may be soothing or counterirritating. Liniments have been used for centuries for sore and stiff muscles and sprains and bruises.

Oils have been used in performing massage since ancient Greek times. Oils serve as a lubricant to minimize uncomfortable skin friction during sliding and kneading techniques. Certain vegetable oils may also add moisture and nutrients to the skin. Commonly used vegetable oils include almond, olive, and grape seed. Mineral oils are sometimes used. They are generally washed out of sheets more easily than vegetable oils. Vegetable oils trapped in sheets can spoil and turn rancid, causing sheets to have an unpleasant odor. However, some consider vegetable oils more healthy for both the giver and the receiver of massage.

Jojoba (pronounced *ho-ho-ba*) is an oil-like substance made from seeds of the jojoba plant found in the North American desert. Native Americans used jojoba for skin and hair care. Many massage practitioners use jojoba either by itself or in combination with lotions, because it is hypoallergenic and healthy for skin, and washes out of sheets easily.

Practitioners choose their oils based on a number of factors. These include properties such as the "feel" of the oil (eg, thick or thin), inherent nutrients, and scent. Unscented oils are available. Grocery stores oils may be used if they are of a high quality and cold pressed. Oils developed specially for massage can be purchased from suppliers.

Lotions are semiliquid substances containing agents for moisturizing the skin or for therapeutic purposes such as reducing itching or local pain. Lotions are designed to be absorbed into the skin, unlike oils, which tend to stay on top of the skin. Lotions are good for situations in which lubrication is desired for a warmup phase, but more friction is desired later in the session. Lotions may also be preferred by receivers who feel too oily after massage with mineral or vegetable oil. Lotions also tend to be more water soluble than oils and are, therefore, more easily washed out of sheets.

Practitioners often experiment with different topical substances and concoct combinations of substances to get the properties that best enhance their work. They frequently mix different oils or lotions and oils.

Some substances are more likely to cause allergic reactions than others. Also, some skin types are more easily irritated than others. Scent can be an important consideration. People going back to work after massage may desire a unscented substance, and men usually prefer different scents than women. Care should be taken in choosing a topical substance for each unique recipient of massage.

▪ SAFETY AND COMFORT OF THE RECEIVER

Positioning the Receiver

Details about the receiver's position on the table, chair, or other surface will be described in the sections on specific techniques and approaches. However, there are some important general guidelines. The receiver should always be in a position that is comfortable and safe. Bolsters may be used for support to certain body areas. The receiver should not have to exert muscular effort to stay in position or to hold draping in place. Various size bolsters or rolled towels may be used to position receivers properly.

For example, in the supine position, a bolster under the knees may take pressure off of the lower back, or a neck roll provide support in the cervical area as shown in Figure 5–3. In the prone position, support is put under the ankles to ease pressure on the lower back, and small cushions may be placed under the shoulders for women with large breasts or men with round chests. See Figure 5–4. In the side-

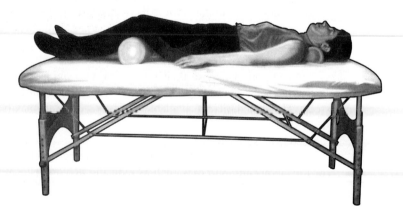

FIGURE 5–3. Placement of bolsters under knees and neck in supine position.

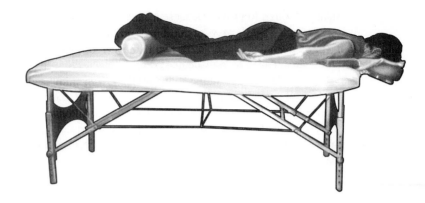

FIGURE 5–4. Placement of bolsters under ankles and shoulders in prone position; head supported by face cradle.

lying position, support should be provided for the superior leg and arm and under the head, as pictured in Figure 5–5.

Draping

Covering the body during massage serves to protect the receiver's modesty, provide clear professional boundaries, and keep the receiver warm. Skill in draping helps the receiver feel safe and allows for maximum relaxation. Draping should be sub-

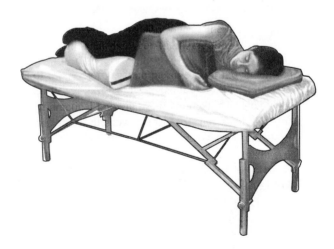

FIGURE 5–5. Placement of bolsters under top leg and arm in side-lying position; head supported with pillow.

stantial enough to provide a sense of safety and modesty. The use of thin sheets or narrow small towels may leave the recipient feeling unduly exposed. A flimsy drape may suggest sexual intent to a receiver. Those with a history of sexual abuse may be particularly sensitive to inadequate draping.

When receivers remove some or all of their clothing, some general guidelines apply. The genitals and women's breasts should be draped at all times. Mutual consent or familiarity between practitioner and receiver are not good reasons to ignore this guideline. Draping can be adjusted to allow access to areas close to the genitals or breasts (eg, attachments to the adductors or pectoralis major), while maintaining clear professional boundaries.

Draping with a sheet provides maximum coverage. The part to be massaged is uncovered and then recovered during the session. Skillful tucking will enhance the security of the drape and prevent inadvertently exposing the receiver. An additional drape for women's breasts may be used when massaging the chest or abdomen.

When the receiver is changing from the supine to the prone position, or vice versa, the sheet should be held in place while the person turns over under it. "Tenting" allows the receiver to turn over and avoid getting wrapped up in the sheet. Care should be taken not to expose the receiver to the practitioner or to others who might be in the room.

Large towels may also be used for draping. The same general guidelines for modesty apply whatever type of drape is used.

In some situations, receivers do not remove their clothes and draping is unnecessary. For example, receivers usually remain clothed during pre-event and post-event sports massage, chair massage, and some shiatsu and other energy-balancing sessions.

■ SELF-CARE FOR THE PRACTITIONER

Physical Aspects of Self-Care

Physical self-care is important for the well-being of the massage and bodywork practitioner. In addition to general health practices, practitioners need to pay special attention to their hands, posture, and body mechanics. Scheduling of sessions should also be taken into consideration.

The hands are the primary vehicle for giving massage. Nails should be clipped so short that they cannot be seen if the hands are held up with the palm toward the face. Rings and bracelets should not be worn, since they might scratch or distract the receiver. Hands should be washed thoroughly before and after every session. This will help protect both the giver and receiver of massage from communicable diseases. Practitioners who smoke should be especially careful to remove odors from their hands. The hands should always be warm and dry before touching the receiver. If necessary, they can be warmed beneath a heat lamp, by hot water, or by rubbing them briskly together. Hands may be dried with a towel or by applying powder to them.

Practitioners can protect themselves from injuries to the hands, arms, and back with conditioning exercises, proper hand position and body mechanics during massage, the use of a variety of techniques, and adequate time for rest between sessions. Common injuries sustained by massage practitioners include tendinitis and tenosynovitis, damage caused by overuse and repetitive strain, and nerve impingement injury (eg, carpal tunnel and thoracic outlet syndromes). A conditioning program should include exercises to strengthen the upper body, especially the hands, wrists, and arms. Flexibility may be maintained through regular stretching.

In applying techniques, strain on finger, thumb, and wrist joints should be minimized. The thumb is especially vulnerable to misuse during specific high-pressure techniques like trigger point work. The wrists suffer when applying pressure with the wrist in a bent position, as might happen in compression techniques. Consider the use of the elbow or a special massage tool to apply direct sustained pressure when working in heavily muscled areas.

Proper posture during sessions will minimize shoulder and back problems. Be sure your table is at the proper height for you. A table too high or too low can cause poor body mechanics and put undue strain on your body. Keep your back straight during the session, and bend your knees instead to lower your body. Martial arts stances are very effective when giving massage. They help take the strain off of your back by using the legs, which are less prone to injury. These stances not only help keep the back straight, but also position you to use body leverage to accomplish deep pressure. Figure 5–6 shows good body mechanics for giving massage, that is bending the knees while keeping the back straight.

Sitting on a chair or stool while working on the head, hands, and feet also helps minimize strain on the body. The height should be adjusted to allow you to keep your back and wrists relatively straight.

Varying techniques during a session will minimize repeated strain on a particular body area. Proper warming up techniques not only prepare the recipient of massage, but may also help warm up the hands and body of the practitioner. There are techniques for relaxing tense muscles that cause less strain to the practitioner's body; for example, positional release techniques and some forms of energy work. Techniques that strain the practitioner's body should be alternated with less stressful techniques to provide a resting phase to a session. At the end of a session, the hands are often hot or feel "charged" with energy. Running cold water on them after washing helps to normalize them.

The number of massage sessions any practitioner can perform safely in one day depends on the type of massage performed, his or her strength and fitness, and the quality of his or her body mechanics. Someone just starting out doing massage must build the strength and stamina to perform the work safely. A sudden drastic increase in the number of sessions performed per week may lead to strain, pain, and possible injury.

The following are guidelines for scheduling sessions for a week. They take into account how much work you can expect to perform and maintain your own health and well-being. Generally, you should schedule *no more than:*

- five 1-hour sessions in one day, if you work four days per week
- four 1-hour sessions in one day, if you work five days per week
- 20 hours per week total

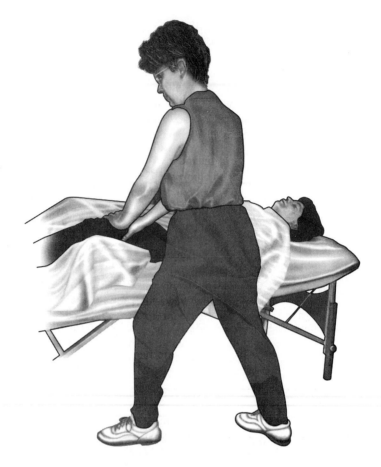

FIGURE 5–6. Good body mechanics for giving massage, bending the knees while keeping the back straight.

Furthermore, you should:

- have 15–20-minute breaks between sessions
- have at least a 30-minute break after three consecutive 1-hour sessions
- do no more than four 1-hour sessions in one day, if the type of massage is strenuous

If you have a private massage practice, you will also need time to clean linens, keep client or patient records, do financial bookkeeping, and perform other chores related to having your own business.

Emotional Self-Care

Emotional self-care is often overlooked, but it is equally important to prevent stress and burnout. Care should be taken to establish and maintain clear professional boundaries. The practitioner's job is to help patients or clients, not to rescue them from their life's problems. It is useful to have a fellow practitioner with whom to discuss upsetting situations. Peer and professional supervision can help you keep clear boundaries and sort out confusing situations that come up in the practitioner–recipient relationship.

■ PERFORMING THE MASSAGE

Length of the Session

The length of a massage session varies and depends on the intent or goals of the session and the context in which it is given. For example, a massage session for general health purposes usually lasts from ½ hour to 1½ hours. This is typical at a health club, spa, or private massage therapy practice. Chair massage given to employees of a business may last 15–20 minutes. Athletes may receive pre-event massage for 15 minutes and general maintenance massage for 30 minutes to 1 hour. Massage that is part of a larger therapy session (eg, physical therapy) may last as little as 10 minutes. Guidelines for session length will be given for each type of massage described later in this book.

Amount of Lubricant

Generally speaking, you should use the least amount of lubricant needed to get the job done. Too much lubricant prevents firm contact, and the hands will only slip and slide over the surface of the skin. This is especially true when doing more specific work on small areas and when friction is used. Too little lubricant can cause skin irritation, especially in people with thick hair on the arms, legs, or chest, and in people with fair skin. More oil may be used in warming up an area with sliding movements and then wiped off for techniques that are best performed with less lubricant. Recipients of massage may benefit from extra lubricant to relieve dry skin. Additional lotion or oil may be applied after massaging a particular body area as a moisturizer.

The face is an area where little, if any, lubricant should be used. Care should be taken not to get oil or lotion in the hair when working on the neck. Recipients may want to wear surgical or shower caps to keep lubricants out of the hair.

Lubricant should be absorbed into the skin, or wiped off of the skin, before clothes are put back on. Some substances can stain clothes, or certain scents may be difficult to wash out. Rubbing with a dry towel will remove most lotions and oils, and alcohol may be used when more thorough removal is desired.

Sequence of Techniques and Routines

Individual techniques are rarely performed in isolation, but are blended into sequences for the desired effects. Generally, warming and superficial techniques are followed by deeper more specific techniques, with finishing ones more superficial and light. Smooth transitions between techniques give a skillful feel to a session.

Routines are regular sequences of techniques performed in almost the same way each time. A routine may also include a regular sequence of body sections addressed during a session. Experienced practitioners usually establish a routine way of working, which they vary depending on the needs of the receiver. Routines are useful to establish a smooth pattern of working and are an effective way to learn new massage techniques. Routines will be presented for some of the different approaches discussed later in this book.

Specificity and Direction

Much of massage is performed in a general way and over larger areas of the body. For example, long sliding strokes are often performed over the whole back, and muscle *groups* are kneaded and stretched as opposed to individual muscles. This more general way of applying techniques is appropriate for effects such as warming an area, eliciting the relaxation response (a total body reaction), or relaxing a muscle group.

When performing deep sliding strokes to a limb, always move in line with the venous flow, that is, movements should be distal to proximal. Moving fluids away from the heart, or against venous flow, can cause backflow of blood, which can damage the valves in the veins.

Lighter sliding movements using superficial pressure may be performed proximal to distal. These are used as return strokes between deep sliding movements to the limbs distal to proximal. They may also be used when finishing an area before going to the next area of the body.

Massage practitioners are said to be working with specificity if they focus their use of techniques on a specific condition and in a small area (eg, relieving a trigger point with thumb pressure, or deep transverse friction on a tendon). This requires thorough knowledge of anatomic structures and good palpation skills.

Pressure, Rhythm, and Pacing

Pressure, rhythm, and pacing are qualities used to describe massage movements. These qualities will vary with the desired effect of the session, of a sequence of techniques, or of a single technique.

Pressure is related to the force used in applying techniques and to the degree of compaction of tissues as the technique is applied. The amount of pressure used in any one situation will depend on the intended effect and the tolerance or desires of the recipient. Generally speaking, when working an area, pressure should be applied lightly at first, then more deeply if desired, then finishing lightly. This allows tissues to be warmed and prepared gradually, and the body to adjust better to the cessation of deep pressure. If too much pressure is used too quickly on a specific area, tissue damage and bruising may result. Too light pressure may cause tickling, and too deep pressure may elicit a tightening-up response. Both effects are undesirable.

Rhythm refers to a recurring pattern of movement with a specific cadence, beat, or accent. Rhythm may be described as smooth, flowing, or uneven. Rhythm is important when applying techniques generally and in sequence, as with sliding movements and kneading. Working specifically is often by nature lacking rhythm, as when you slow down to press a trigger point or acupressure point. Each massage practitioner has his or her own rhythm for working, which is developed over time. A smooth, flowing, and regular rhythm helps to elicit relaxation in the receiver. An uneven rhythm may be stimulating, or in some cases distracting, to a receiver. Once a rhythm is established, it should not be interrupted. Try to avoid breaking contact with the skin once a session has begun, or do so with as little loss of rhythm as possible. Establishing a pleasant rhythm is part of the art of massage.

Pacing refers to the speed of performing techniques. Generally, a slower pace is more relaxing, while a faster pace more stimulating. Choice of pace depends on the desired effect.

▪ SUMMARY

General principles for giving massage include guidelines about the professional relationship, the physical environment, safety and comfort of the receiver, self-care for the practitioner, and the specifics of performing the massage. The focus of these principles is to provide massage that is effective and safe for both giver and receiver.

Massage practitioners should maintain a professional demeanor including dress, cleanliness, and language. The relationship between giver and receiver should be understanding and sympathetic, but never personal. The practitioner needs to be knowledgeable about the psychosocial implications of touch, including issues around culture, gender, and personal touch histories. The amount of talking that occurs should enhance, not detract from, the session, and personal information about the receiver should be held confidential. The intent is to create a safe, comfortable, and healing atmosphere.

The physical environment ideally includes massage tables or chairs suited to the practitioner's needs. Other important factors are comfortable room temperature, good air quality, appropriate lighting and sound, modest dressing arrangements, and overall cleanliness and neatness of the area. Topical substances such as liniments, oils, and lotions may be chosen to enhance the therapeutic effects of the massage. Bolsters, pillows, and other props may be used to position receivers safely and comfortably. Draping is used to protect receivers' modesty, provide clear professional boundaries, and keep them warm.

Physical and emotional self-care practices help practitioners maintain their own wellness while caring for clients and patients. Massage sessions should be scheduled to provide enough time for rest and recovery for the practitioner. Keeping clear professional boundaries and receiving peer or professional supervision are two emotional self-care approaches to help prevent stress and burnout.

The length of a massage session depends on the setting and the needs of the recipient and varies from 10 minutes to 1½ hours. The amount of lubricant used, if any, is related to the desired effects. Generally speaking, use the least amount of lubricant needed to get the job done effectively. Individual massage techniques are blended into sequences and routine ways of working to provide organization to a session. Specificity, direction, pressure, rhythm, and pacing are factors that vary depending on the desired results when performing massage techniques.

■ REFERENCE

Montagu, A. (1978). *Touching: The human significance of the skin,* 2nd ed. New York: Harper & Row.

II

Classic Western Massage

Classic Western Massage Techniques

Classic Western massage is the most common type of massage found in the United States today. It has been the basis for most of the therapeutic applications of massage found in physiotherapy since the late nineteenth century and is described in various texts on natural healing. Swedish massage is a form of classic Western massage popularized in spas, public baths, and health clubs in the mid-twentieth century.

Explanations about the effects of classic Western massage are usually based in Western concepts of anatomy and physiology and Western notions of health and disease. The techniques of classic Western massage are recognized as valuable for improving circulation of blood and lymph, relaxing muscles, improving joint mobility, inducing general relaxation, and promoting healthy skin.

Classic Western massage techniques are methods of soft tissue manipulation developed in Europe and the United States over the past two centuries. The five technique categories commonly used to describe Western message are: effleurage, petrissage, friction, tapotement, and vibration. These categories were used by Mary McMillan at the beginning of the twentieth century (1921).

Effleurage is sliding or gliding movements; petrissage is lifting, pressing, and squeezing movements; friction involves rubbing two surfaces across one another; tapotement is percussive; and vibration causes oscillation in tissues. Touch without movement is also found in classic massage, but does not fit neatly into any of the five traditional categories. Two forms of touch without movement found in classic texts are passive touch and direct static pressure (Kellogg, 1929).

The categories of classic massage are useful for thinking about how techniques are performed, their physiological effects, and common uses. Keep in mind that there are an endless number of variations of massage techniques, and that the ones presented in this text are merely representative of many possibilities.

■ EFFLEURAGE

Effleurage techniques slide or glide over the skin with a smooth continuous motion. Pressure may be light to moderate, as when applying oil or warming an area, or may be deep, as when facilitating venous return in heavily muscled areas. Experienced practitioners can perform effleurage in many different ways to suit the body area and to evoke specific effects.

Effleurage is perhaps the most versatile of the classic techniques and is used most frequently. For example, effleurage is usually used to begin a session, especially when oil or lotion is applied. It accustoms the receiver to the touch of the practitioner. It is used as a connecting or transition technique. It is often performed as a break from more specific techniques, to move gracefully from one area to another, to conclude work on an area, or to end the session.

While performing effleurage, a practitioner skilled in palpation can assess the general condition of the soft tissues and the firmness and shape of the musculature. Sensitive fingers may find areas of tension or holding. In some cases where pain is present, it may be the only technique employed.

Effleurage can affect the recipient's body and mind in a variety of ways. The qualities of pressure, pacing, and rhythm may be varied for different effects. For example, when effleurage is performed with moderate pressure, slowly and smoothly on the back, it may stimulate the parasympathetic nervous system and evoke the relaxation response. It enhances venous return in the limbs when performed with moderate to deep pressure moving distal to proximal. Deep effleurage may also provide a passive stretch to a muscle group.

Variations of Effleurage

Basic sliding effleurage is performed with the palms and fingers of the hands, the thumbs, fists, or forearms. When using the palms, the hands mold to the surface of the body part, providing full contact as shown in basic effleurage of the leg in Figure 6–1. The thumbs may be used in small places like between the metatarsals of the foot as in Figure 6–2. More pressure may be applied using the forearms or fists in broad places like the back and hamstrings. See Figure 6–3.

Shingles effleurage refers to alternate stroking, first one hand then the other in continuous motion, with the strokes overlaying each other like shingles on a roof. One hand always remains in contact with the receiver as the other hand is lifted. This gives the feeling of unbroken contact. Shingles effleurage is commonly applied to the back with hands parallel to the spine and to the direction of movement as shown in Figure 6–4. It may also be performed with hands perpendicular to the spine and to the direction of movement.

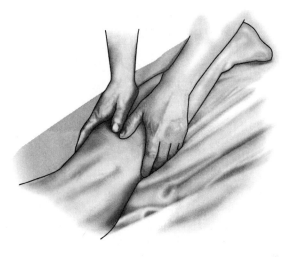

FIGURE 6–1. Basic sliding effleurage using the palms of the hands provides full contact with the leg.

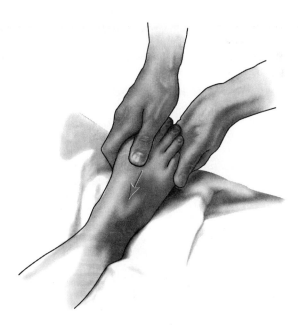

FIGURE 6–2. Basic sliding effleurage using the thumb gets into the small spaces between the metatarsals of the foot.

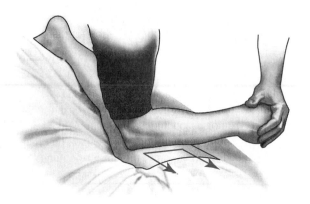

FIGURE 6–3. Basic sliding effleurage of the hamstrings using the forearm.

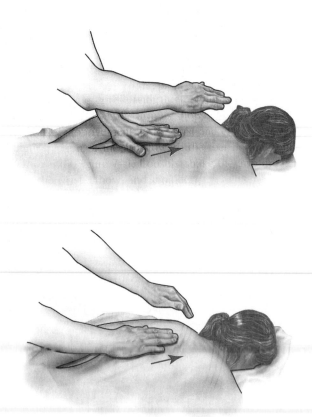

FIGURE 6–4. Shingles effleurage with hands parallel to the spine and to the direction of movement.

Bilateral tree stroking traces a pattern reminiscent of branches growing out from both sides of the trunk of a tree. It is usually performed on the back starting with the hands on either side of the spine, and moving laterally across the shoulders or around the sides as far as you can reach. This movement is repeated as you progress to cover the entire back. It may be performed standing at the head and progressing from the shoulders toward the hips as shown in Figure 6–5. It may also be done standing at the side moving from hips to shoulders.

Three-count stroking of the trapezius is performed in three strokes, alternating hands with each movement. Count one begins at the origin of the lower trapezius and moves toward its insertion in the shoulder. Count two begins just as the first stroke concludes, moving from the origin of the middle trapezius toward the insertion. As soon as the first hand has completed its slide over the lower trapezius, it lifts and crosses over to the origin of the upper trapezius to begin count three. Count three moves laterally to the insertion to complete the sequence. Figure 6–6 shows how the stroke is performed from the opposite side. The entire three-count sequence is repeated several times. This particular method of stroking the whole trapezius is rhythmic and relaxing when well done. It must be timed so that in spite of the lost contact as each hand is raised, the receiver feels unbroken contact.

Horizontal stroking is usually applied to broad, rounded areas like the thigh, abdomen, or lower back. The movement is across the width of the body part, rather than over the length. Horizontal stroking may be considered a hybrid form of effleurage and petrissage because in addition to sliding, there may be a lifting and pressing motion.

To perform horizontal stroking on the lower back, stand facing the table at the side of the receiver near the waist. Place your hands lightly on the receiver's back, one hand on each side with the fingers of both hands pointing away from you, as shown in Figure 6–7. Slide both hands toward the spine using firm pressure, and then continue the movement all the way to the other side. One hand will move forward and one hand backward, crossing at the spine. The motion is then reversed without changing the position of the hands. As the hands slide from side to side, they execute a lifting and pushing together of the soft tissues. No pressure should be placed over the spinous processes as the hands pass over them. Greatest pressure comes with the lift and push together of the tissues as the hands move upward and inward to meet and cross over.

Mennell's superficial stroking is very light effleurage usually performed on a limb, moving in one direction either centripetally (distal to proximal) or centrifugally (proximal to distal) but never in both directions. To perform it on the arm with the recipient prone, slide your hand from the recipient's wrist to the shoulder while maintaining full contact and using the lightest pressure possible. See Figure 6–8. Return to the starting position through the air just over the skin surface in a controlled even rhythm. Take the same time to perform the return movement as the stroke that contacts the receiver. This is a gentle relaxing technique.

Nerve strokes are another very light effleurage movement. They are performed with the fingertips gently brushing the skin. They may also be done on top of the drape. Nerve strokes can go in any direction and are often used when finishing a

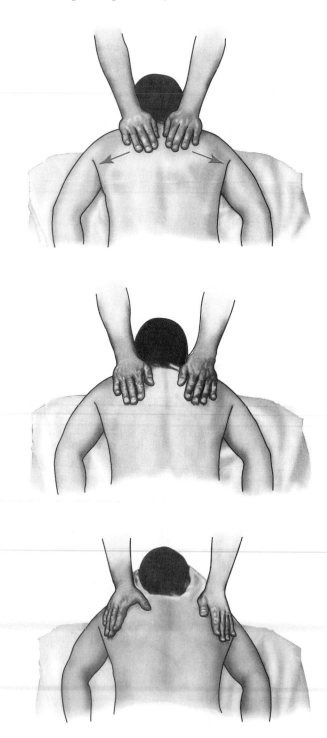

FIGURE 6–5. Bilateral tree stroking across the back.

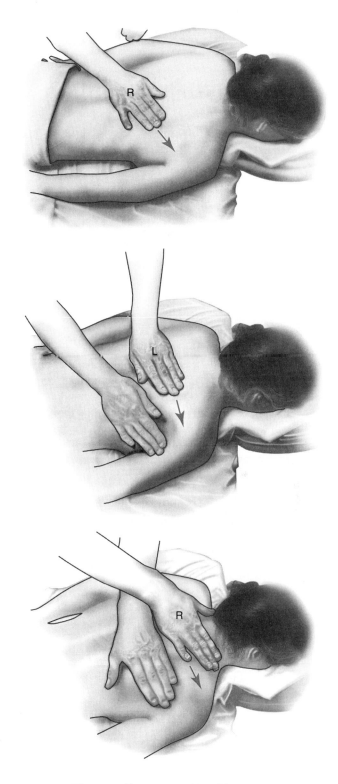

FIGURE 6–6. Three-count stroking of the tapezius.

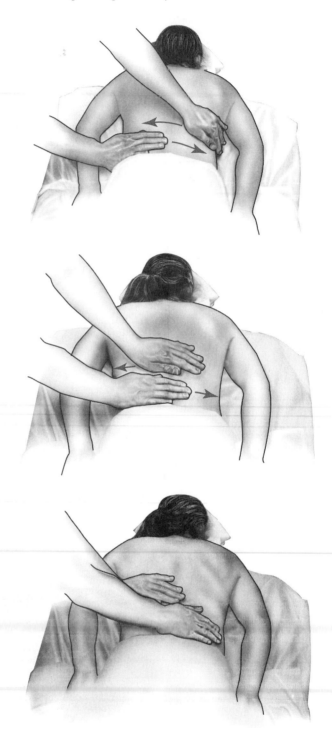

FIGURE 6–7. Horizontal stroking across the lower back.

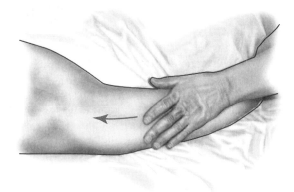

FIGURE 6–8. Mennell's superficial stroking over the arm with the recipient prone.

section of the body or when ending the session. A few seconds of nerve strokes are usually enough to create a relaxing effect.

Knuckling is an effleurage variation taught by Hoffa in which the pressure is first applied with the back of the fingers in a lose fist, gradually turning the fist over as it slides over the skin, and finishing with the palm of the hand. See Figure 6–9. Hoffa describes knuckling further.

> *Gradually bring the hand from plantar [flexion] to dorsal [hypertension] flexion. Pressure is not continuous, but swells up and down, starting lightly and becoming stronger, then decreasing again in pressure. The hand must not adhere to the part but*

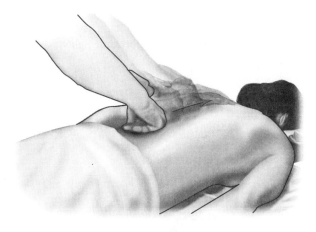

FIGURE 6–9. Knuckling performed on the back.

should glide over it lightly. Knuckling should only be used where there is enough room for the hand to be applied.

Sedating effleurage of the back is very effective in evoking the relaxation response and may be used for concluding a session if the intent is deep relaxation or sleep. The movement consists of long sliding strokes directly over the spine that start at the base of the skull and go all the way to the coccyx. Hands alternate. As one hand is about to complete its motion near the coccyx, the other hand begins the next stroke starting at the base of the skull. Pressure must be light but firm and the rhythm monotonous. Pressure that is too light might stimulate rather than sedate. This gives the recipient the feeling of continuous contact, with one hand beginning the next stroke before the other hand finishes.

Keep the motion going for a minute or two to help the recipient relax completely. A tingling sensation may be felt in the arms and legs as relaxation occurs. Some recipients may fall asleep. If this technique is applied for more than two or three minutes, it tends to stimulate rather than relax so it should not be continued for too long.

▪ PETRISSAGE

Petrissage techniques lift, wring, or squeeze soft tissues in a kneading motion or press or roll the tissues under or between the hands. Petrissage may be performed with one or two hands depending on the size of the muscle or muscle group. There is minimal sliding over the skin except perhaps in moving from one area to another when using lubricant. The motions of petrissage serve to "milk" a muscle of accumulated metabolites (waste products), increase local circulation, and assist venous return. Petrissage may also help separate muscle fibers and evoke muscular relaxation.

Before performing petrissage, prepare and warm an area, usually with effleurage. Use only a small amount of oil or lotion when warming up the area, since too much lubricant will make it difficult to grasp the tissues during petrissage. If you are working without lubricant, light compressions may be used to warm an area.

Care should be taken to avoid pinching or bruising the tissues and to not work too long in one area. Adjust the amount of pressure used to match the condition of the recipient. Muscular and physically strong receivers will enjoy harder pressure, while less pressure should be used for smaller or frail individuals.

Variations of Petrissage

Basic two-handed kneading is performed by lifting, squeezing, and then releasing soft tissues with hands alternating in a rhythmical motion. Graham (1884) described the fingers and hands as slipping on the skin during kneading, while Kellogg (1929) discouraged letting the hands slide. In basic kneading, tissues are lifted with the whole hand in firm contact rather than with just the fingertips, as shown in Figure

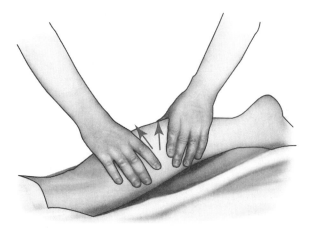

FIGURE 6–10. Basic two-handed kneading. Tissues are lifted with the whole hand in firm contact.

6–10. The movement is a lifting away from the underlying bone. Two-handed kneading works well on the larger muscles of the arms, shoulders, and legs.

One-handed kneading may be used on smaller limbs, for example, arms and children's legs. Place your hand around the part, picking up the muscle mass using the whole hand. The kneading movement may be described as circular—grasping the tissues on the up motion, and relaxing the hand on the down motion without losing contact. As with two-handed kneading, the rhythm should be slow and regular. Progression to a new position should follow three or four repetitions in the same place. In general, the movements should be performed distal to proximal, and effleurage may be interspersed with petrissage or may follow it, to enhance venous return.

The biceps is a good place to practice one-hand kneading. Grasp the biceps with one hand as shown in Figure 6–11. Let the muscle belly fit firmly into the palm of the hand while the thumb and fingers apply pressure and lift as they begin the kneading motion.

Alternating one-hand kneading may be used to work flexors and extensors at the same time. For example, on the upper arm, grasp the biceps with one hand and the triceps with the other hand. Alternate lifting and squeezing first the biceps and then the triceps in an even rhythm. See Figure 6–12. Perform this technique rapidly when stimulation is desired.

Circular two-handed petrissage is best performed on broad flat areas like the back. This technique may be applied to one side of the spine after warming the area using deep effleurage. Stand facing the receiver from the side and near the hips and be ready to move along toward the head while performing the technique. Place both hands firmly on one side of the receiver's back, with the hand nearest the hips ready to start the movement over the upper portion of the gluteals. Each hand will describe a counterclockwise circle, timed so that when the hands pass each other, the

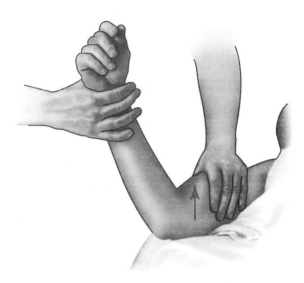

FIGURE 6–11. One-handed kneading. Tissues are lifted with the whole hand in firm contact.

soft tissues are picked up and pressed between the hands. The hands are almost *flat* as they shape themselves to the contours of the back. Pick up tissues between the hands (not with the hands) as they pass each other as shown in Figure 6–13. After about three repetitions of this technique in one place, slide the lower hand up to where the upper hand has just been working, while the upper hand slides to a new position closer to the head. Eventually, the technique progresses from lower back to upper back, ending over the shoulders. This technique may also be performed on the forehead using the thumbs.

Alternating fingers-to-thumb petrissage is very useful for following the direction of the fibers of the more superficial muscles such as the trapezius. In this technique, the soft tissues are pressed between the thumb of one hand and the first two fingers of the other hand. The hands alternate back and forth with an even rhythm.

To perform the technique, the fingers of one hand pick up the tissues and press them against the opposite thumb. At the same time, the thumb is moving toward, and pressing the tissues against, the fingers of the opposite hand. See Figure 6–14. This same motion is repeated alternating hands and working from the distal to the proximal (or lateral to medial) aspects of each muscle.

Skin rolling is a technique in which the skin and subcutaneous tissue are picked up between the thumb and the first two fingers and gently pulled away from the deeper tissues. Once the skin is pulled away, the thumbs may push forward, lifting the tissues in a smooth continuous motion and causing a rolling effect. Skin rolling stretches the underlying fascia and increases superficial circulation. It is often performed on the back, but may be applied to almost any part of the body. Figure 6–15 shows skin rolling on the back.

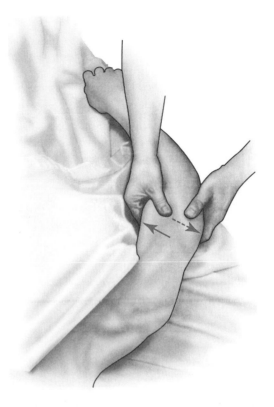

FIGURE 6–12. Alternating one-handed kneading. Alternate lifting and squeezing biceps and triceps in an even rhythm.

In *compression* techniques, tissues are pressed or rolled against underlying tissues and bone in a rhythmic motion. The effects are similar to other petrissage techniques as the tissues are squeezed under the hands. Figure 6–16 shows compression using the palm of one hand, while the other hand provides additional force from above. Note that the heel of the top hand is placed so that it does not put pressure on the wrist of the bottom hand. The compressing force is applied through the palms, as you lean into the movement with your body weight. Avoid using just your arms and shoulders to perform compression techniques. A variation useful in working the buttocks is compression with a fist.

Rolling is a form of petrissage performed on the limbs. The limb is grasped lightly on the opposite sides with the palms of both hands. The muscles of the limb are rolled against one another as the hands press in and perform an alternating back-and-forth motion. Rolling progresses from distal to proximal to facilitate venous return. The larger your hands are in proportion to the limb, the easier rolling will be to perform.

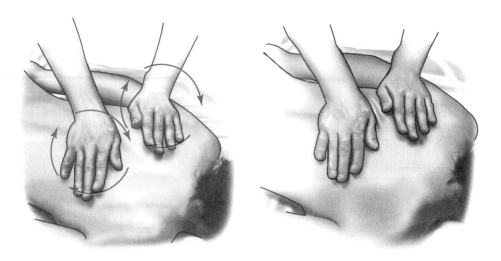

FIGURE 6–13. Circular two-handed petrissage. Tissues are picked up between the hands as they pass each other.

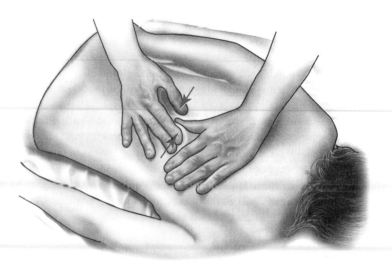

FIGURE 6–14. Alternating fingers-to-thumb petrissage. The soft tissues are pressed between the thumb of one hand and the fingers of the other hand.

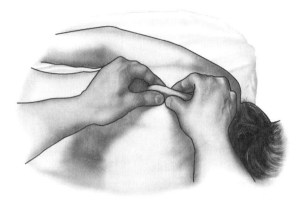

FIGURE 6–15. Skin rolling. Superficial tissues are picked up and gently pulled away from deeper tissues.

▪ FRICTION

Friction is performed by rubbing one surface over another repeatedly. For example, the hand is used to rub the skin for superficial warming, as in a traditional rubdown. The resistance to the motion provided by the surface causes heat and stimulates the skin.

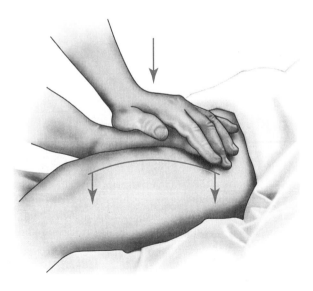

FIGURE 6–16. Compression using reinforced palm. The heel of the top hand is placed so that it does not put pressure over the wrist of the bottom hand.

Friction may also be created between the skin and deeper tissues. In *deep friction,* the practitioner's fingers do not move over the skin, but instead move the skin over the tissues underneath. Deep friction addresses one small area at a time and adds specificity to the massage by affecting specific structures such as a particular section of a muscle or tendon. Cross-fiber, parallel, and circular friction are common forms of deep friction.

Superficial Warming Friction

Practitioners use friction to create heat in an area by rubbing the skin briskly with the palms of their hands. This is called *superficial warming friction,* and the heat is generated by the friction between the giver's hands and the receiver's skin.

Variations of warming friction use different parts of the hands to create the friction and may use greater pressure to affect deeper tissues such as when using the knuckles (Figure 6–17) and in *sawing* (Figure 6–18). Warming friction is best done "dry" or with little lubricant, since oil or lotion reduces the amount of resistance between the two surfaces and thus reduces the amount of friction.

Deep Friction

Deep friction is used to create movement between the deeper tissues and helps keep them from adhering to one another. For example, tissues of the musculoskeletal system are designed for smooth and efficient movement and should slide over each other without sticking. With lack of movement, stress, or trauma to an area, muscle fibers may stick together or tendons stick to tissues they come in contact with. Deep friction can help keep tissues separated and functioning smoothly.

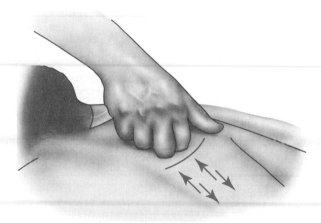

FIGURE 6–17. Warming friction using the knuckles. The first two knuckles move back and forth on the skin to create friction, and from spot to spot over the area to be warmed.

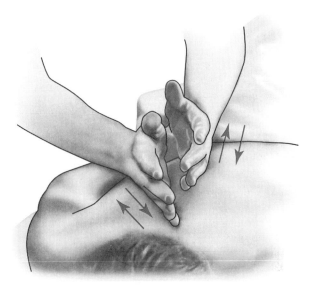

FIGURE 6–18. Warming friction created with a "sawing" motion. The sides of the hands move back and forth on the skin to create friction, and from spot to spot over the area to be warmed.

Deep friction may also be used to create movement in tissues around joint spaces such as the ankle, reach into small spaces like the suboccipital region, or be used in areas that lack muscle bulk such as on the head. Areas that don't lend themselves well to petrissage (eg, at tendonous attachments) may be massaged with deep friction.

Deep friction may be performed in a cross-fiber, parallel, or circular motion. Cross-fiber refers to deep friction applied across the direction of the fibers, while parallel friction is applied in the same direction as the fibers. Circular friction is performed using circular movements, which move the underlying tissues in many directions. Figure 6–19 shows cross-fiber friction being applied to the paraspinal muscles.

Deep friction is performed with the tips of the fingers, the thumb, or the heel of the hand, depending on the size of the surface to be covered. For example, small tendons in places such as the wrist or around the ankle may be frictioned with the fingertips. In Figure 6–20, circular friction is applied with the heel of the hand to free up the broad iliotibial band on the side of the leg.

Before deep friction is applied, the area must be warmed up thoroughly, usually with effleurage and petrissage. The lubricant used in the warming-up phase may have to be wiped off before performing friction, to allow the practitioner's hands to move the skin without sliding over it. Deep friction is a three-dimensional technique. Practitioners must be keenly aware of the depth at which they are working, and the depth of the tissues they wish to affect. If the tissues are just beneath

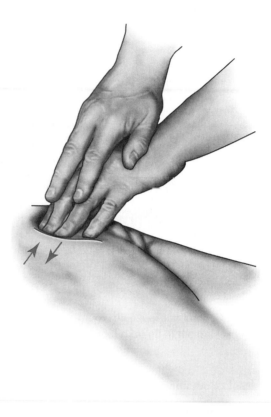

FIGURE 6–19. Cross-fiber friction to the paraspinal muscles. The fingertips create friction by moving the skin over the deeper tissues.

the skin, then lighter pressure may be effective. If the tissues are deep or under other tissues, then you must "work through" the more superficial tissues. It is helpful to visualize the tissues in cross-section and to develop palpation skills that will allow you to feel the layers of tissue. Care must be taken in applying deep pressure. Do not try to "muscle through" more superficial tissues, but instead soften them layer by layer. This process takes patience and sensitivity.

Friction Used in Injury Recovery

Deep transverse friction is a specific type of cross-fiber friction that is applied directly to the site of a lesion. It is used to facilitate healthy scar formation at an injury site. The mechanical action across tissues causes broadening and separation of fibers. Deep transverse friction encourages a more parallel fiber arrangement of scar tissue and fewer cross-connections that limit movement.

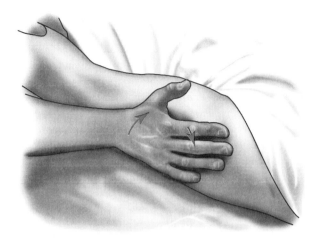

FIGURE 6–20. Circular friction to the broad iliotibial band. The heel of hand creates friction between the skin and deeper tissues, and between the tendon and underlying muscles.

James Cyriax popularized the use of deep transverse friction used in rehabilitation. In the *Illustrated Manual of Orthopedic Medicine* (1993), the following principles were given for treating muscle and tendon lesions:

- The fingers and skin move together to affect deep tissues.
- The effect of friction is most important, not the amount of pressure used.
- The movement must be over the precise site of the lesion.
- The tissue must be in the appropriate tension.
- Do 6 to 12 sessions of 20 minutes each on alternate days for best results.

In addition to promoting healthy scar formation, circular and cross-fiber friction around an injury site can help keep normal tissues from adhering to the scarred area. Such adhering of tissues may cause chronic pain or inflammation. This is especially important where there is a large wound, such as in a cesarean section or other surgery.

■ TAPOTEMENT

Tapotement consists of a series of brisk percussive movements following each other in rapid, alternating fashion. Tapotement has a stimulating effect and is pleasant to receive if performed skillfully. The most common classic forms of tapotement are hacking, rapping, cupping, clapping, slapping, tapping, and pincement.

The movement of tapotement is light, rapid, and rhythmic. The hands should "bounce off" of the surface as they make contact, lightening the impact. The recipients should not feel like they are taking a beating, but should feel pleasantly stimulated. The percussive sound itself can be pleasing and can add to the therapeutic effect. Different hand positions create different sounds, and different parts of the body sound different when struck. Quacking and squishes described below are nontraditional forms of tapotement that make distinctive, interesting sounds. Tapotement takes a certain rhythmic ability and much practice to master. The effort to learn it, though, is well worthwhile for the diversity it can bring to your work. Experiment with varying rhythms and hand positions for different effects.

Tapotement is often used in finishing either a section of the body, a side of the body, or the session itself. Because it is stimulating, tapotement is useful in situations in which the receiver must be alert when leaving the session. For example, it may be used if the receiver must drive directly after a session or go back to work. Athletes benefit from tapotement before a competition. Some people simply like the tingling and alive feeling that tapotement can leave with them.

While performing tapotement, the amount of force to use and the degree of stiffness of the hands depends on the area receiving the technique. Heavily muscular areas like the back and thighs can withstand more force, while more delicate areas like the head need a light touch. When performing tapotement over a broad area, as in ending a session with tapotement over a whole side of the body, the amount of force used will vary as you move from one section to another.

Variations of Tapotement

Hacking is performed with the hands facing each other, thumbs up. The striking surface is the ulnar surface of the hand and sometimes the sides of the third, fourth, and fifth fingertips. See Figure 6–21. The wrists, hands, and fingers should be held loosely during the rapid percussion movement. Alternate hitting with the left and

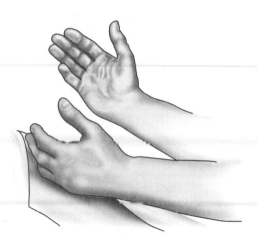

FIGURE 6–21. Hacking. Tapotement performed with the ulnar side of relaxed hands.

right hands. Performed correctly, the effect of hacking is one of pleasant stinging and stimulation.

To practice hacking, shake your hands letting the wrists, hands, and fingers relax and "flip up and down." No attempt should be made to hold the fingers together or the hands and wrists in any particular position. If relaxation is complete, you will notice that the hands fall into a neutral plane of motion that neither supinates nor pronates the forearms. Move the hands rapidly alternating one up and one down keeping the hands relaxed and shaking them. Practice on the back moving from the hips to the shoulder, and then back to the hips again. Never hit hard over the kidneys.

A similar movement, called *rapping,* may be performed using lightly closed and loosely held fists. The fists may be held palms down as in rapping on a door as shown in Figure 6–22. In side-rapping (sometimes called *beating*), the striking surface is the ulnar side of the fist. Keep the force of the blows light and "rebounding" in effect rather than jarring.

Cupping and *clapping* are applied with the same rhythmic, rapidly alternating force. For both techniques, cup the hand so that the thumb and fingers are slightly flexed, and the palmer surface contracted. The thumb is held tightly against the first finger. For *cupping,* strike the body surface with the outside rim of the cupped hand, keeping the palm contracted as shown in Figure 6–23. There will be a hollow sound. A sight vacuum is created with each blow, which some believe may loosen broad flat areas of scar tissue or fascial adhesions. Cupping is also used for loosening congestion in the respiratory system.

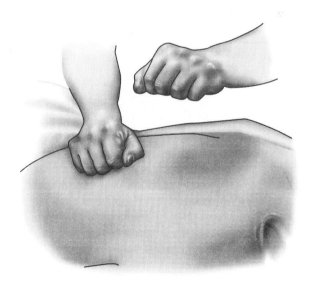

FIGURE 6–22. Rapping. Tapotement performed with the knuckles of a loosely closed fist, as if rapping lightly on a door.

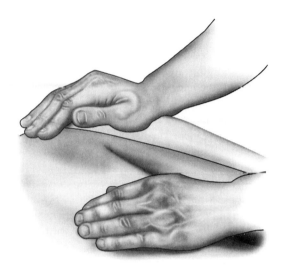

FIGURE 6–23. Cupping. Tapotement performed with the outside rim of a cupped hand.

Let the palm contact the body surface for *clapping*. This produces a less hollow sound and provides a broader contact surface. *Slapping* is performed with an open hand, the fingers held lightly together. Strike gently and briskly with the palmer surface of the fingers, rather than with the whole hand.

Tapping is done with the ends of the fingers. Sharp light taps are done either with the edge of the fingernails or padding of the fingers. See Figure 6–24.

Pincement is a rapid, gentle movement in which superficial tissues are picked up between the thumb and first two fingers. It might be described as "plucking." A rhythm is established alternating left and right hands. See Figure 6–25.

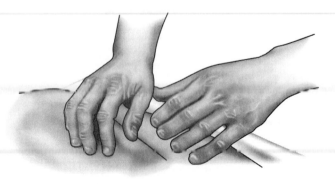

FIGURE 6–24. Tapping. Tapotement performed with the fingertips of a relaxed hand.

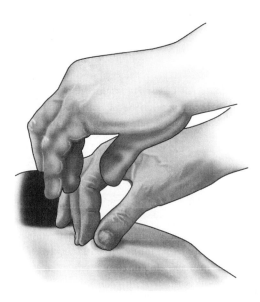

FIGURE 6–25. Pincement. Tapotement performed by gently picking up superficial tissues between the thumb and first two fingers with a light rapid movement.

Quacking is done with the palms together and fingers loosely apart. The striking surface is the lateral edges of the tips of the fourth and fifth (little) fingers as shown in Figure 6–26. As the fingers hit the bony surface, they come together making a quacking sound.

Squishes are done with the hands loosely folded, making an air pocket with the palms. The striking surface is the back of one of the hands. As the back of the hand hits, the palms push out the air between them, creating a "squishing" sound.

▪ VIBRATION

Vibration may be described as an oscillating, quivering, or trembling motion, or movement back and forth or up and down performed quickly and repeatedly. The vibration may be fine, and applied to a small area with the fingertips. Or it may be coarse, and involve shaking a muscle belly back and forth.

Vibration over the abdomen is sometimes used to stimulate the organs of digestion and elimination. Coarse vibration, in the form of jostling, may be used to help a recipient become aware of holding tension, to bring greater circulation to a muscle, and to help it relax. Fine *vibration* techniques impart an oscillating motion to the soft tissues and have a stimulating effect. They may also numb or relax specific muscles.

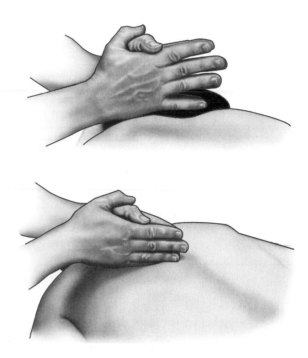

FIGURE 6–26. Quacking. Tapotement performed with the hands together and fingers loosely apart. Fingers come together as the little finger strikes, making a "quacking" sound.

Electric vibrators may be used to impart fine vibration to tense muscles. The motion of vibration can often be sustained for a longer period of time with a machine than if performed by hand. There are many types of hand-held vibrators appropriate for muscle relaxation. Some impart a coarser vibration, others a finer oscillation. One type of vibrator straps to the back of the hand and causes vibration in the fingers. This allows the practitioner to stay in direct contact with the receiver and perform another technique such as light effleurage or friction. A standard hand-held vibrator is shown in Figure 6–27. A still finer vibration may be created by sound waves. There are devices that impart a lower frequency wave than ultrasound and are within the scope of practice of most practitioners.

Variations of Vibration

A *fine vibration* or trembling motion is imparted through the fingertips, but generated by the forearm. To practice fine vibration, place one hand on a muscle with the fingertips slightly apart. The trembling movement comes from the whole forearm, through the elbow, and the wrist and finger joints are kept in a fixed position. The elbow should be slightly flexed. This vibrating motion should be more in and out than side to side. The fingers remain in contact with the same spot during the vibra-

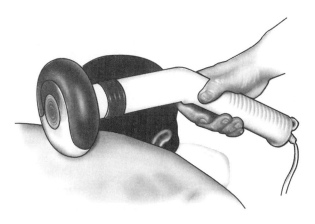

FIGURE 6–27. Fine vibration applied with a hand-held electric vibrator.

tion and are then lifted off of the skin and replaced to a new spot. Heavy pressure should be avoided. Fine vibration on the abdomen is shown in Figure 6–28.

Light effleurage with vibration may be used for a soothing effect. While performing a light effleurage movement, add a sight vibration back and forth with the fingertips. Pressure can be so light that there is slight contact between the hand and the skin. It is a light brushing movement. In cases of hypersensitive nerves, this technique has been credited with having a soothing effect.

Shaking is a coarse form of vibration that can assist muscular relaxation. For example, a muscle such as the biceps or gastrocnemius may be grasped with one hand and shaken gently back and forth. Figure 6–29 shows shaking of the muscles of the leg. The leg is bent at a 90 degree angle to help create slack in the muscles facilitating the shaking movement.

In shaking the upper leg, two hands are used, one on each side of the leg. In this case, the shaking movement is back and forth from hand to hand. This is also called *jostling*. It is helpful at times to shake the entire limb gently to mobilize the surrounding joints and encourage relaxation and "letting go" of the whole area.

■ TOUCH WITHOUT MOVEMENT

Techniques that involve *touch without movement* are difficult to fit neatly into the five classic categories, since those categories are defined by movement itself. Nevertheless, various forms of touch without movement have been used in Western systems of massage. In the early twentieth century, J. Harvey Kellogg used seven categories to describe the "procedures of massage," which included the five classic ones plus touch and joint movements.

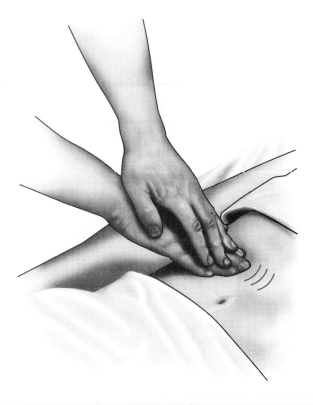

FIGURE 6–28. Vibration applied with fingertips to the abdomen.

Touch without movement is not casual or social touch, but is skilled touch with intention. Kellogg cautions that this is not ordinary touch, but "touch applied with intelligence, with control, with a purpose; and simple as it is, is capable of producing decided physiological effects" (p. 52).

Passive touch is simply laying the fingers, one hand, or both hands lightly on the body. Passive touch may impart heat to an area, having a calming influence on the nervous system, or as some believe, help balance energy. Historically, the effects of passive touch have been attributed to "hypnotic" or "electrical" effects, "magnetism," and "subtle qualities of manner, a peculiar softness of the hand, or other personal quality not easy to describe" (Kellogg, 1929, p. 53). The use of passive touch to balance energy is more fully developed in systems of massage outside of classic Western systems. Passive touch is often used to end a session, or before turning over. It is used effectively for its calming effects when applied to the feet or to the head, as shown in Figure 6–30.

Direct static pressure, or simply *direct pressure,* may be applied with a thumb, finger or fingers, elbow, or knuckles. Tissues are compressed using light to heavy pressure. Simple direct pressure can be considered a form of compression without the rhythmic movement and has also been called "static friction." Direct static pres-

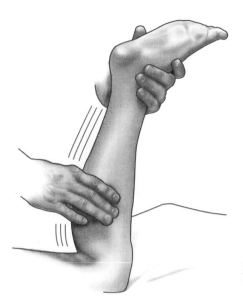

FIGURE 6–29. Shaking the muscle belly of the gastrocnimius for a course vibration.

sure to various areas or points is known to relieve pain and diminish congestion. Pressure applied with enough force to cause blanching is followed by vasodilation upon release of pressure, thus improving local circulation. Direct pressure to a hypertonic muscle often helps the muscle to relax. Figure 6–31 shows direct pressure to the suboccipital muscles to help relieve tension headache.

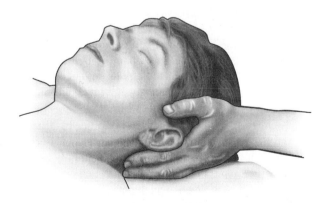

FIGURE 6–30. Passive touch holding the head. Sometimes used to close a session.

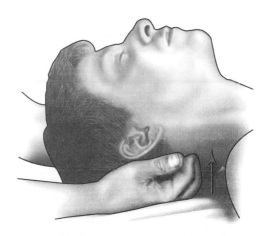

FIGURE 6–31. Direct pressure to suboccipital muscles. Fingers press up into the muscle attachments along the occipital ridge.

Pressure should be applied carefully to avoid bruising or damaging tissues. Direct pressure is often preceded by warming the area with effleurage or compressions and followed with effleurage to "smooth-out" the area or transition to another place.

Direct static pressure has been used for centuries. Theories about how it works have evolved over the years and include the concepts of zone therapy, motor points, stress points, reflex points, trigger points, and acupressure points. The intentions of practitioners using direct static pressure may differ, and the amount of pressure used, location of areas pressed, and duration of pressure may also vary.

▪ SUMMARY

Classic Western massage is a synthesis of various popular systems of massage developed in Europe and the United States in the nineteenth and twentieth centuries. It organizes the many possible variations of soft tissue manipulation into five categories of techniques called effleurage, petrissage, friction, tapotement, and vibration. Effleurage is sliding or gliding movements; petrissage is lifting, pressing, and squeezing movements; friction involves rubbing two surfaces over one another; tapotement is percussive; and vibration causes oscillation in tissues. Techniques involving touch without movement do not fit neatly into the five classic categories, but have been used in many Western systems of massage throughout history. Two forms of touch without movement commonly used are passive touch or holding and direct static pressure.

Each of the many techniques presented has a variety of uses and effects. Massage practitioners should understand these so that the techniques can be applied effectively in a massage session. Reading about the techniques and studying the illustrations can help you understand the main concepts involved. However, skill in performing the techniques can only be acquired through practice, and with guidance from an experienced practitioner.

▪ REFERENCES

Beard, G., & Wood, E. C. (1964). *Massage: Principles and techniques.* Philadelphia: W. B. Saunders.

Cyriax, J. H., & Cyriax, P. J. (1993). *Illustrated manual of orthopedic medicine,* 2nd ed. Boston: Butterworth & Heinemann.

Graham, D. (1884). *Practical treatise on massage.* New York: Wm. Wood and Co.

Hoffa, A. J. (1900). *Technik der massage,* 3rd ed. Verlagsbuchhandlung, Stuttgart: Ferdinand Enke. As translated by F. M. Tappan and Ruth Friedlander.

Kellogg, J. H. (1929). *The art of massage: A practical manual for the nurse, the student and the practitioner.* Battle Creek, MI: Modern Medicine Publishing Co.

McMillan, M. (1921). *Massage and therapeutic exercise.* Philadelphia: W. B. Saunders.

7

Joint Movements

Classic Western massage traditionally includes joint movements, as well as soft tissue manipulation. Pehr Ling's original system of medical gymnastics, developed in Sweden in the early 1800s, included passive movements of the soft tissues and joints (Roth, 1851). The term "Swedish movements" was commonly used in the United States to refer to various joint movements up through the 1950s.

Joint movements are traditionally categorized as active (ie, free, assistive, and resistive) and passive (McMillan, 1925). Free active movements are performed entirely by a person without assistance from a practitioner. In assistive movements, recipients initiate the movement, while practitioners help them perform the movement. In resistive movements, practitioners offer resistance to the movement thereby challenging the muscles used. Passive movements refer to movements initiated and controlled by the practitioner, while the recipient remains totally relaxed and passive.

Joint mobilizations are passive movements performed within the normal range of joint movement. They can easily be integrated into a massage routine. They cause movement of the soft tissues around and within joints, freeing up the motion at the joints involved. Massage techniques may be applied to muscles while the associated joint is being mobilized.

Stretching is a type of passive joint movement that is performed to the limit of the range of motion. It is used to increase flexibility at the joint, as it elongates the muscles and connective tissues that cross the joint. Stretching may also be used for muscle relaxation.

Practitioners use joint movements for a variety of reasons including to stretch surrounding tissues, increase joint range of motion, stimulate production of synovial fluid, increase kinesthetic awareness, stimulate muscle relaxation, and build muscle strength. Some contemporary systems of bodywork, such as Trager® (referred to as psychophysical integration), use joint movements to affect the nervous system, reeducate muscles, and integrate function. Receivers can also learn to let go of tension they are unconsciously holding onto during passive joint movement. Joint movement adds a kinetic dimension to a massage session and provides diversity of technique.

Joint movements, both active and passive, have been used for decades to help improve posture and body alignment. Stretching can improve the function of an area such as the shoulder or hip by increasing the flexibility around a joint.

Joint manipulations or *adjustments* (sometimes called *chiropractic adjustments*) are *not* within the scope of this text. By joint manipulations and adjustments, we mean techniques that take a joint beyond its normal range of motion and that are specific attempts to realign a misaligned joint, usually using a thrusting movement. They should be performed only by those trained to do so within their legal scope of practice. "Cracking" necks and backs and "popping" toes are potentially dangerous and should not be performed as part of classic Western massage.

In this chapter, we will describe simple passive joint movements that fall under the categories of nonspecific joint mobilizations and stretching. These movements may be incorporated into a general massage session or might be used for specific therapeutic goals.

■ GENERAL PRINCIPLES FOR JOINT MOVEMENTS

Practitioners should be familiar with the bony structure and muscles that move each joint. Together these determine the movements possible at the joint. Normal range of motion refers to the degree of movement commonly found at a joint and is useful knowledge to generally assess the degree of flexibility at a joint. Knowing the normal limitations to movement at each joint will decrease the likelihood of inadvertently damaging a joint or the surrounding tissues, and increase safety for the recipient.

Caution is advised in cases of abnormality of the bony structure, hypermobility, recent injury, and diseases of the joints such as bursitis and arthritis. A past trauma may have caused some unusual conditions around a joint, including shortening or loss of muscle tissue, scarring in connective tissues, and abnormal joint structure. Sometimes "hardware," such as metal pins and plates, is present from past injuries. Joint replacements are becoming more common, and movement around artificial joints may be restricted. Hip replacements are important to know about, especially in the elderly. Take the time to learn about the condition from the recipient, from available medical records, or from the recipient's physician to ensure a safe application of joint movements. Remember that massage and joint movements are contraindicated when inflammation is present.

Palpation skills are very important for learning about how joints move. Practitioners can learn much about the condition of the joint and surrounding tissues from the kinesthetic feel of the movement. Sensing things like "drag" and "end feel" offer clues to restrictions to normal range of motion, areas of tightness, patterns of holding, and the limits of stretches.

The stretches described in this chapter are passive movements applied as *static stretches*. Avoid sudden, forceful, or bouncing movements while performing the stretches. Move the part being stretched into position and hold at the limit of movement, which is determined by feeling for the point of resistance. Use feedback from the recipient for safety. The recipient should feel the stretch, but not feel pain. Hold for 10–15 seconds, and then try to increase the stretch. The muscles will often relax after a short time allowing further stretch (30–45 seconds overall).

Breathing may be used to help the recipient relax during a stretch. The body is more relaxed during exhalation than during inhalation, and holding the breath causes tension in the musculature and restricts movement. So it is better to stretch a muscle on the exhalation. Once you and the recipient are in position to apply a stretch, ask her to "take a deep breath and then let it out slowly." During the exhalation, apply the stretch.

The following is a summary of the general guidelines for performing passive joint movements:

- Stay within the normal range of motion of the joint.
- Qualities of movement for mobilizations are smooth, free, and loose.
- Warm surrounding tissues before stretching.
- Use breathing to enhance a stretch.
- Stay within the comfort range of the recipient.
- Be aware of abnormality of joint structure and adapt movements accordingly.

▪ JOINT MOVEMENT TECHNIQUES

Neck

STRUCTURE AND MOVEMENT. The "neck" is a general term for the region between the head and the trunk. It includes the seven cervical vertebrae and the surrounding soft tissues. The cervicals are the smallest, most delicate vertebrae and are designed to allow for a lot of movement but not bear a lot of weight. They are arranged vertically with an anterior convex curve.

The musculature in the neck region is complex with most deeper, smaller muscles entirely within the neck, and many larger and more superficial muscles with attachments often superior or inferior. The bony and muscular structures allow a variety of movements including flexion, extension, hyperextension, lateral flexion, and rotation.

MOBILIZATIONS. Neck mobilizations may be performed when the recipient is lying supine. The mobilizations occur between the cervical vertebrae and in the suboccipital region. All of the following examples may be performed with the practitioner seated at the head of the recipient. It is useful to have an adjustable stool or chair on wheels so that you can get in good position, for both leverage and self-care.

Simple neck mobilizations may be performed by lifting the head slightly off the table and moving it into lateral flexion, rotation, forward flexion, and hyperextension. Be sure to have a firm grip on the head. You may have to remind the recipient to relax, since it takes great trust to let someone hold and move your head. You may also assure them that you will not "crack" their neck, and that such manipulations are not part of these mobilizations. Keep the movements small at first and gradually increase the range of motion as the recipient allows.

Finger push-ups may be used to produce gentle movement between the cervical vertebrae. First warm up the neck muscles with effleurage and circular friction along each side. Straighten the neck, so that the recipient is directly face-up. Simply place the fingers at the base of the neck on either side, palms up, and push up on the tissues applying direct static pressure. Move your hands about an inch at a time along the neck, pressing up at each spot as you move along. You will feel movement between the vertebrae and notice movement at the head. Variations of finger push-ups include alternating pressing from side to side. The rhythm would be to press right, press left, move along; press right, press left, move along; repeating the sequence along the neck moving toward the head.

The *melt-down* is a variation of the finger push-up applied in the suboccipital region. Place your hands, palms up, under the recipient's head, with fingers along the suboccipitals. Lift the head with the hands, and then lower the wrists to the table, while leaving the head balanced on the fingertips. Usually within 5–10 seconds, the neck muscles relax, the suboccipital tissues "melt," and the head hyperextends. You will notice the recipient's head falling back, and your fingers will be deep into the suboccipital space. This pressure usually feels good to the recipient. Finish by gently pulling on the occiput to straighten any hyperextension remaining from the movement.

A *wavelike movement* may be created in the neck by simply applying deep effleurage on both sides at the same time, moving from the base to the suboccipital region. You exaggerate the natural curve of the neck by pressing up as you slide along. The neck will return to its normal curve as you finish the movement. See Figure 8–21. At the end of the movement, give a gentle pull on the occiput to straighten any hyperextension remaining from the movement. The *wave* is a good technique to use to detect tension in the neck. The wavelike motion will not occur if the recipient is unconsciously holding tension in the neck or if the neck muscles are shortened and tight.

STRETCHES. Massage and simple mobilizations are used to warm up the neck thoroughly before applying stretches. The following stretches may be performed when the recipient is lying supine on a table.

A stretch in *lateral flexion* helps lengthen the muscles on the sides of the neck. Place the head in position to one side at a point where you feel the tissues just starting to stretch. The head placement, either face up or turned to the side, will determine which muscles are stretched most. Place one hand on the shoulder and the other on the side of the head. You can create a gentle stretch of tissues by pushing the head and shoulders in opposite directions as shown in Figure 7–1. Guide the recipient to exhale as you apply the stretch. The head will move to a position of

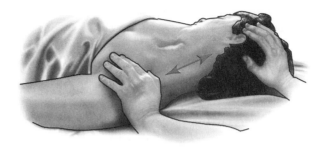

FIGURE 7–1. Stretch of trapezius and cervical muscles with neck in lateral flexion.

greater lateral flexion as the upper trapezius relaxes and lengthens. Repeat on the other side.

Range of *rotation* may be enhanced with a simple stretch. Position the head face-up so that the neck is straight. Then rotate the head to one side keeping the neck vertically aligned. Gently push the head into greater rotation, stretching the neck muscles. Repeat on the other side.

Position the head face-up to stretch the neck in *forward flexion*. Lift the head with one hand, and with the other hand, reach under the head and across to the tip of the shoulder. The head rests on the forearm. Reach under that arm with the free hand and place it on the other shoulder. The head should be cradled safely at the place where the forearms cross as shown in Figure 7–2. Slowly stretch the neck into forward flexion. Stand during this movement for best leverage.

The cross-armed stretch may also be performed with the head rotated. This will stretch neck muscles at a different angle. After forward flexion, return to the

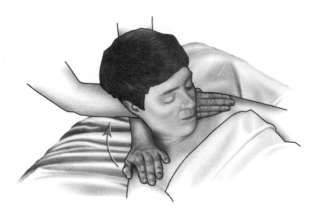

FIGURE 7–2. Cross-arm stretch of cervical muscles with neck in forward flexion.

starting position and turn the head to one side. Repeat the forward flexion to each side with the head in rotation. For safety, be sure that the stretch is pain free.

Shoulder Girdle

STRUCTURE AND MOVEMENT. The shoulder girdle is a complex region that can be defined in many ways. For our purposes, the shoulder girdle will be defined as including the glenohumeral, acromioclavicular, and scapulocostal joints. The glenohumeral joint is classified as a ball-and-socket joint, and the acromioclavicular joint as diarthrodial nonaxial. The scapulocostal juncture may be described as a gliding joint of the scapula with the rib cage separated by muscles and a bursa (Cailliet, 1981, p. 2).

The shoulder girdle is the most mobile area of the body. Movements possible in the shoulder girdle include the upper arm movements of flexion, extension, hyperextension, abduction, adduction, rotation, and horizontal flexion. Movements of the scapulae themselves include elevation, depression, upward and downward rotation and tilt, and retraction and protraction. The entire shoulder girdle is structured to accomplish circumduction.

MOBILIZATIONS. Shoulder girdle mobilizations may be performed with the recipient in either the supine, prone, side-lying, or seated position. Mobilization of the joints of the shoulder may be accomplished indirectly by movement of the arm or by movement of the scapula.

To mobilize the shoulder girdle with the recipient in the supine position, take hold of the hand and lift and wag the arm as shown in Figure 7–3. While *wagging* the arm, there will also be movement at the wrist and elbow. *Shaking* is performed by creating a slight traction of the arm toward the feet holding onto the hand and leaning back as shown in Figure 7–4. Loosely shake the arm up and down. Movement will be felt at the wrist, elbow, and shoulder.

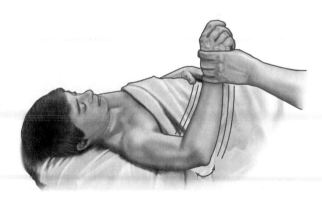

FIGURE 7–3. Wagging for arm and shoulder mobilization.

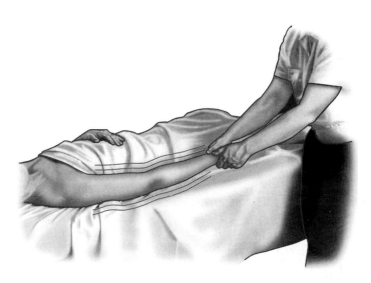

FIGURE 7–4. Shaking for arm and shoulder mobilization.

Direct mobilization of the shoulder may be accomplished by holding onto the upper arm with one hand close to the glenohumeral joint and the other hand at the tip of the shoulder. Simply move the shoulder through the full range of motion possible in the supine position. The quality of movement should be smooth, free, and loose. This same technique is effective in the prone, side-lying, and seated positions. Figure 7–5 shows shoulder mobilization with the recipient supine.

With the recipient prone, the scapula may be mobilized using pressure applied at the top of the shoulder. Position the recipient's arm on the table with elbow bent and hand near the waist. Then place your hand on top of the shoulder near the tip and pressing lightly toward the feet. The scapula will move and lift if the attached muscles are relaxed as shown in Figure 7–6. Don't force the movement, but encourage relaxation by gentle motions and reminding the recipient to let go of tension in the area. Once the medial border lifts, you may apply effleurage to massage the muscles that attach there.

STRETCHES. Use massage and mobilizations to warm up the shoulder girdle before stretching. Shoulder girdle stretches are effective in the supine, prone, and side-lying positions. The muscles of the shoulder girdle are stretched primarily with movements of the upper arm.

In the supine position, a stretch in *horizontal flexion* may be performed by moving the arm over the chest. This elongates the muscles that attach to the medial border of the scapula, including the rhomboids, as well as the posterior shoulder muscles. Hold onto the recipient's lower arm near the wrist with one hand, while

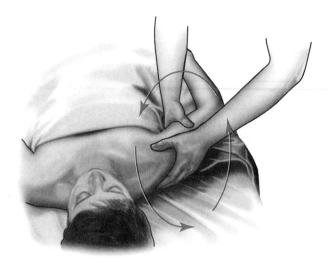

FIGURE 7–5. Direct mobilization of the shoulder with recipient in supine position. Passive shoulder roll.

the other hand reaches under to the medial border of the scapula. Stretch the arm over the chest and enhance the stretch by gently pulling back on the scapula at the same time. See Figure 7–7.

A very pleasant stretch may be applied with the recipient's arms extended overhead. This stretch may be performed one arm at a time or both arms at the same time. For a two-arm stretch, simply place the arms overhead, grasping the forearm

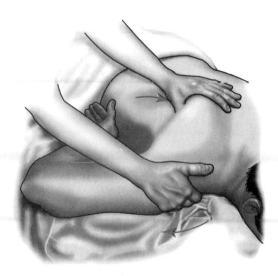

FIGURE 7–6. Move and lift the scapula by pulling back at the shoulder.

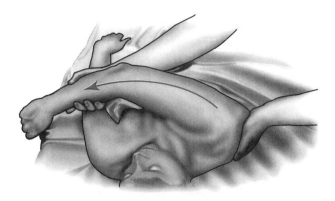

FIGURE 7–7. Stretching the shoulder muscles with arm in horizontal flexion.

near the wrist. Lean back to create the stretch at the shoulder as shown in Figure 7–8. This technique stretches all of the muscles of the shoulder girdle, including the latissimus dorsi and pectoral muscles.

A similar stretch may be applied with the recipient seated in a massage chair. Grasp the forearm with both hands and move the arm overhead to a position in line with the angle of the body. You should be facing in the same direction as the recipient. Lift the arm upward and give it a gentle shake as shown in Figure 7–9.

Elbow

STRUCTURE AND MOVEMENT. The elbow is formed by the junction of the distal end of the humerus and the proximal ends of the radius and the ulna. Movements of the humeroulnar joint are limited to flexion and extension. The bony structure of the

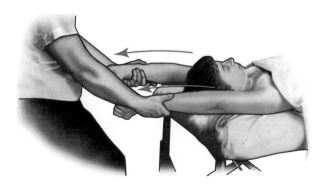

FIGURE 7–8. Stretching the shoulder muscles with arms overhead. Lean back to create the stretch using your body weight.

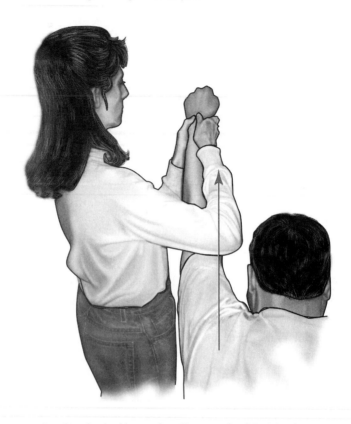

FIGURE 7-9. Stretching the shoulder muscles with arm overhead. Recipient in a massage chair.

joint further limits the range of motion in extension. What we think of as the point of the elbow is the olecranon process of the ulna.

The movements of pronation and supination of the forearm (palm-down and palm-up) occur as the head of the radius rotates over the surfaces of the capitulum of the humerus and the radial notch of the ulna. At the same time, the distal ends of the radius and ulna glide over one another.

MOBILIZATIONS. Mobilizations at the elbow are limited by the structure of the joint. *Wagging* of the arm as described above offers some mobilization at the elbow. You may also pronate and supinate the forearm by holding the hand and turning it alternately palm-up and palm-down.

To perform a simple mobilization at the elbow, bend the arm at the elbow so that it is perpendicular to the table. Hold the arm just below the wrist. Trace a circle with the hand creating movement at the elbow as shown in Figure 7–10.

STRETCHES. Stretches of muscles that cross the elbow are accomplished largely by stretching the whole arm as in the overhead stretch of the shoulder described above.

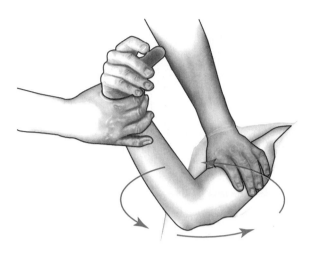

FIGURE 7–10. Circle the lower arm thus creating movement at the elbow.

If the biceps muscles are shortened, the stretch is created by simply straightening out the arm at the elbow.

Wrist

STRUCTURE AND MOVEMENT. The wrist joint is formed by the union of the slightly concave surface of the proximal row of carpal bones with the distal end of the radius and the midcarpal joint. What people commonly call the "wrist bone" is actually the distal end of the ulna. Movements possible at this juncture include flexion, extension, hyperextension, radial and ulnar deviation (side-to-side movement), and circumduction.

MOBILIZATIONS. Mobilizations at the wrist are best performed with the recipient supine. The soft tissues in the wrist area may be warmed up with small sliding effleurage movements with the thumbs prior to mobilizations and stretching. A useful starting position for basic mobilizations and stretching is achieved by clasping the recipient's hands, palms facing and fingers interwoven. The recipient's elbow is bent and may be resting on the table. In the hand clasp position, you may take the hand through its entire range of motion at the wrist including flexion, extension, hyperextension, side-to-side in radial and ulnar deviation, and circumduction. Keep the movement well within the possible range of motion.

A light, quick mobilization may be performed at the wrist with a *waving* movement. Hold just above the recipient's wrist (palm down) with both of your hands, the thumbs on top and index fingers below. Use the remaining fingers to cause the hand to *wave,* by pressing up against the heel of the hand quickly and repeatedly, letting gravity help it fall between times. Movement at the wrist also occurs during less specific mobilizations including wagging the arm as shown in Figure 7–3, and supination and pronation of the forearm.

STRETCHES. Flexion and hyperextension are the major stretches performed at the wrist. Figure 7–11 shows stretching the flexors of the forearm by hyperextending at the wrist. Press down gently on the palm side of the fingers to create the stretch. Now flex the hand at the wrist and press down on the back side of the hand to create a stretch of the extensors of the forearm as shown in Figure 7–12. During these stretches, be careful to approach the limit of motion slowly.

Hand

STRUCTURE AND MOVEMENT. Joints within the hand and above the wrist include the metacarpophalangeal juncture (ie, knuckles) and the small joints between phalanges. The second through fifth fingers each have three phalanges with two joints, while the thumb has just two phalanges with one joint. The joint between the carpal and metacarpal of the thumb is designed to allow freer movement than similar junctures of the carpals and metacarpals. Movement may also occur between metacarpals. Movements of the fingers include flexion, extension, abduction, and adduction. The hand as a whole is capable of holding and grasping objects.

MOBILIZATIONS. Perform mobilizations of the joints of the hands very carefully, matching the force used to the size and strength of the hand you are working with. Warm the muscles in the recipient's hands with effleurage and light frictions before performing mobilizations and stretches.

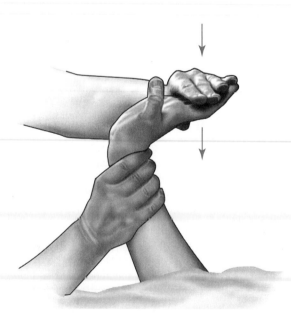

FIGURE 7–11. Stretching the flexor muscles of the forearm by hyperextending the wrist.

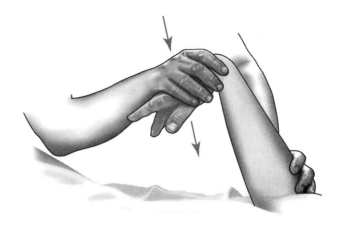

FIGURE 7–12. Stretching the extensor muscles of the forearm by flexing the wrist.

Mobilization of the knuckles, one at a time may be achieved making *figure eights*. Hold the recipient's hand with one of your hands, his fingers pointing toward you, palm-down. With your other hand, grasp the fifth (little) finger firmly near the knuckle and move in a small figure eight pattern two or three times, mobilizing the joint. See Figure 7–13. Repeat for each knuckle joint.

A similar, but lighter, mobilization of the knuckles may be achieved by grasping the fingers more distally. Perform the figure eights as described above.

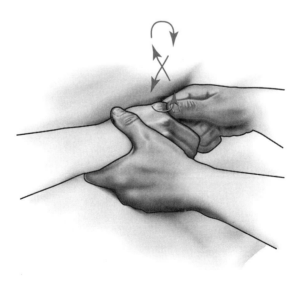

FIGURE 7–13. Figure 8's at the knuckles of the hand.

You can mobilize the tissues between the metacarpals with a *scissoring* motion. With the recipient's palm down, take hold of knuckles of the fifth and fourth fingers as shown in Figure 7–14. Simply move one knuckle up and the other down at the same time, alternating in a scissoring motion. Repeat along all of the knuckles.

STRETCHES. There are a few simple stretches for the joints of the hand. Perform them slowly and with care. The fingers can be hyperextended at the knuckles. Interlace your fingers with the recipient's, palm to palm, placing the tips of your fingers just below the recipient's knuckles. Gently press between the metacarpals, bending the fingers into hyperextension. This movement may also cause the metacarpals to spread out, stretching the tissues between them.

Taking the whole hand into hyperextension can stretch all of the flexor muscles within the hand and the wrist flexors in the forearm. Hold the forearm with one hand and, with the other hand, press back on the phalanges causing hyperextension at the knuckles and at the wrist. Gently stretch the tissues of the hand and the forearm. See Figure 7–11.

The extensor muscles in the forearm can be stretched by flexing at the wrist. With the recipient's elbow resting on the table, let the hand relax naturally into flexion. Place your palm on the back of the hand and gently press down to stretch the wrist extensors. See Figure 7–12.

Chest

STRUCTURE AND MOVEMENT. The "chest" is a common term for the area on the front and sides of the upper body generally defined by the ribs, sternum, and clavicle. It is the

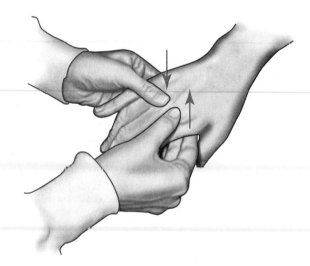

FIGURE 7–14. Scissoring motion to create movement between the metacarpals of the hand.

part of the thorax accessible when lying supine. The entire thorax, including the chest, expands and contracts with the inhalation and exhalation of breathing. The pectoral muscles are located on the chest.

MOBILIZATIONS. The rib cage may be mobilized by gently rocking it from the side. Stand facing the side of the table in line with the rib cage. Put one hand on top of the other and place them on the rib cage as shown in Figure 7–15. Gently rock the rib cage by repeatedly pushing and then letting up the pressure in a rhythmic manner. Move around on the rib cage to mobilize different areas. You will feel the elastic quality of the rib cage as it springs back after you push.

If you can reach far enough with your arms, you can mobilize the chest from both sides. Facing the head of the table, reach over with one hand to the far side of the chest, fingers pointing down toward the table. Place the other hand on the near side, fingers pointing up. See Figure 7–16. Gently rock the rib cage by alternating pulling with the far hand and pushing with the near hand. Establish a smooth rhythm to encourage relaxation of the surrounding musculature.

STRETCHES. There are no highly movable joints on the chest itself. However, the pectoral muscles of the shoulder girdle attach there. Use the overhead stretch of the arms as shown in Figure 7–8 to lengthen the pectorals.

Hip

STRUCTURE AND MOVEMENT. The hip joint is a typical ball-and-socket joint formed by the articulation of the head of the femur with the deep cup-shaped acetabulum of the pelvis. The large muscles that move the hip joint are located primarily on the thigh

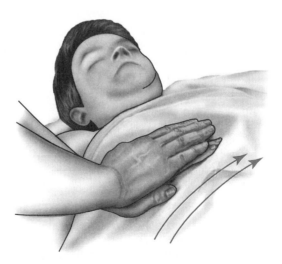

FIGURE 7–15. Placement of hands for mobilizing the rib cage from one side.

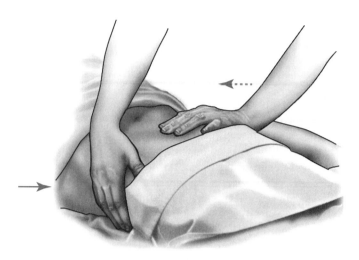

FIGURE 7–16. Placement of hands on both sides of the rib cage for mobilization.

and the buttocks. The iliopsoas is a strong hip flexor that attaches to the lumbar vertebrae and inner surface of the ilium and the lesser trochanter of the femur. Movements possible at the hip joint include flexion, extension, hyperextension, abduction, adduction, diagonal abduction and adduction, outward and inward rotation, and circumduction.

MOBILIZATIONS. Most hip mobilizations are performed with the recipient in the supine position. Mobilizations are an excellent way to affect the deeper muscles that move the hip.

With the recipient supine, remove the bolster from under the knees. The legs should be straight and slightly apart. Stand facing the thigh at the side of the table. Gently rock the leg into rotation by placing the hands palms down on the top of the thigh and pressing down and away. See Figure 7–17. The leg will usually rotate back, especially if the gluteals are tight. The foot will wag from side to side if performed properly. Repeat with a rhythmic rocking motion.

To move the hip through its full range of motion, bend the leg, placing the foot in one hand, and using the other hand for support at the knee. See Figure 7–18. Let the knee trace a circle as the hip flexes, adducts diagonally, extends, abducts diagonally, and goes round again in circumduction. The movement should be smooth and loose.

STRETCHES. The muscles that move the hip can be stretched in many directions. The following are a few simple yet useful stretches for the hip joint.

A stretch for the gluteals may be applied with the hip in flexion by pressing the knee toward the chest (supine position). See Figure 7–19. The hamstrings may be stretched with the leg straight and in flexion as shown in Figure 7–20. To enhance

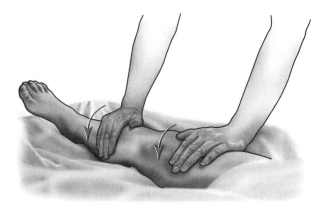

FIGURE 7–17. Rocking the leg to create rotation in the hip joint.

the stretch and involve all of the gluteal and leg muscles, dorsi flex the foot while you bring the leg perpendicular to the table, and then as far toward the chest as possible.

Diagonal adduction of the thigh while lying supine will also stretch the gluteals. Bring the knee toward the chest, and then let it cross the body diagonally as shown in Figure 7–21. The shoulders remain flat on the table, while the supine twists and the hip muscles stretch. This is also a good stretch for the lower back.

To stretch the adductors, separate the legs, abducting one so that you can stand between it and the table as shown in Figure 7–22. Face the head and place your hand on the leg remaining on the table. Use your body to move the outside leg into abduction as far as possible.

The flexors may be stretched from the prone or side-lying position. With the recipient prone, stand at the side of the table facing the head. Bend the leg at the knee and grasp the thigh from underneath. The lower leg can rest against your shoulder. Lift the knee off the ground, putting the hip into hyperextension. You may anchor the hip with the other hand. This stretch takes some strength and is most easily performed if the recipient is smaller than you are.

The stretch into hyperextension can be more easily performed with the recipient in side-lying position. Stand behind the recipient facing the table at the hip. Cradle the upper leg with one arm while you stabilize the trunk with the other. Pull the upper leg back into hyperextension as shown in Figure 7–23. Because you are pulling the leg back, instead of lifting it up, this technique is more efficient and takes less strength. It primarily stretches the quadriceps and iliopsoas muscles.

Knee

STRUCTURE AND MOVEMENT. The knee is classified as a hinge joint and is formed by the articulation of the distal end of the femur with the proximal end of the tibia. A large sesamoid bone embedded in the connective tissues that cross the joint forms the

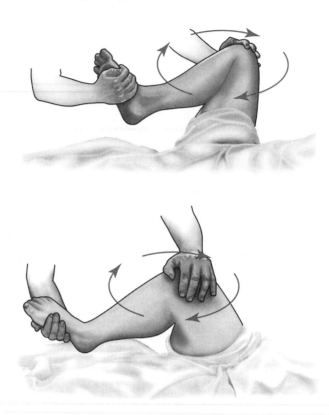

FIGURE 7–18. Taking the hip through its full range of motion.

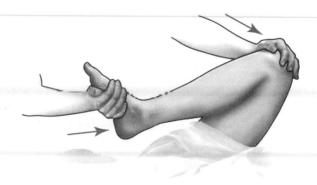

FIGURE 7–19. Stretching the gluteals by bringing knee to chest.

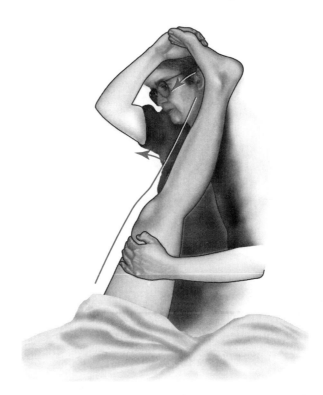

FIGURE 7–20. Stretching the hamstrings with straight leg flexion.

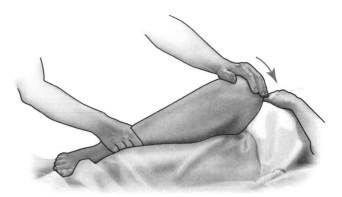

FIGURE 7–21. Stretching the muscles of the hip and lower back with diagonal adduction of the bent leg.

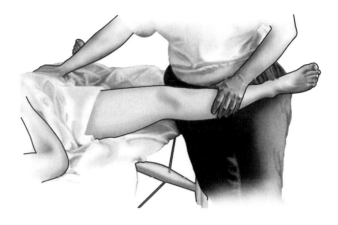

FIGURE 7–22. Stretching the adductors of the leg. Use body weight to move leg into abduction.

knee cap or patella. The major movements of the knee joint are flexion and extension. Some minor inward and outward rotation of the tibia is possible when the knee is flexed in a non-weight-bearing situation.

MOBILIZATIONS. The knee joint is best mobilized with the recipient in the prone position. For a simple mobilization, stand facing the side of the table at the knee. Pick up the leg near the ankle with both hands, so that the lower leg is perpendicular to the table. Lift the leg slightly off the table and wag it back and forth. This also mobilizes the hip joint.

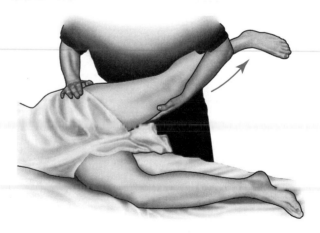

FIGURE 7–23. Stretching the hip flexors with the recipient side-lying.

Another simple mobilization at the knee involves tossing the lower leg back and forth from hand to hand. This "leg toss" technique helps the recipient learn to relax and let go of tension in the legs. After the leg toss, you may perform a different knee mobilization by circling the lower leg. Place one hand on the thigh to steady it and grasp the lower leg near the ankle with the other hand. Make small circles with the lower leg. Stay well within the small range of this circular motion.

STRETCHES. A few of the stretches for the hip joint, performed with a straight leg, also stretch muscles that cross the knee. See Figures 7–20 and 7–22. An additional stretch for the knee extensors can be created with the recipient in the prone position by bringing the heel of the foot toward the buttocks. See Figure 7–24.

Ankle

STRUCTURE AND MOVEMENT. The ankle is a hinge joint formed by the junction of the talus with the malleoli of the tibia and fibula. The structure is bound together with many ligaments for stability. The tendons of muscles of the lower leg that attach to the foot all pass over the ankle. They are bound neatly at the ankle by a band of connective tissue called the retinaculum. Movements possible at the ankle include dorsiflexion (flexion), plantar flexion (extension), pronation (eversion and abduction), and supination (inversion and adduction).

MOBILIZATIONS. When the recipient is prone, the ankle may be accessed by lifting the lower leg so that the foot comes off the table. For a dorsiflexion mobilization, stand at the feet facing the end of the table. Lift one leg and place both hands on the foot,

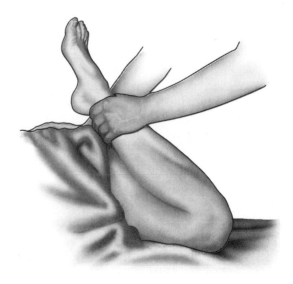

FIGURE 7–24. Stretching the quadriceps by bringing the heel of the foot toward the buttocks.

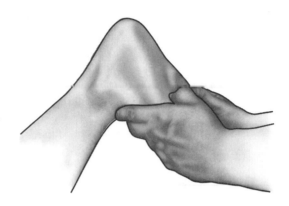

FIGURE 7–25. Dorsiflexion of the foot with direct pressure to bottom of foot with the thumbs.

thumbs on the bottom of the foot. Lean into the foot with the thumbs in the arch, moving the foot into dorsiflexion as shown in Figure 7–25. Repeat the mobilization several times in a rhythmic manner, changing the location of the thumbs to affect different spots on the feet.

With the lower leg lifted so that it is perpendicular to the table, the ankle can be put through a full range of motion. Grasp the bottom of the foot from above and move the ankle through dorsiflexion, pronation, plantar flexion, and supination in a circular movement. This is also an excellent position from which to apply simple dorsiflexion and plantar flexion as shown in Figure 7–26.

With the recipient supine, the ankle can be mobilized by placing the heels of the hands on the foot just under the malleoli of the tibia and fibula (ankle bones) and pressing in alternation one side and then the other. The movement is rapid and causes the heel of the foot to move from side to side at the articulation of the talus and malleoli of the tibia and fibula. See Figure 8–12.

STRETCHES. Stretches at the ankle are primarily performed in dorsiflexion and plantar flexion and may easily be done with the recipient prone or supine. Stretches may be applied from any of the positions mentioned for mobilizations. Simply move the foot into dorsiflexion or plantar flexion and take it to the limit of range of motion. Figure 7–26 shows the ankle and foot stretching in plantar flexion. This movement helps elongate the foot flexors located on the front of the lower leg and may be felt across the top of the foot.

Foot

STRUCTURE AND MOVEMENT. The foot may be described as an elastic arched structure made up of 26 bones and designed for support and propulsion. A foot has 7 tarsal bones (ie, calcaneus, talus, navicular, cuboid, and 3 cuneiforms), 5 metatarsals, and 14 phalanges. There is a longitudinal arch, which extends from the heel to the heads of the 5 metatarsals, and a transverse arch, which extends side to side formed by the

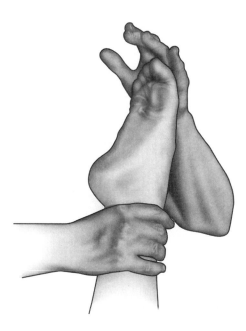

FIGURE 7–26. Stretching the flexors of the foot in plantarflexion. Lower leg perpendicular to the table.

anterior tarsal bones and the metatarsals. The intertarsal joints are irregular joints and allow slight gliding movements, and the interphalangeal joints of the toes are hinge joints that allow for flexion and extension.

MOBILIZATIONS. The mobilizations for the feet are similar to those for the hands. They are best performed with the recipient supine. The soft tissues in the feet may be warmed up with small sliding effleurage movements with the thumbs or fingers, and compressions with the fist on the bottom of the foot.

Hold the foot steady with one hand and with your other hand, grasp the fifth (little) toe firmly near the knuckle and move in a small figure eight pattern two or three times mobilizing the joint. Repeat for each knuckle joint. You can mobilize the tissues between the metatarsals with a *scissoring* motion. Take hold of knuckles of the fifth and fourth toes. Simply move one knuckle up and the other down at the same time, alternating in a scissoring motion. Repeat for all of the metatarsals.

Sometimes the toes curl under due to shortening of the toe flexors that are located on the bottom of the feet. The toes can be mobilized into extension using effleurage along the underside of the toes. This is usually performed with the thumbs. Do not "pop" or pull on the toes forcefully straightening them out, which is uncomfortable to most recipients and dangerous.

STRETCHES. There are a few stretches for the intrinsic tissues of the foot itself. As described above, you can plantar flex the foot from either the prone or supine posi-

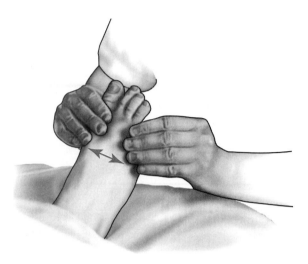

FIGURE 7–27. Creating space between metatarsals by pulling sides of foot away from each other.

tions, stretching the tissues on the top of the foot, including the extensor muscles. The toes alone may easily be stretched back at the ball of the foot or pressed forward for a stretch. The foot may be spread stretching the spaces between the metatarsals, and the muscles that run across them. Simply grasp both sides of the foot and pull in opposite directions, widening the foot and stretching related tissues as shown in Figure 7–27.

You may also interlock your fingers between the toes of the foot. This in itself is usually enough to spread the toes and metatarsals into a stretch. See Figure 7–28.

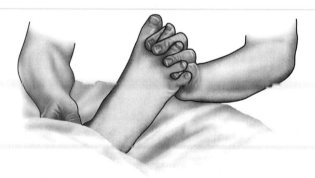

FIGURE 7–28. Creating space between metatarsals by interlocking fingers with recipient's toes.

It will be ineffective if your hands are too small in relation to the recipient's foot, and may be painful if your hands are relatively big.

Since the foot is a small part of the body with many joints, it can be massaged thoroughly rather quickly combining soft tissue techniques with mobilizations and stretches. Joint movements help recipients regain a sense of their feet as having moving parts and help sharpen their kinesthetic sense. This is important especially for those who live in cultures where shoes are worn all day.

■ SUMMARY

Classic Western massage traditionally includes joint movements as well as soft tissue manipulation. Joint movements may be categorized as active (free, assistive, resistive) and passive. During passive joint movements the practitioner initiates and controls the movement, while the recipient remains totally relaxed and passive.

Joint mobilizations are passive movements performed within the normal range of joint movement. Stretching is a type of passive joint movement that is performed to the limit of the range of motion and is used to increase flexibility at a joint. Mobilizations and stretches can be easily integrated into a massage routine.

Joint manipulations or adjustments are not within the scope of this text. These are techniques that take a joint beyond its normal range of motion and are specific attempts to realign a misaligned joint, usually using a thrusting movement. Joint manipulations and adjustments should be performed only by those trained to do so within their legal scope of practice. This text focuses on simple passive joint movements, which fall under the categories of nonspecific joint mobilizations and stretching.

General guidelines for performing passive joint movements safely are as follows: stay within the normal range of motion of the joint; qualities of movement for mobilizations are smooth, free, and loose; warm surrounding tissues before stretching; use breathing to enhance a stretch; stay within the comfort range of the recipient; be aware of any abnormality of joint structure and adapt movements accordingly.

The areas of the body for which passive joint movements are effective are the neck, shoulder girdle, wrists, hands, chest, hips, knees, ankles, and feet. Practitioners should have a practical knowledge of the structure of and the movement possible at each joint to ensure the safety of the recipient during passive joint movements.

Practitioners use joint movements for a variety of reasons including to stretch surrounding tissues, increase joint range of motion, stimulate production of synovial fluid, increase kinesthetic awareness, induce muscle relaxation, and build muscle strength. Some contemporary systems of bodywork, such as Trager® (referred to as psychophysical integration), use joint movements to affect the nervous system, reeducate muscles, and integrate function. Receivers can also learn to let go of tension they are unconsciously holding onto during passive joint movement. Joint movement adds a kinetic dimension to a massage session and provides diversity of technique.

■ REFERENCES

Cailliet, R. (1981). *Shoulder pain,* 2nd ed. Philadelphia: F. A. Davis.

McMillan, M. (1925). *Massage and therapeutic exercise.* Philadelphia: W. B. Saunders.

Roth, M. (1851). *The prevention and cure of many chronic diseases by movements.* London: John Churchill.

Classic Full-Body Massage

Classic full-body massage is typically performed in sessions lasting from 30 minutes to 1½ hours. These sessions are generally wellness oriented. Their purpose is to improve circulation, relax the muscles, improve joint mobility, induce general relaxation, promote healthy skin, and create a general sense of well-being.

A classic full-body session usually includes all of the classic massage techniques, some touch without movement, and passive joint movements. Oil, lotion, or other lubricant is used. Although each practitioner combines and blends various massage techniques in different ways, there are some general guidelines for giving a full-body massage. These guidelines address draping, sequence of body parts, order of techniques, continuity, rhythm, pacing, and specificity.

▪ GENERAL GUIDELINES

DRAPING. Recipients should be draped with a sheet or large towel, and body parts skillfully uncovered and recovered as needed. Genitals and women's breasts should be covered at all times.

SEQUENCE OF BODY PARTS. In a full-body massage session, recipients generally lie prone or supine for the first part of the massage, and then turn over for the second part. Whether they start prone or supine is a matter of preference for the practitioner and the recipient. Sometimes the side-lying position is used, such as with pregnant women.

There are no hard and fast rules for sequence, but it should facilitate a smooth flow from one part of the body to the next. The following are two suggestions for sequences in a full-body routine.

- If a session starts with the recipient in the prone position, a commonly used sequence of body sections would be the back, buttocks, and legs. Then turn over to the supine position with a sequence moving from legs, to arms and shoulders, neck, chest and abdomen, and ending with the head and face.

- If the session starts with the recipient in the supine position, a commonly used sequence of body sections would be head and face, neck, shoulders and arms, chest and abdomen, legs and feet. Then turn over to the prone position with a sequence moving from legs to buttocks and ending on the back.

The advantages of starting in the prone position include that it may feel safer to a recipient new to massage, back massage triggers the relaxation response sooner, and it allows those who need to be more alert at the end of the session to finish face-up. An advantage of starting in the supine position is that the practitioner can massage the head, face, and neck right away, which is good for recipients who do a lot of desk or computer work.

ORDER OF TECHNIQUES. For each part of the body, start with effleurage to apply oil or other lubricant. Continue with effleurage to warm the area and to facilitate venous return, using lighter and then deeper pressure. Effleurage on the limbs should always be performed moving distal to proximal, unless the pressure used is very light. Follow with petrissage for general loosening. Use deep friction, vibration, and direct pressure as appropriate for more specific work. Finish with effleurage and/or tapotement.

When ending work on a specific part of the body, the prone or supine side, or the entire session, some thought should be given to finishing techniques. Finishing techniques may be used to reconnect parts of the body that have been worked on more specifically or to further sedate or stimulate the recipient. Effleurage and tapotement are the usual finishing techniques that can be used to create a sense of wholeness. Light effleurage, sometimes called nerve strokes, is more soothing, while tapotement is more stimulating. Passive touch in the form of simple holding at the head or feet is calming and is sometimes used to end a session.

CONTINUITY. A full-body session should flow smoothly. A sense of flow is achieved through an orderly sequence and smooth transitions from one part of the body to the next. Skill in draping, including uncovering and recovering, can add to the sense of smooth transitions.

A practitioner should take care when establishing touch at the beginning of a session, and then create a sense of continuous touch throughout the session. Establishment or removal of touch should never be abrupt. This does not mean that you may never take your hands off a recipient during a session, but that doing so should be kept to a minimum and be done as imperceptibly as possible.

RHYTHM, PACING, AND SPECIFICITY. The rhythm of a classic full-body massage session may be described as smooth and even, and the pacing as moderate in speed. Trying to perform a full-body session in half an hour will necessitate a faster pace with less attention to detail. A session focusing on general relaxation will be slower paced and usually minimize or eliminate stimulating techniques such as tapotement. If the recipient requests more attention to certain parts of the body such as the back and neck, then those areas would receive more time and specific techniques, while the rest of the body would receive less specific massage.

▪ CLASSIC FULL-BODY MASSAGE ROUTINE

There is no one best way to perform a classic full-body massage session. Practitioners usually develop their own style and sequences into routine ways of working. These routines typically change with experience and according to the individuality and need of the recipients. Today's eclectic practitioners may use a classic full-body routine as a starting point and then integrate contemporary techniques as appropriate to accomplish the goals of the session.

The following is an example of a one-hour full-body routine that may be used to practice the various classic Western massage techniques on different parts of the body. By having an established sequence and order of techniques, the practitioner is free in the learning stages to focus on various skills, including good body mechanics, draping, specific techniques, smooth transitions, continuity, rhythm, and pacing.

It is impossible to describe every single movement you will make during this routine. It will often "feel right" to add a few effleurage strokes as connectors or to soothe an area. Use this routine as a starting point to practice classic massage techniques, and feel free to add variations of techniques as you become more attuned to the work. Most of the techniques described are illustrated in Chapters 6–9. To lengthen the routine you may insert techniques from Chapters 6, 7, and 9 as appropriate.

Prone Position (25 minutes)

Before leaving recipients alone to undress in private, request that when you return they be covered with the drape and lying face-down on the table. Show them how the face cradle works, and position a bolster approximately where their ankles will be. Before you start the session, adjust the position of the face cradle and the bolster for safety and comfort.

Back (15 minutes). Uncover the back down to the waist. Standing at the head, begin applying oil or lotion on the back. Bilateral tree stroking is a good technique to use to apply oil. The movement should be smooth and eventually cover the entire back and sides. Use light to moderate pressure. Repeat three or four times.

Without losing contact, move to one side of the recipient. Stand at the hip and face the head. Work this side of the back entirely before moving to the other side.

Perform the "shingles" effleurage technique along the near side of the spine. Fingers point toward the head. Use moderate to deep pressure. Fully warm the erector muscles of the spine. Perform circular friction with the fingertips along the erector muscles moving from the sacrum to the neck. To apply deeper pressure, use both hands, placing one hand on top of the other as shown in Figure 8–1.

Perform effleurage with the thumbs on the lower back between the iliac crest and the last three ribs to massage the quadratus lumborum. Repeat this technique in two or three strips moving out laterally from the spine. Use moderate to deep pressure.

Reconnect the lower back with the shoulder with a few light "shingles" effleurage strokes. Then perform a deeper effleurage over the upper back and shoulder. Place one hand over the other to apply greater pressure, and use a circular movement around the shoulder as shown in Figure 8–2. Perform circular two-handed petrissage over the entire trapezius. Follow with basic kneading to relax the upper trapezius. Kneading with one hand works better with smaller recipients as shown in Figure 8–3. Begin finishing this side of the back with three-count stroking of the trapezius. Follow with horizontal stroking of the back moving from lower back to shoulders.

Transition to the other side by performing light effleurage from waist to shoulders as you walk around the head of the table. Repeat the entire sequence on the other side beginning with shingles effleurage.

When both sides of the back have been massaged, redrape the back. Finish the entire back with rapping tapotement using moderate pressure.

Lower Limbs and Buttocks (10 minutes). Undrape one leg up to the waist, being careful not to expose the natal cleft. Tuck the drape securely under the leg and at the waist.

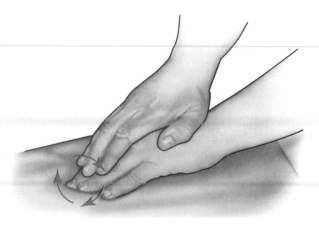

FIGURE 8–1. Circular friction along erector muscles using fingertips.

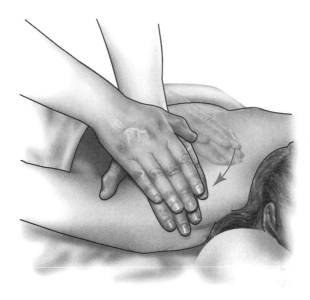

FIGURE 8–2. Deep effleurage over upper back and shoulder.

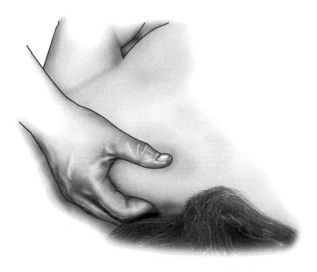

FIGURE 8–3. Basic one-hand kneading of upper trapezius.

Stand at the side of the table facing the head. Apply oil or lotion to the entire leg and hip with basic sliding effleurage using light to moderate pressure. Follow the curves of the leg in a continuous motion from foot to hip. Be sure to touch both sides of the leg. The inside hand will slide onto the back of the leg below the attachments of the adductors and follow the outside hand around the hip. Coordinate the movements of your hands so that as the outside hand starts to return down the leg, it is followed by the inside hand. See Figure 8–4. Both hands return to the ankle with a light sliding motion.

Note: Your hands should never touch or come unreasonably close to the genital area. Care should be taken when working on the inside of the leg to maintain ethical and comfortable boundaries. Skillful draping in this area will help to create a feeling of safety for both the recipient and the practitioner.

The lower limb and hip are massaged in this order: buttocks, upper leg, lower leg. Warm up the buttocks muscles using deep circular effleurage, one hand on top reinforcing the other as shown in Figure 8–5. Follow with compressions using the fist to reach deep gluteal muscles. Moderate to deep pressure may be used on these large muscles. Be sure to work the attachments along the iliac crest. Finish with circular effleurage as you started, using either the hand-over-hand position or the fist.

Two or three basic sliding effleurage strokes to the entire leg and hip help create a smooth transition to the upper leg. Perform deep effleurage with alternating fists on the hamstrings, from above the popliteal fossa to the attachments on the ilium as shown in Figure 8–6. Continuing with one fist, perform effleurage along the iliotibial band and the tensor fascia lata muscle moving from the knee to the ilium. This broad band of fascia and muscle can accept moderate to deep pressure.

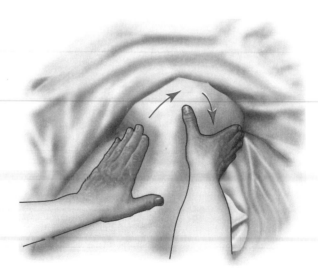

FIGURE 8–4. Applying oil to the entire leg, prone position.

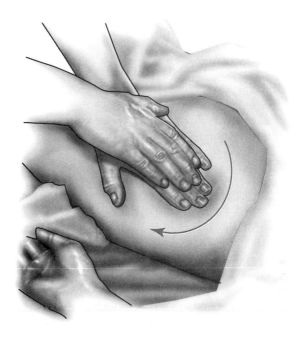

FIGURE 8–5. Deep effleurage to the gluteals using reinforced fingertips.

Warm up the adductors with basic sliding effleurage using the palms. Reach to the medial side of the thigh, and then pull up and around to the back of the thigh in a smooth sliding motion. Alternating hands, move from the knee to just below the attachments of the adductors. Be mindful of the cautions mentioned above when working the inside of the leg.

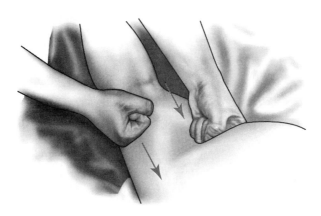

FIGURE 8–6. Deep effleurage to hamstrings using fists.

Perform basic two-handed kneading on the upper leg, including the back and both sides. Figure 8–7 shows kneading the adductors of the upper leg. Finish with effleurage distal to proximal, first to the upper and then to the entire leg.

Use two-handed kneading to massage the lower leg. Finish with basic sliding effleurage to the lower leg, following the gastrocnemius to the attachments on either side of the knee. Perform horizontal stroking to the upper and lower legs, starting on the upper leg. Finish with a few basic effleurage strokes from ankle to hip. Redrape the leg. Finish this leg with nerve strokes from the buttocks to the ankle.

Move to the other side and repeat the entire leg sequence. Finish the back side of the body with the recipient fully draped. Place one hand on the back and the other hand on a lower leg, and gently rock the body. Switch hands from one leg to the other leg. This should take only 5–10 seconds.

Turning Over

Ask the recipient to turn over. Assist by anchoring the drape with your leg against the side of the table and holding the other side of the drape up. This is called "tenting." Have the recipient roll away from you. This will prevent the drape from getting wrapped up around the recipient during the turn over. Lower the drape.

Note that the recipient was out of your sight as he or she turned over under the "tent." If there is more than one session going on in the room, be sure that you do not expose the recipient to others.

Supine Position (35 minutes)

Lower Limbs (10 minutes). Uncover one of the lower limbs and tuck the drape securely. Apply oil to the entire limb using basic sliding effleurage.

Perform deep effleurage to the thigh using both hands. Follow this with two-handed kneading. Jostle the thigh muscles, causing passive movement in the hip and knee joints as shown in Figure 8–8. Use horizontal stroking to lift and compress

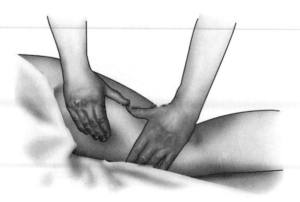

FIGURE 8–7. Two-handed kneading to adductors of the thigh.

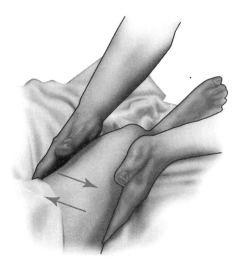

FIGURE 8–8. Jostling the thigh muscles, supine position.

the thigh muscles. Finish work on the thigh with effleurage using both hands, distal to proximal.

Perform effleurage to the entire limb as a transition, followed by effleurage of the lower leg only. Apply circular friction around the knee using the heels of the hands as shown in Figure 8–9.

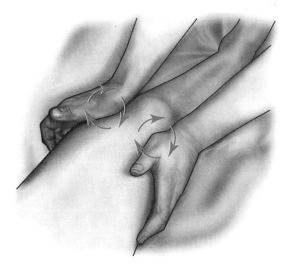

FIGURE 8–9. Circular friction around knee using heels of hands.

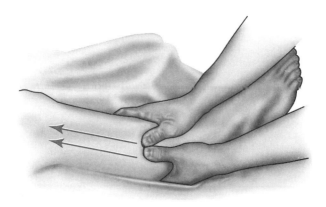

FIGURE 8–10. Thumb stripping along tibialis anterior.

Apply deep effleurage with the thumbs to tibialis anterior. Perform this thumb stripping on the lateral side of the lower leg from just above the ankle to the attachment on the lateral condyle of the tibia. You will complete two to four strips depending on the size of the muscle. See Figure 8–10. Follow the thumb stripping with direct pressure along the tibialis anterior, moving about one inch at a time proximal to distal. Reinforce the thumb to apply more pressure as shown in Figure 8–11.

Slide down the lower leg and perform circular friction around the ankle with the fingertips. Then mobilize the ankle using the heels of the hands. The foot will wiggle back and forth as shown in Figure 8–12.

Effleurage between the metatarsals using the thumb. Slide along the bottom of the foot with the fist from the ball of the foot to the heel, as shown in Figure 8–13,

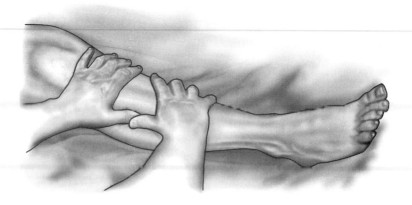

FIGURE 8–11. Direct pressure along tibialis anterior using thumbs.

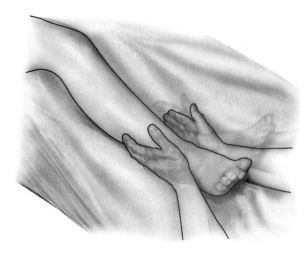

FIGURE 8–12. Ankle mobilization using the heels of the hands. Foot moves from side to side.

using moderate to deep pressure. Finish massage of the foot with slapping tapotement using the back of the hand.

Finish the entire limb with light effleurage moving distal to proximal, followed by nerve strokes moving proximal to distal. Redrape the leg.

Uncover the other limb, and repeat the entire sequence. After both legs have been massaged, and before moving to the upper body, some nerve strokes over the redraped legs may be used as a finishing and transition technique.

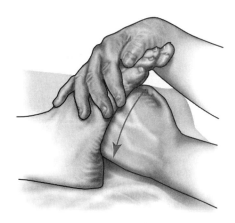

FIGURE 8–13. Effleurage to bottom of foot using the fist.

Arms and Shoulders (10 minutes). Uncover one arm and shoulder. Apply lubricant to entire upper limb using basic sliding effleurage moving distal to proximal. The movement should flow from the hand to the shoulder, including around the deltoid muscle.

Perform alternating one-hand petrissage to the upper arm. Squeeze the biceps side, then the triceps side, alternating in a rhythmical motion. Be sure to petrissage the entire upper arm from the shoulder to the elbow.

Mobilize the shoulder by grasping the upper arm with both hands just below the shoulder and moving the joint in a circle. This is a passive shoulder roll, in which the shoulders are brought forward, elevated, rolled back, and then depressed. Move both clockwise and counterclockwise.

After a few light effleurage strokes to the entire limb as a transition, perform one-hand effleurage to the lower arm as an additional warm-up using moderate to deep pressure. Knead the muscles of the lower arm, particularly near the elbow. Follow with thumb stripping to the flexor and extensor muscles on the lower arm, from the wrist to their attachments near the elbow. See Figure 8–14.

Interlock your fingers with the recipient's and press gently with your fingers to the back of his or her hand to mobilize the joints at the knuckle. Keeping the fingers interlocked, mobilize the wrist taking it through its normal range of motion. Apply effleurage to the back of the hand between metacarpals using your thumb. Then lightly squeeze along each finger moving proximal to distal. Turn the hand over so that it is palm up. Apply effleurage to the palm of the hand with your thumbs moving distal to proximal as shown in Figure 8–15. Grip the hand on the little finger and thumb sides, palm down, and gently squeeze the hand while broadening the palm and separating the metacarpals.

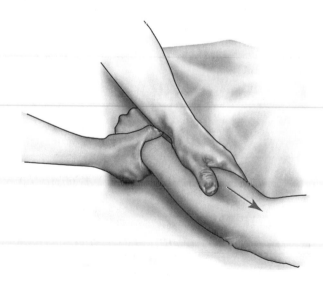

FIGURE 8–14. Thumb stripping along extensor muscles of the lower arm.

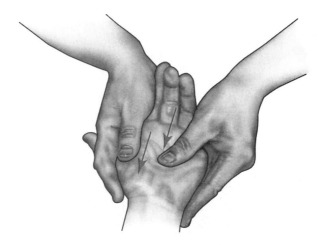

FIGURE 8–15. Effleurage to palm of hand using thumbs.

Use basic sliding effleurage from hand to shoulder to kinesthetically reconnect the arm. Lift the arm, holding just below the wrist, and perform effleurage on the pectoral muscles with a loose fist moving lateral to medial and stopping at the breast tissue. See Figure 8–16.

A basic sliding effleurage stroke may be performed over the sternum between the breasts as shown in Figure 8–17. Use good judgment in applying this stroke with women. It may be advisable to omit the technique if the woman has large

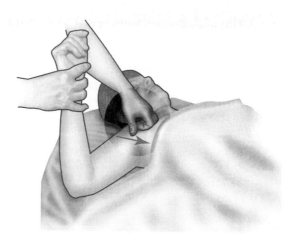

FIGURE 8–16. Effleurage to pectoral muscles using loose fist.

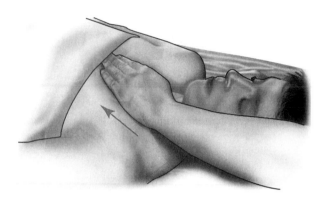

FIGURE 8-17. Basic sliding effleurage over sternum using palm of hand.

breasts or if she might feel it as an invasion of her boundaries. Err on the side of omission, and ask permission if in doubt.

Finish with basic sliding effleurage to the entire upper limb using moderate pressure. Redrape the arm and shoulder. Repeat the entire sequence on the other arm.

Abdomen (5 minutes). The abdomen is a sensitive area for many people. If the recipient is new to massage, or new to you, ask permission to work in this area. Explain to women that the breasts will be draped. You might want to explain the purpose of massaging the abdomen. Find out if they have eaten within the past hour, and skip the area if that is the case. People experiencing constipation or gas in the bowels may be sensitive to pressure; however, massage of the abdomen may help relieve those conditions.

Cover a woman's breasts with an additional drape before you pull back the larger drape to the iliac crest exposing the abdomen. Do not expose the pubic area.

Begin by gently laying a hand on the abdomen to establish contact. Perform effleurage moving clockwise in a circular pattern. Use the fingertips of one hand, while the other hand rests on top. See Figure 8–18. Move in a large circle along the bottom of the ribs and around the outline of the pelvis, followed by smaller, then even smaller concentric circles. Check with the recipient to make sure the pressure is comfortable.

Perform vibration to the area with the fingertips moving from place to place in a clockwise pattern. Take care in areas that recipients report as feeling sore. Petrissage the abdomen with a flat hand, palm down, using an undulating or wavelike motion. Push in first with the heel of the hand, and then roll onto the fingertips. The soft tissues of the viscera are stimulated with the rhythmic compression. Move from place to place on the abdomen.

Repeat circular effleurage moving clockwise as a transition. Follow with horizontal stroking of the abdomen. Finish the area with passive touch in the center of

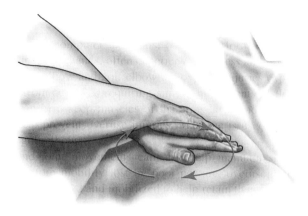

FIGURE 8–18. Effleurage in circular pattern applied to abdomen.

the abdomen. Remove your hand and recover the recipient to the shoulders with the larger drape. The breast drape may remain in place for warmth or may be removed at this time.

Neck and Shoulders (5 minutes). You may sit at the head of the recipient to work on the head and shoulders. Establish contact by mobilizing the shoulders with a "cat paw" movement, alternating pushing one side and then the other as shown in Figure 8–19.

Apply lubricant to both sides of the neck (one hand on each side), performing effleurage along the trapezius from the shoulder tips to the occipital ridge. Turn the

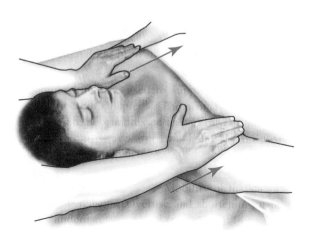

FIGURE 8–19. "Cat paw" motion to gently mobilize shoulders. Alternate hands pushing on shoulders.

head slightly to one side and perform effleurage with the fist on the upper trapezius from the occipital ridge to the shoulder as shown in Figure 8–20. The upper trapezius will stretch mildly.

Continuing on the left side, use circular friction along the occipital ridge and the neck to warm the deeper muscles of the region. Start with the suboccipitals (medial to lateral) and then down the cervicals to the base of the neck. Follow this with thumb stripping to the deep cervicals from the occiput to the base of the neck. Finish the left side with effleurage back and forth from the tip of the shoulder to the occiput. Turn the head slightly to the left, and repeat the sequence to the right side.

Create a wavelike neck mobilization. Place the hands palms-up at the base of the neck, one on either side of the spine, with fingertips pressing up on the cervical muscles. Draw the fingers toward the occiput, maintaining pressure upwards. The cervical vertebrae will rise and fall as the fingers pass underneath. If the muscles are relaxed, this will create a wavelike motion in the neck. See Figure 8–21.

Finish with effleurage to both sides of the shoulders and neck. Start the movement at the tips of the shoulders and draw the hands toward the base of the neck and up to the occiput. Mobilize one shoulder at a time, holding the head with one hand and pushing on the tip of the shoulder with the other hand. Cradle the head briefly in both hands to end this section.

Face and Head (5 minutes). Use very little or no lubricant on the face. Ask the recipient what he or she prefers. Lotion may offer an acceptable solution; however, the entire face and head sequence can usually be performed quite well without using lubricant.

Place the hands gently on the face with fingertips at the jaw. Draw the hands toward the temples in an effleurage stroke using the full palm-side of the hands as shown in Figure 8–22. Repeat two or three times. Perform circular friction with the

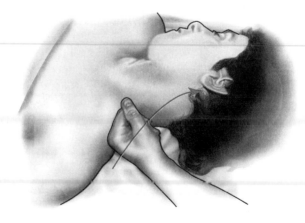

FIGURE 8–20. Effleurage to upper trapezius using fist.

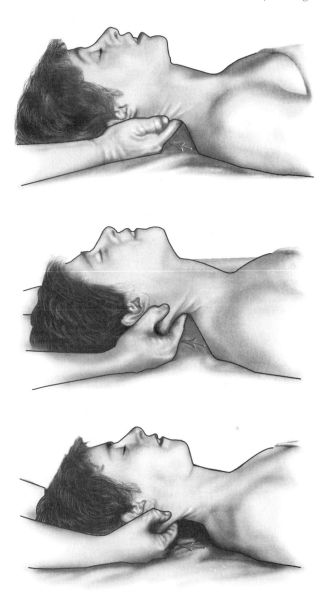

FIGURE 8–21. Wavelike neck mobilization. Draw the fingers toward the occiput while maintaining pressure upwards.

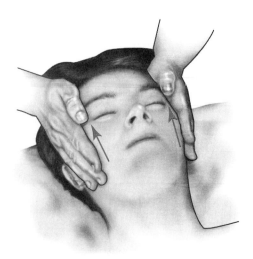

FIGURE 8–22. Effleurage to face using palms.

fingertips over the masseter and then the temporalis muscles. Stroke the muscles of the forehead using effleurage with the thumbs moving medial to lateral.

Petrissage the forehead using a circular motion of the thumbs. The movement is timed so that the tissues are lifted and pressed as the thumbs move by one another. This is similar to the two-handed circular petrissage described in Chapter 6.

Stroke alongside of the nose with the thumbs and continue the effleurage movement along the cheekbones. Press up under the cheekbones with the fingertips using light to moderate pressure.

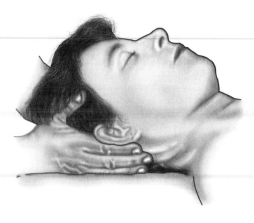

FIGURE 8–23. Cradling the head to finish the session.

Loosen the scalp with circular friction over the entire hair area. A relaxed scalp will have a greater degree of movement than a "tight" scalp. Loosening the area will improve blood supply to the skin and hair follicles.

Finish the entire session by cradling the head as shown in Figure 8–23. Hold for a few seconds until you can feel the recipient completely relax.

■ SUMMARY

A classic full-body massage lasts from ½ to 1½ hours and includes massage of the back, legs, abdomen, arms, neck, and head. The recipient is typically unclothed and draped with a sheet for modesty. The practitioner blends the five classic techniques, touch without movement, and joint movements into a particular sequence to create a routine. Oil or lotion is used to enhance movement over the skin and to prevent chaffing.

The order of techniques for each part of the body usually includes a warm-up with effleurage, followed by petrissage, and then specific work as appropriate using techniques like deep friction, vibration, or direct pressure. Work on a particular area is concluded with finishing techniques to reconnect, smooth out, and gradually lighten touch. Finishing techniques typically include either light effleurage, tapotement, or touch without movement (holding).

Classic full-body massage is typically wellness oriented. Its purpose is to improve circulation, relax the muscles, improve joint mobility, induce general relaxation, promote healthy skin, and create a general sense of well-being.

Application to Parts
of the Body

Practitioners may want to focus more time and attention on a particular part of the body. This could be due to recipient request; the judgment of the practitioner from observation, palpation, or information from a health history form; or a specific referral from a health care provider. Extended sessions in a smaller area provide an opportunity for more focused attention to specific muscles and other structures.

■ WHOLENESS AND MEANING

Note that even though the following sections of this chapter focus on different parts of the body, a real body is not so easily divided. There is layering of tissues and function. For example, while the upper trapezius is in the cervical region, the whole trapezius extends down the spine through the thoracic region. Another example is that in working with someone with rounded shoulders, you would want to address all anterior muscle shortening, as well as in the pectorals. More than just the most obvious muscles may be involved. You cannot isolate a region entirely and be effective. Work in a specific area will necessarily flow into the surrounding sections and sometimes to the entire body.

Another consideration is that different parts of the body have special significance in human terms. Their meaning is determined by what they allow us to do and to be in this world, their social and emotional associations, and their specific use in a particular person's life (eg, a musician's hands or a runner's legs). Practitioners should keep in mind that they are not just working on shoulders or legs, but that they are dealing with human beings who give their bodies, and parts of their bodies, meaning. As you interact with the recipient, be aware that you are not just touching a body—you are touching a person.

The following are descriptions of single techniques and sequences of techniques that may be integrated into the classic full-body massage illustrated in Chapter 8. The face and head, cervical region, back, buttocks, lower extremities, upper extremities, chest, and abdomen are the sections presented. A discussion of the meaning of each specific part of the body in human terms is followed by the benefits of massage, anatomy, cautions, and technique applications.

■ HEAD AND FACE

Much of our consciousness as human beings is focused in the head and face. It is the center for thinking and processing information. Our senses of sight, hearing, taste, and smell are housed here. The structures for bringing food into our bodies are here. We communicate with others through the structures of speech, and our faces convey our feelings and emotional states through facial expression. The muscles of the face are part of the process of thinking, as seen in furrowed brows and frowns of concentration. Relaxing the muscles of the head and face helps bring clarity of mind and release of mental and emotional stress.

Applications of Massage

Massage can help release tensions in the face and head acquired in daily living. This may be an area of tension for people whose jobs involve a lot of thinking or require extensive use of the eyes. Reading, writing, looking at a computer monitor, and doing activities that require fine hand–eye coordination such as needlework or drawing put strain on the muscles of the face, especially around the eyes. People who wear eyeglasses may feel strain from the weight of the glasses on the nose and ears.

Emotional distress may also lead to tension in the face and head. Worry and anxiety may create tension in the forehead and temporal area. Habitual clenching of the jaw can cause tension in the masseter and temporalis muscles and the TMJ pain syndrome. While crying can lead to a healthy release of emotions, it can also create strain around the eyes. Holding back emotions, and "holding back the tears," is actually accomplished by tension in the face, throat, and diaphragm.

The muscles of the face and head may also be affected by certain pathologies, such as stroke and Bell's palsy. Face and head massage can help relieve the tension present in these conditions.

Anatomy

The musculature of the face and head is complex and includes muscles of expression, mastication, and movement. Some muscles are skeletal muscles that create movement, such as the masseter. The muscles of expression in the face are embedded in the cutaneous tissue and move the skin itself, such as in wrinkling the forehead, frowning, and smiling. These muscles are relatively thin and more delicate than skeletal muscles. Some of the major muscles of facial expression are pictured in Figure 9–1.

Techniques

The following techniques may be integrated into the basic massage of the face and head described in Chapter 8. They provide more specific attention to the facial muscles, skin, and scalp.

Always ask the recipient if they are wearing contact lenses, since some of these techniques may dislodge them. A general rule is to avoid movements around the orbit, or over the eyes, if a person is wearing contact lenses.

Squeeze to Eyebrows. The tissues in the eyebrow area become tense in people who squint, are sensitive to light, or use their eyes a lot in their work (eg, computer work, reading, or activities that require fine hand–eye coordination). Congestion in this area often accompanies tension headache. The corrugator supercilii muscle, which draws the eyebrow downward and medially, is located there. Gently squeeze the tissues between the thumb and the forefinger, beginning at the nose and moving laterally to the outside edge of the eye orbit. See Figure 9–2. Pressure should be light to moderate.

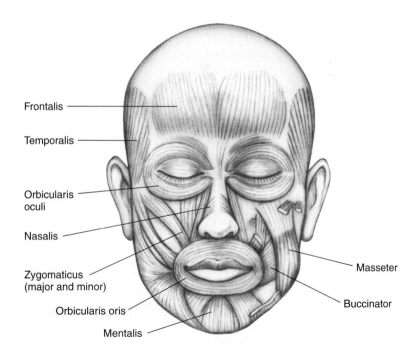

Frontalis

Temporalis

Orbicularis oculi

Nasalis

Zygomaticus (major and minor)

Orbicularis oris

Mentalis

Masseter

Buccinator

FIGURE 9–1. Major muscles of facial expression.

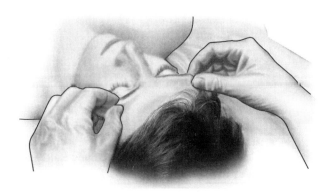

FIGURE 9–2. Gentle squeezing of tissues along eyebrow line.

Effleurage Over the Eyelids. This technique is similar to the common gesture of rubbing the eyes when tired. It massages orbicularis oculi, the sphincter muscle of the eyelids. Gently, using very light pressure, stroke the closed eyelids with your thumbs as shown in Figure 9–3. The movement is medial to lateral. Stroke once near the top, once in the middle, and once near the bottom of the eyelid.

Thumb Slides Along the Nose. People who wear glasses often rub or squeeze the tissues between the eyebrows at the bridge of the nose to relieve pressure where the glasses sit. Procerus, a small muscle located there, draws the medial angles of the eyebrows downward and produces transverse wrinkles over the bridge of the

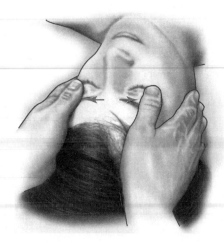

FIGURE 9–3. Very light effleurage over eyelids with the thumbs.

nose. Those with sinus congestion may also feel tenderness in the external tissues of the upper nose area.

Using light to moderate pressure, slide a thumb over the procerus muscle, and then use both thumbs to slide along the outline of the nose from the eyes to the little depression at the base. See Figure 9–4.

Direct Pressure Along the Zygomatic Arch. Pressure to the zygomatic or cheekbone area will sometimes help relieve congestion there. Perform effleurage with the fingertips along the underside of the zygomatic arch starting at the base of the nose and moving laterally. Apply direct pressure to the little depression at the base of the nose, and then moving laterally as before, press up and under the zygomatic arch with the index and third fingers. See Figure 9–5. Use light to moderate pressure. The area will be tender if the sinuses are congested.

Massage Around the Mouth and Jaw. There are a number of muscles around the mouth and jaw, which create movement for eating, speaking, and expression. For example, chewing, sipping, whispering, singing, smiling, frowning, and sneering all involve muscles around the mouth and jaw. Muscles that aid in mastication include the masseter, pterygoid muscles, and the temporalis.

Begin specific work around the mouth and jaw with effleurage using the thumbs to outline the upper lip (ie, moustache area) and then the lower lip as shown in Figure 9–6. Knead the tissues on the chin and along the jawline with the thumb and first two fingers. Deep circular friction is effective on the strong jaw muscles such as the masseter.

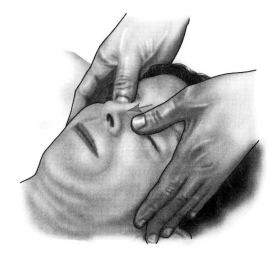

FIGURE 9–4. Thumb slides along side of nose.

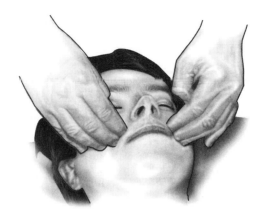

FIGURE 9–5. Direct pressure under zygomatic arch with the fingertips.

Massaging the Ears. The ears are made of soft cartilage and have many curves and folds. People who wear glasses, clip-on earrings, or any heavy earrings usually enjoy massage to the ears. They may be massaged between the thumb and index finger. Follow the curves to rub the entire ear, including the ear lobes. As you approach the outer edges of the ear while rubbing, give a gentle pull to stimulate the area as shown in Figure 9–7. Perform circular friction all around the base of the ears to massage the small auricular muscles attached there. See Figure 9–8.

Mobilization of the Scalp. The skin that covers the top of the head (ie, the scalp) can be moved freely on most people. Stress can lead to tension in the muscles of the head, causing the scalp to be less mobile. Mobilizing the scalp has similar effects to

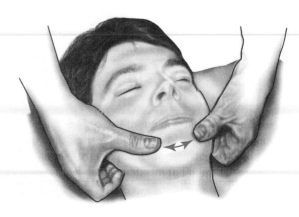

FIGURE 9–6. Thumbs outline the lower lip.

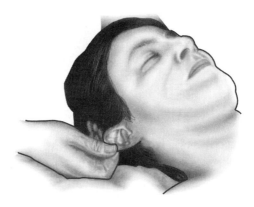

FIGURE 9–7. Gentle pull on the ears.

skin rolling, which frees the underlying fascia and increases superficial circulation. Since circulation to hair follicles is increased, this helps promote healthy hair.

The scalp can be mobilized using a frictionlike technique in which fingers placed on the scalp move the skin over the underlying muscle and bone. As the skin moves, the fingers stay in place as shown in Figure 9–9. Mobilize the entire scalp, including the back of the head. The pressure used is much lighter than deep friction, since the object is simply to move the scalp.

The hair may also be used to move the scalp. Grasp the hair close to the skin and use it as a handle to move the scalp back and forth. This works best with thick hair. It will not work if the recipient has hair that is too thin or too short to grasp.

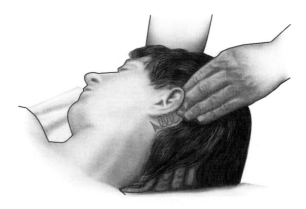

FIGURE 9–8. Circular friction around the base of the ears.

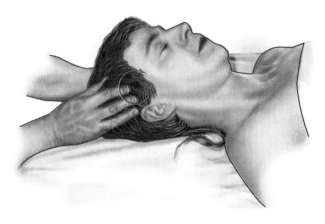

FIGURE 9–9. Mobilizing the scalp with the fingertips. The skin moves over underlying muscle and bone.

Muscles on the Head. There are several broad thin muscles on the head. Some of these move the scalp, for example, the occipitofrontalis and temporoparietalis. The large temporalis muscle, found above the ears, elevates the mandible and aids in mastication. These muscles are massaged somewhat in the process of mobilizing the scalp as described above. Deeper pressure may be applied using circular friction with the fingers.

Passive Touch Over the Eyes. Placing the hands gently on the face with palms over the eyes can be soothing. It is similar to the self-comforting gesture of holding your face in your hands. See Figure 9–10. Pressure should be very light.

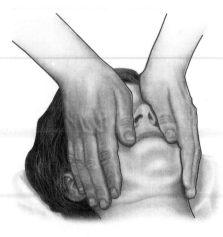

FIGURE 9–10. Passive touch over eyes with the palms of the hands.

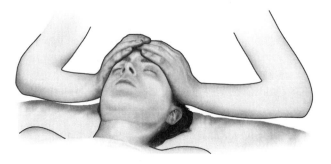

FIGURE 9–11. Pressing the sides of the head with the palms of the hands.

Pressing or Holding the Sides of the Head. Pressing the sides of the head near the top as shown in Figure 9–11 can help relieve tension. Use the full hand, and press in with moderate to heavy pressure depending on the recipient. Slowly release the pressure. Actually, it is the sensation of pressure, and then letting go, which is relaxing. Simply holding the head as described in Chapter 8 can be relaxing and is a good finishing technique. Pressure should be light, since the idea is to give the impression of holding, not pressing.

▪ CERVICAL REGION

The cervical or neck region is "pivotal" in many senses of the word. It links the head with the torso and houses the delicate spinal cord. Nerves and blood vessels going to the brain pass through the cervical region. It contains the muscles that hold the head in position during upright posture and movement in different planes. It is the pivot point for the head and provides the structure and musculature that allows us to access sensation as we turn our heads to look, listen, smell, and taste.

Applications of Massage

Poor posture and body mechanics can lead to excessive tension in the neck. The "head forward" posture and poor sitting posture at workstations are two common sources of chronic neck tension. A cold draft on the back of the neck or sleeping in a cramped position can sometimes cause neck stiffness. Long airplane or automobile rides can also leave neck muscles painful and stiff.

Stressful life situations may aggravate cervical tension and may literally be a "pain in the neck." A major cause of tension headache is hypertonicity of the cervical muscles, which refer pain into the head. Trigger point work on the cervical and upper back muscles may be integrated into a classic massage routine for effective relief of tension headache. The contraction of muscles and pain in the neck region from whiplash or wryneck (torticollis) may be relieved with massage.

Anatomy

The major muscles in the neck include the upper trapezius, splenius capitis and cervicis, semispinalis capitis and cervicis, longissimus capitis, levator scapulae, sternocleidomastoid (SCM); and the deeper smaller muscles of the suboccipitals (rectus capitis posterior major and minor, oblique capitis superior and inferior), multifidi and rotatores. Generally speaking, the more superficial muscles are larger and thicker, and the deeper ones are smaller and thinner. Some of the deeper muscles of the posterior neck are shown in Figure 9–12.

Techniques

The following techniques may be integrated into the basic massage of the neck described in Chapter 8. When working in the cervical area, attention should be given first to relaxing the superficial muscles, allowing better access to the deeper muscles. The area should be thoroughly warmed up before deeper techniques are performed.

Endangerment sites in the cervical region include the anterior neck and the arteries and veins supplying the brain. The carotid artery and jugular vein are located

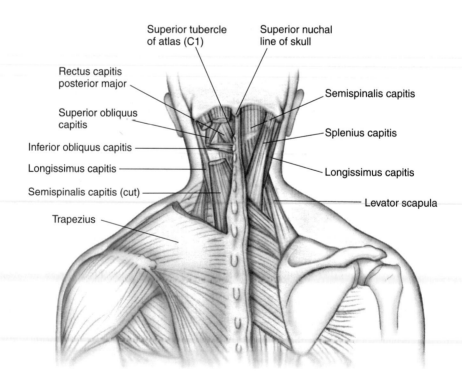

FIGURE 9–12. Deep muscles of the posterior neck.

on the sides of the neck. These areas should be avoided in the elderly or anyone with a history of atherosclerosis, that is, hardening of the arteries.

Direct Pressure to the Cervicals. With the recipient in the supine position, direct pressure may easily be applied to the cervical muscles on either side of the spine. The index and third fingers may be used to apply moderate pressure upward as shown in Figure 9–13. Pressure may be applied to both sides simultaneously, or back and forth from one side to the other. Start at the base of the neck and apply the direct pressure to one spot then the next, moving toward the suboccipital area. A slight mobilization of the neck will occur.

Deep Pressure to the Suboccipitals. With the recipient in the supine position, direct pressure may be applied to the suboccipital muscles using all of the fingers. Place the fingers along the suboccipitals and simply apply pressure upward. The chin will elevate, and the head will fall back slightly into a mild hyperextension.

Deeper pressure may be applied to the suboccipital muscles with the thumb. This is a useful technique when working with stiff or tense neck muscles. Cradle the head in one hand and rotate it away from the side you are working on. With the thumb of the other hand, slowly apply pressure into the suboccipital space. You can deepen the pressure by carefully accentuating the natural extension of the head that occurs. See Figure 9–14. Direct pressure may be alternated with deep cross-fiber friction for a thorough and deep massage of the suboccipitals. This should be followed by stretching, as described in Chapter 7, for more lasting effects.

Direct Pressure to Thoracic Attachments While Supine. Some of the muscles of the neck attach to the thoracic spine or ribs. Direct pressure to these attachments can help improve flexibility of the neck. When performing passive forward flexion of the neck, you can sometimes feel a resistance at the lower attachments of the cervi-

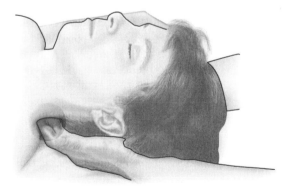

FIGURE 9–13. Direct pressure to posterior cervical muscles using fingertips, recipient supine.

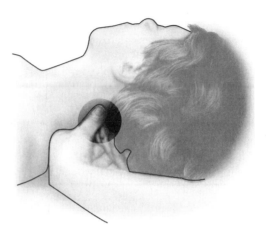

FIGURE 9–14. Direct pressure to suboccipitals with the thumb, recipient supine.

cals. These attachments are effected during upper back massage, but may also receive attention with the recipient in the supine position.

Reach under the trunk, palms up, to about the fourth thoracic vertebra, and place the fingers on both sides of the spine. Press up at one spot, and then the next, moving upward toward the base of the neck. The weight of the trunk will offer resistance and allow deep pressure to be applied.

A variation of this technique is to use the same hand placement, but slide the fingers along the spine using deep pressure. The slide will help stretch tissues. Note that these techniques applied with the receiver supine take considerable strength on the part of the practitioner and should be performed only by those with strong flexors in the hands and wrists.

Neck Massage in the Prone Position. The cervical muscles may be massaged when the recipient is in the prone or seated position. If using an adjustable face cradle, tilt it down so that the neck is slight stretched. This creates more space in the neck.

Effleurage with the thumb may be used to warm the cervical muscles. Perform effleurage from the base of the neck to the suboccipitals. This may be followed by kneading with one or both hands as shown in Figure 9–15.

Once the muscles are warmed up, the thumb, or the fingers if you are standing at the head of the table, may be used to apply direct pressure. Pressure may be applied at an angle into the suboccipital space and toward the top of the head. Care should be taken not to apply so much pressure that the recipient's face feels smashed into the face cradle. Direct pressure with the thumbs or elbow may be applied over the thoracic attachments of the cervicals.

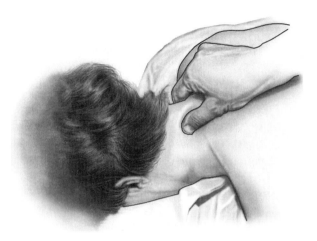

FIGURE 9–15. One hand kneading to posterior cervicals, recipient prone.

▪ BACK

"Spend more time on my back" is a frequent request of recipients of massage. The back is the core area for maintaining upright posture and a place of attachment for the movements of the arms and legs. It is a heavily muscled area that works hard and is prone to tension, aches, and stiffness. Poor body mechanics when sitting, lifting, playing sports, or during physical activities such as gardening can cause backache.

The back is a place where worry and anxiety are frequently held and is sometimes experienced as Atlas did when carrying the weight of the world on his shoulders. A bent-over posture evokes the image of weakness, discouragement, and defeat; a straight back presents the image of strength, self-confidence, and vigor.

Applications of Massage

Soothing back massage is associated with the qualities of nurturing, sympathy, and deep relaxation. Perhaps because the nerves of the parasympathetic nervous system exit the posterior vertebrae, the relaxation response is easily triggered during massage of the back. Back massage is often used to help people go to sleep.

Deep massage of the back muscles can help release tension held there and relieves the stiffness and soreness that accompanies heavy physical labor. Joint movements improve the mobility of the scapulae (ie, shoulder blades), enhancing movement in the shoulder girdle. Tension in the upper trapezius can refer pain into the head. Massage of this area, commonly called "massaging the shoulders," can help relieve tension headache.

Anatomy

It is important for practitioners to develop a three-dimensional concept of the back. This includes the recognition that the "back" is the posterior portion of the torso, which also has sides. The back is thick, with layers of muscles from large broad superficial muscles to the tiny deep muscles of the spine. The scapulae, or shoulder blades, located on the upper back, are an integral part of the shoulder girdle. They glide over the posterior ribs and have numerous muscular attachments, which generate the free movement of the shoulder complex. Practitioners work at various depths of penetration during massage of the back.

The large superficial muscles of the back include the trapezius and latissimus dorsi. Spinal muscles include the erector spinae (iliocostalis, longissimus, spinalis), the deep posterior spinal muscles (multifidi, rotatores, interspinales, intertransversarii, and levatores costarum), and the semispinalis thoracis. Muscles surrounding the scapulae include subscapularis, upper trapezius, posterior deltoid, supraspinatus, infraspinatus, teres major and minor, levator scapulae, and the rhomboids on the medial border. The quadratus lumborum is in the lower back, with attachments on the last rib, the transverse processes of the upper four lumbar vertebrae, and the iliac crest.

Techniques

The following techniques may be integrated into the basic back massage described in Chapter 8. They include techniques that allow more focused attention to specific muscles that move the spine and techniques for the back in general (eg, skin rolling, and for relaxation). Specific massage and movements for the shoulder girdle are covered in more detail in the section on the upper extremities.

Skin Rolling. Skin rolling is an excellent technique to help relieve tension in the back. It helps restore elasticity to the subcutaneous connective tissues and improves superficial circulation. Skin rolling is performed by lifting the cutaneous tissues from the underlying muscles. It should be performed after a general warm-up of the area. It may be applied sequentially by lifting the tissues in one place and then the next, eventually covering the entire back. It may also be performed in strips using a continuous motion, by lifting the tissues and, without letting go, sliding the hands along the back in a line. The tissues are lifted as the hands slide along by the pressure between the thumbs and fingers. Skin rolling is also described in Chapter 6, Figure 6–15.

Warming Friction of the Back. Warming friction may be used to create heat in any relatively flat area. It is effective over the erector muscles on either side of the spine, over the rhomboids, and on the muscles covering the scapulae. Lubricant will reduce the effect of the friction and so should be used sparingly or wiped off before performing warming friction.

Sawing friction is performed with the little-finger side of the hands, palms facing each other. The hands are moved back and forth in a sawing motion, sliding over the skin and creating friction on the skin. Deeper pressure will create friction in deeper tissues. The skin will appear red as the superficial blood vessels dilate. Sawing friction is also described in Chapter 6, Figure 6–18.

Warming friction may also be performed with the knuckles. Figure 6–17 in Chapter 6 shows knuckling friction over the erector muscles of the thoracic region.

Effleurage Between the Ribs. Effleurage of the intercostals with the fingertips helps relax these tiny muscles. This facilitates easier and deeper breathing by allowing the rib cage to expand more. Find the intercostal spaces using palpation skills, and slide the fingers in the spaces moving from the spine laterally and around the sides of the rib cage. See Figure 9–16.

Sequence for the Lower Back. The muscles of the lower back can get stiff and sore from sitting for long periods of time, especially in chairs or car seats with poor lumbar support. The following sequence of techniques helps relax the muscles of the lower back and relieve general fatigue of the area.

Warm up the entire back with effleurage and circular friction as described in the full-body classic Western massage in Chapter 8. For the lower back portion of the routine, insert the following five-part sequence of techniques.

Once the lower back is warmed up, apply effleurage with the thumbs using moderate to deep pressure (ie, thumb stripping) to the quadratus lumborum in the space between the iliac crest and the twelfth rib. Place one thumb on top of the other for support. The first strip is applied just laterally to the spinous processes. Each strip is performed just laterally to the one before. See Figure 9–17.

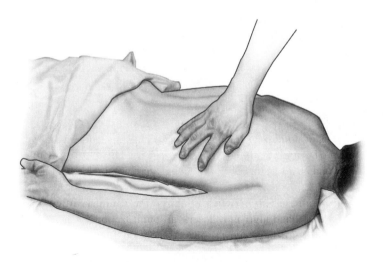

FIGURE 9–16. Effleurage of intercostals using fingertips, recipient prone.

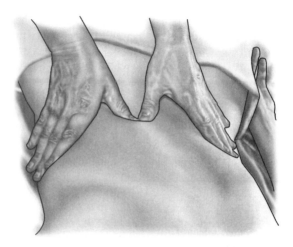

FIGURE 9–17. Thumb stripping along lower back on quadratus lumborum.

Follow this with circular friction to the erector muscles, also using the thumbs. Apply direct pressure with the thumbs to the erector muscles using moderate to heavy pressure. Begin at the iliac crest and press in at about one-inch intervals along the muscles, up to about the last rib. See Figure 9–18.

Use knuckling friction to the erector and quadratus lumborum muscles to further warm and bring blood to the lower back. Finish with thumb stripping using moderate to deep pressure. Use effleurage on the entire back to kinesthetically reconnect the lower back to the rest of the body.

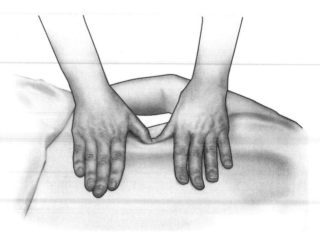

FIGURE 9–18. Direct pressure to erector muscles in the lower back using the thumbs.

Back Massage for Relaxation. If the purpose of the back massage is relaxation, either avoid specific painful work on the back altogether, or spend at least five to seven minutes after painful work on lighter, soothing techniques. Use long flowing effleurage strokes with moderate to slow continuous motion. The movement should feel "seamless." Vary the pattern to avoid boredom. Mix up vertical, circular, and horizontal patterns of effleurage. Some petrissage of the shoulder may be integrated for variety. Avoid tapotement, and finish either with nerve strokes or passive touch over the scapulae.

Back massage has been used in hospitals and nursing homes for those having trouble falling asleep. Chapter 6 contains a description of sedating effleurage of the back.

▪ BUTTOCKS

The large muscles of the hip region help support the entire body and provide the power for locomotion. They are the most important and the most stressed muscles in many sports. They are the perch points of the sitting posture, the most common position for today's students and desk workers.

The hips and buttocks can be a source of sexual appeal, and also a source of poor self-image, particularly in women. In this culture, there is an embarrassment associated with this region. For those physically or sexually abused as children, it is often a region of remembered pain and suffering. Practitioners should take great care when working in this region to create a feeling of safety and modesty.

Applications of Massage

Sports and fitness participants are often stiff and sore in the hip area from the strain of physical activity. On the other hand, those who are more sedentary may also experience stiffness from lack of movement. Tight buttocks muscles can impinge on the sciatic nerve and cause leg pain. Soft-tissue manipulation and joint movements improve circulation to the area, relax muscles, and improve mobility at the hip joint. The elderly may benefit from improved hip mobility and, therefore, improved locomotion.

Anatomy

The more superficial muscles of the hip region are the large gluteals (maximus, medius, minimus), which run superior and inferior. The smaller deeper hip rotators include the piriformis, gemelli, quadratus femoris, obturator internus and externus. The deeper muscles run medial to lateral as shown in Figure 9–19.

Techniques

The following techniques may be integrated into the basic massage of the lower limbs and buttocks described in Chapter 8. Some practitioners massage the buttocks as part of a back routine, while others include the buttocks in a lower limb se-

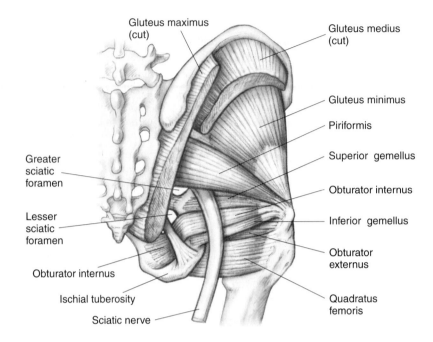

Gluteus maximus (cut)

Gluteus medius (cut)

Gluteus minimus

Piriformis

Superior gemellus

Greater sciatic foramen

Obturator internus

Inferior gemellus

Lesser sciatic foramen

Obturator externus

Obturator internus

Ischial tuberosity

Quadratus femoris

Sciatic nerve

FIGURE 9-19. Deep muscles of the buttocks.

quence. Since most of the attachments are on the ilium and femur and create movement in the thigh, it makes sense to treat the buttocks when massaging the lower limbs.

Use of the Elbow and Forearm. Because you must work through the large superficial muscles to reach the smaller deeper muscles, it is useful to use the elbow or forearm to apply some techniques to the buttocks. You can apply more pressure and avoid straining the hands. However, care should be taken not to use too much pressure, and palpatory sensitivity should be developed so that you can feel the condition of the tissues as you would with your hands. The elbow or forearm is not used to "muscle through" the tissues, but to apply more pressure skillfully.

The elbow or forearm may be used for broad strokes, and the point of the elbow (olecranon process) for more specific techniques such as direct pressure to a spot. The elbow or forearm may be used to apply effleurage, direct pressure, and circular or transverse friction. Figure 9–20 shows direct pressure to the deep gluteals using the elbow.

Use of the Fist. The fist is useful for applying deep pressure during compressions or effleurage on the large muscles of the buttocks. Figure 9–21 shows compressions applied to the gluteals using the fist. One advantage of this over using the palms is

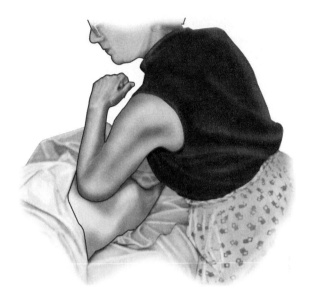

FIGURE 9–20. Use of elbow to apply direct pressure to deep buttocks muscles.

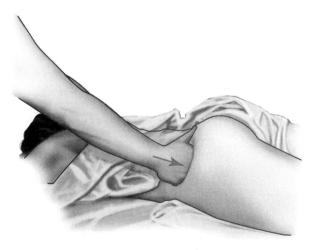

FIGURE 9–21. Compression to the gluteals using the fist. Note the straight wrist position.

that the wrist can be kept straight, thus avoiding potential wrist damage when applying deep pressure.

Direct Pressure to Gluteal Attachments. Direct pressure to the gluteal attachments helps relax the muscles and facilitates a better stretch. Use the thumbs, knuckles, or elbow to press along the attachments along the iliac crest and sacroiliac junction. Follow with effleurage to the area using the fist.

Mobilizations and Stretching. A thorough treatment of the muscles of the buttocks should include both massage and joint movements. Mobilizations and stretching help condition the deep rotators of the hip joint, which are difficult to reach directly with massage. While massage of the buttocks is necessarily performed with the recipient prone, most joint movements are done supine. If one of the major goals of the session addresses mobility in the hips, it may be useful to begin prone to warm up the muscles, and finish supine for the joint movements described in Chapter 7.

▪ LOWER EXTREMITIES

The lower extremities are the principal means of locomotion for bipedal human beings. They afford us a great degree of independence as we can get from one place to another on "our own power." Loss or diminished use of the legs, through disease, accident, or old age, can result in greater dependence and loss of freedom. Having "a spring in your step" is a sign of vitality and positive outlook. Athletes depend on their legs to play their sports, and walking has become the premier fitness activity today.

In most cultures, shoes are worn for protection, and also confine the feet. It feels good to free the feet and kick off your shoes after wearing them all day. Going barefoot or wearing sandals is a sign of leisure and relaxation. It seems that if your feet hurt, you hurt all over. Foot massage is valued as a pleasurable treat.

Applications of Massage

People who stand long hours in their jobs often experience stress and pain in the legs and feet. Women in this culture tend to wear shoes with little support, and often wear high heels, which puts the feet and legs in a strained position. Those who sit a lot typically have problems with loss of leg strength, muscle shortening, and poor circulation. With age there is loss of strength, flexibility, and "spring," and muscles are more frequently stiff and sore. Massage and stretching can help the legs and feet feel and function better by improving circulation, joint mobility, and muscle relaxation.

Anatomy

For purposes of massage, the lower extremities may be thought of in three sections, that is, thigh, lower leg, and feet. In the prone position, the buttocks are often included with the lower extremities. There are three large joints in the lower extremities (ie, hip, knee, and ankle), and several small joints within the feet.

The major muscles of the anterior thigh include the quadriceps (rectus femoris, vastus intermedius, vastus lateralis, vastus medialis), and sartorius. Muscles found on the medial thigh include the adductors, that is, adductor brevis, adductor longus, adductor magnus, gracilis, pectineus. High on the lateral thigh is tensor fasciae latae. The posterior thigh includes the hamstrings, that is, biceps femoris, semi-membranosus, semitendinosus. The iliopsoas (ie, psoas and iliacus muscles), act on the hip joint, but, for the purposes of massage, are palpated in the abdomen. See Figure 9–22.

The muscles of the lower leg act largely on the ankle joint and include the anterior muscles (tibialis anterior, peroneus tertius, and the extensors), the lateral muscles (peroneus longus and brevis), and the posterior muscles (gastrocnemius, soleus, tibialis posterior, and the flexors).

There are many small muscles intrinsic to the feet, most of which are on the plantar side or bottom. The plantar muscles include a superficial layer (ie, abductor hallucis, flexor hallucis longus, flexor digitorum brevis, abductor digiti minimi brevis), a middle layer (ie, lumbricales, flexor digiti minimi brevis, quadratus, flexor digitorum longus), and a deep layer (adductor hallucis, interossei plantares, flexor hallucis brevis, ligamentum plantarum longum). The plantar aponeurosis is a super-

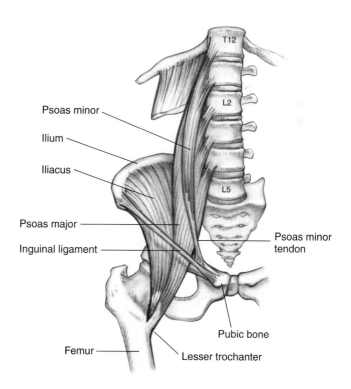

FIGURE 9–22. Iliopsoas muscle.

ficial strong fibrous band of fascia that runs from the heel to the ball of the foot and binds the longitudinal arch. It is the central part of a broad band of fascia that covers the muscles on the plantar side of the foot. The dorsal surface of the foot is fairly bony. The extensor digitorum brevis and the dorsal interossei are accessible to massage.

Techniques

The following techniques can be integrated into the basic massage of the lower extremities described in Chapter 8. Detailed attention is given to the feet, lower leg, and thigh.

One of the major endangerment sites is in the lower extremities, the popliteal fossa located behind the knee. Care should be taken not to apply pressure in this area. However, attachments of muscles may be followed around the area.

Avoid deep pressure over varicose veins, especially likely in older recipients. Do not massage the legs if blood clotting or phlebitis is present.

Avoid irritating bunions found at the base of the great toe. Watch for athlete's foot and other fungal infections that may be spread through touch. Avoid massaging feet with active infections.

Foot Massage. A thorough foot massage can make you feel good all over. It touches all of the small intrinsic muscles of the feet, as well as attachments of muscles of the lower leg, and mobilizes the many joints found there. It relaxes the muscles, improves circulation, and restores feeling to a part of the body encased in shoes most of the time.

The following foot massage routine uses techniques described in more detail in Chapters 7 and 8. The sequence includes soft-tissue manipulation and joint movements for the complex musculoskeletal structure of the foot.

Begin by applying lubricant to the foot and ankle. Special lubricants are available for the feet that contain cooling substances such as peppermint and menthol. Be sure to cover the whole foot and around each toe.

Mobilize the ankle using the heels of the hands. Using your thumb, apply basic sliding effleurage between the metatarsals on the dorsal surface of the foot, and then mobilize the space between metatarsals with a scissoring action. Mobilize each metatarsal-phalangeal joint with figure eights, and then gently petrissage each toe with a gentle squeezing action along the length of the toe moving proximal to distal. Do one length squeezing top and bottom, and then another squeezing the sides. Do not snap or pull the toes.

Sometimes the toes are curled under into flexion, and sometimes the tendons of the extensors are shortened, causing the toes to be hyperextended at the first joint. In either case, you may spend a little time straightening the toes with effleurage, thumb on top and index finger below.

Use the fist to apply broad pressure to the bottom of the foot. Hold the dorsal surface of the foot with one hand while the other applies the pressure. You may shape the foot around the fist, stretching the top of the foot and accentuating the longitudinal and transverse arches. Basic sliding effleurage may also be applied to the bottom of the foot with the fist. More specific pressure may be applied to the bottom of the foot with the thumbs. Pressing points on the bottom of the foot is thought to improve energy flow to the rest of the body according to acupressure theory, and improve circulation to corresponding body parts according to reflexology. It also helps relax the small muscles found there. Figure 9–23 shows some areas on the bottom of the feet to press to stimulate healthy function of different parts of the body.

Space can be created between metatarsals by holding on to the sides of the foot and pulling the hands away from each other or by interlocking your fingers with the recipient's toes. These techniques help relieve the feeling of the feet being squeezed inside of shoes.

Finish by slapping the bottom of the foot with the back of your hand. This should create a pleasant stimulating sensation. To finish, hold the feet. Repeat the entire sequence on the other foot.

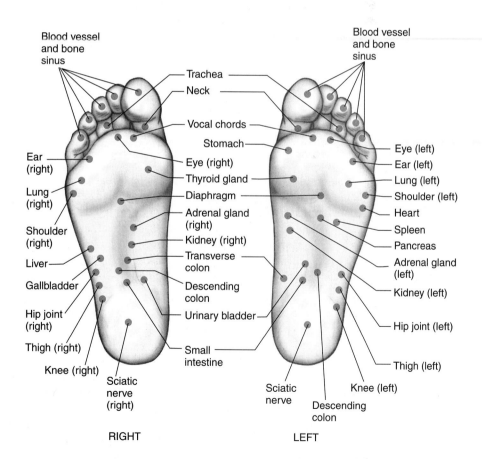

FIGURE 9–23. Areas to press on bottom of feet to stimulate healthy function of different parts of the body.

Enhancing Mobility in the Lower Extremities. Mobility in the lower extremities may be restricted for a number of reasons. Overuse and shortening of muscles in athletes and physical workers, underuse and aging, recuperation from an extended illness or injury, or a sedentary lifestyle can all contribute to stiff joints and lack of fluid movement in the lower limbs.

For best results, all the muscles of the hips, thighs, lower legs, and feet should be thoroughly massaged with effleurage and petrissage and lengthened with stretching; major tendons should be loosened with friction to the point of attachment; and joints taken through their full range of motion. Direct pressure along muscles and tendons has been known to help loosen them. The following techniques may be added to the basic full-body massage described in Chapter 8 to further enhance mobility in the lower extremities.

HIPS. After general massage of the buttocks, mobility at the hip joint may be further enhanced by pressing specific pressure points along the sacroiliac joint, the iliac crest, and around the trochanter at the hip joint. This may be done with the thumbs, an extended knuckle, or the elbow. Figure 9–24 shows the points to be pressed.

When the recipient is supine, take the upper leg through a full range of motion. The hip may be stretched by bringing the knee to the chest, out to the side in abduction, and across the body in adduction.

THIGHS. After general massage of the thigh, perform deep effleurage along each major muscle, including the adductors, to the point of proximal attachment. Figure 9–25 shows the technique for reaching the proximal adductor attachments. You may perform cross-fiber friction near the point of attachment for further effect. Get permission from the recipient to work the attachments in the groin area, and provide secure draping of the genitals.

Perform circular friction over the muscle attachments at the knee, first with the heels of the hands, and then with the fingertips. These attachments are frequently sore to the touch. Cross-fiber friction may be performed over areas in which the tissues seem to be adhering.

LOWER LEGS. Perform general massage of the lower leg in the prone position as described in Chapter 8. Loosen the Achilles tendon using direct pressure along its length, especially at the point of juncture with the muscle. See Figure 9–26. The tendon may be further loosened by moving it back and forth with the fingers after creating slack in it by slightly plantar flexing the foot. Perform joint mobilizations at the ankle and stretch the muscles of the lower leg.

FEET. The thorough foot massage described above may also be performed.

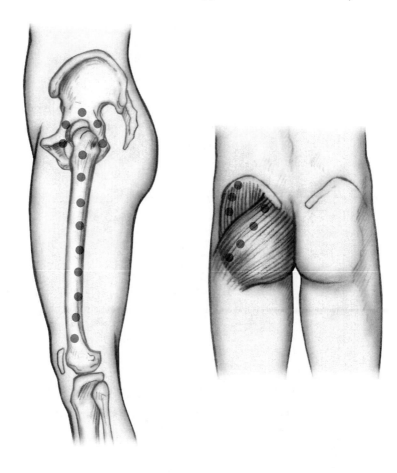

FIGURE 9–24. Points to press to improve mobility of the hip joint.

▪ UPPER EXTREMITIES

It has been theorized that upright posture was an adaptation in the evolution of human beings to free us to use our hands for grasping and manipulating objects. Everyday activities such as cooking and eating, personal grooming, cleaning the house, and gardening are performed using the arms and hands. Hobbies and sports and most work activities also depend on the upper extremities.

The upper extremities are also important in communication. Some ethnic groups are known for using their hands to augment verbal expression. To be friendly or affectionate we shake hands, give pats on the back, and hug. Loss of the use of the arms or hands can be personally and socially devastating.

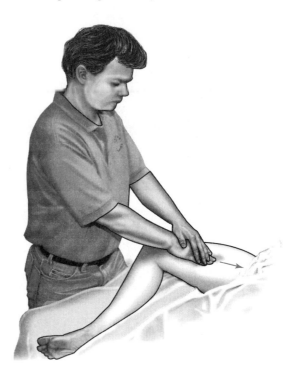

FIGURE 9–25. Position for reaching proximal adductor attachments. Be sure draping is secure.

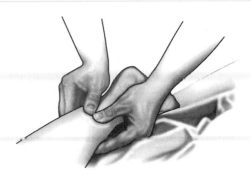

FIGURE 9–26. Direct pressure to Achilles tendon.

Applications of Massage

People who work at computer terminals, or who perform other repetitive move-ments with the arms and hands, often experience tightness and soreness in the upper extremities. Tennis elbow and golf elbow are overuse injuries experienced in those sports and also from activities requiring similar movements of the arms. Massage and stretching can help keep muscles of the arms and hands relaxed and in good condition and help prevent overuse injuries. Massage is used with ice and rest to treat tennis and golf elbow.

Massage and joint movements can also help maintain shoulder flexibility. They can help restore mobility lost by poor posture, overuse, aging, or accident. The hands can be massaged and mobilized to help retain their function in old age.

Anatomy

For purposes of massage, the upper extremities may be thought of in four sections, that is, the shoulders, upper arms, forearms, and hands. The shoulders may be ad-dressed as part of the upper back during massage since the shoulder blades are lo-cated there. Functionally, however, the shoulder blades are part of the shoulder gir-dle and designed to facilitate use of the arms and hands. The joints of the upper extremities include the complex shoulder girdle, the elbows, wrists, and several small joints in the hands.

The muscles that move the shoulder include pectoralis major and minor, del-toid, subscapularis, supraspinatus, infraspinatis, teres major and minor, serratus an-terior, levator scapulae, rhomboid major and minor, and trapezius. Latissimus dorsi is located on the back, but functions primarily to move the upper arm.

Muscles of the upper arm and forearms include the biceps brachii, triceps brachii, brachialis, the smaller muscles of pronation and supination (pronator teres, pronator quadratus, supinator), anconeus, coraco brachialis, and brachioradialis. The anterior forearm also contains the wrist flexors and palmaris longus, while the posterior forearm contains the wrist extensors. There are many small muscles intrin-sic to the hand that move the fingers and thumbs.

Techniques

The following techniques may be used to supplement the basic massage of the upper extremities described in Chapter 8. The primary movers of the scapulae are located on the back and are best addressed as part of a back massage when the re-cipient is prone. The upper arms, forearms, and hands are most easily accessed and mobilized when the recipient is supine.

Enhancing Mobility of the Shoulder Girdle. Mobility of the shoulder girdle may be restricted for a number of reasons. Overuse and shortening of muscles in athletes and physical workers, underuse, aging, and recuperation from a shoulder injury can all contribute to loss of mobility in the shoulder.

A general approach to enhancing shoulder mobility would include warming of the superficial and deeper muscles of the upper back and upper arm with effleurage and petrissage, followed by deep friction on muscles, on tendons, and at attachments. Direct pressure on muscles and tendons, particularly at tender or trigger points, has been known to help muscles relax and lengthen.

The shoulders and upper arms should be mobilized and taken through their full range of motion. Care should be taken not to force movement, potentially damaging tissues. Mobility that has been restricted for some time will take time to regain. The following techniques may be added to the basic full-body routine described in Chapter 8 to further enhance mobility of the shoulder girdle.

PRONE. After general massage of the upper back, create a deeper warming by knuckling or sawing friction between and over the shoulder blades. How much pressure you use will be determined by the size and sensitivity of the recipient. The more heavily muscled the receiver, the more pressure you will use to affect deeper tissues.

Deep effleurage along upper trapezius and over the levator scapula will help loosen those muscles further. It may be useful to then apply vibration to the upper trapezius with an electric vibrator.

Direct pressure along the upper trapezius, and along the medial border of the scapula may help relax these muscles. Apply pressure slowly, meeting the resistance offered by the tissue, then move along to another spot at about one-inch intervals. The reinforced thumb-over-thumb technique may be used for the large upper trapezius as shown in Figure 9–27.

With the receiver in the prone position, a gentle mobilization of the shoulder may be created by simply lifting the upper arm above the elbow, letting the forearm hang down to the floor, and swinging the forearm back and forth like a pendulum. This creates movement in the glenohumeral joint, as well as in the scapula. To create a larger and more controlled movement, place the recipient's arm along-

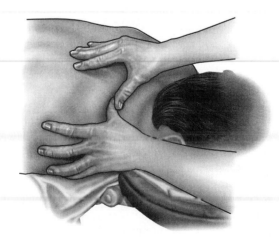

FIGURE 9–27. Direct pressure along upper trapezius with thumbs, recipient prone.

side the body on the table. Grasp the upper arm just below the glenohumeral joint and move the shoulder superior and inferior, and then in a circle in a passive shoulder roll.

The scapula may be isolated for movement by placing the recipient's hand behind the back, which causes the scapula to lift away from the rib cage. Take care not to force this position, which may cause some discomfort. See Figure 9–28. You may modify this position by placing the hand next to the body with the elbow bent as shown in Figure 7–6. In either position, the scapula may be mobilized by placing a hand near the tip and on top of the shoulder and pressing lightly toward the feet. The other hand is placed at the inferior border of the scapula, assisting in the movement. The scapula will lift and move if the attached muscles are relaxed.

SUPINE. Subscapularis may be accessed with the recipient supine. Stand at the side near the shoulder and face the table. Bring the recipient's lower arm across the chest with the upper arm perpendicular to the table. This will expose the underside of the scapula somewhat. Locate the subscapularis in the axilla (ie, armpit) and press into the subscapularis muscle with the fingertips as shown in Figure 9–29. This is usually very tender, so proceed gently.

Mobility in the shoulder girdle may be restricted anteriorly by the pectoral muscles and the anterior deltoid. After general warming, apply deep effleurage to these muscles. Direct pressure along length of the pectorals at ½-inch intervals may help to loosen them further. Care should be taken since the pectorals will likely be sore if hypertonic. Follow the more specific massage with stretches of the upper arm across the body and overhead.

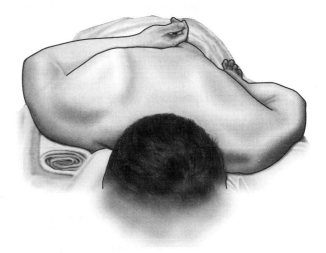

FIGURE 9–28. Placing the recipient's hand behind the back causes the scapula to lift up.

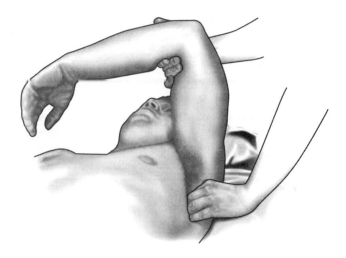

FIGURE 9–29. Accessing the subscapularis, recipient supine.

OVERUSE OF HANDS AND FOREARMS. The muscles of the forearms create movement at the wrist and the hands. Certain occupations and activities tend to stress these muscles and produce chronic tension in them. Regular specific massage of the hands and forearms can help prevent overuse injuries in this area. A complete prevention program would also include regular resting time, stretching and self-massage, and structurally safe performance of the movements. Massage therapists themselves are prone to such overuse.

Warm the forearms and hands with the general massage described in Chapter 8. Add deep stripping effleurage with the thumbs to the anterior and posterior forearms following the long muscles from the wrist to their attachments at the elbow. See Figure 9–30. Apply deep circular friction to the attachments at the elbow. Direct pressure along the belly of the muscles of the forearms may help them relax. Mobilize the wrist joint and stretch the forearm muscles by flexing and hyperextending at the wrist.

To finish each side, perform the hand massage and joint movements described in Chapters 7 and 8. This will affect the forearm muscles that attach on the hand as well as muscles intrinsic to the hand itself.

▪ CHEST AND ABDOMEN

The front of the body includes the chest and the abdomen. These areas are usually addressed separately during massage. However, they are connected for certain functions such as respiration and movements involving forward trunk flexion.

The expansion and contraction of the chest as we breathe is evidence of life. Because it is the location of women's breasts, the chest is associated with both nur-

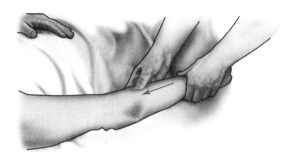

FIGURE 9–30. Deep stripping effleurage with the thumb to the forearm.

turing and sexual appeal. The chest is also associated with strength and power, as when the pectorals are well developed in men.

In the United States, women's breasts are kept covered in public and, therefore, should be draped at all times to maintain modesty and proper professional boundaries. Practitioners can access the pectoral muscles and intercostals of women working around a small drape. When working on women with large breasts, it may be difficult to get to the muscles underneath. Except in medical situations where lymph drainage is desired, it is general practice to omit massage of the breast tissue itself.

The abdomen is a relatively vulnerable area extending from the diaphragm to the pubis. It contains the viscera, that is, the internal organs of digestion, elimination, and reproduction. It lacks the bony protection afforded the lungs and heart in the chest. The abdomen is contained and supported principally by the abdominal muscles. It is the soft belly exposed in humans because of our upright posture.

The word "visceral" has come to mean deeply felt, instinctive, or having to do with elemental emotions. This area is sensitive for many people and should be approached with care.

Anatomy

The chest is generally defined by the rib cage, sternum, and the muscles of the shoulder girdle that attach to them. The prominent muscles of the chest are pectoralis major and minor. Muscles located on the chest with the primary function of respiration include the diaphragm (separates the chest from the abdomen) and intercostals.

The abdomen lies between the thorax or chest and the pelvis. The abdominal cavity contains the stomach, liver, spleen, pancreas, small and large intestines, kidneys, bladder, reproductive organs in females, and other visceral organs. The abdominal muscles surrounding and supporting the viscera include the rectus abdominus and internal and external obliques.

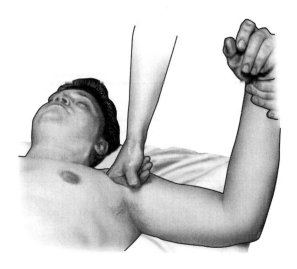

FIGURE 9–31. Compressions over anterior deltoid with loose fist.

Applications of Massage

Poor posture, long periods of sitting at a desk, and carrying objects in the arms can all lead to shortening of the muscles of the chest and abdomen. A chronic slumped posture can inhibit the functions of the visceral organs, lead to back and neck tension and fatigue, and restrict breathing. Massage can help stretch and lengthen shortened anterior muscles that are the result of and contribute to chronic slumped

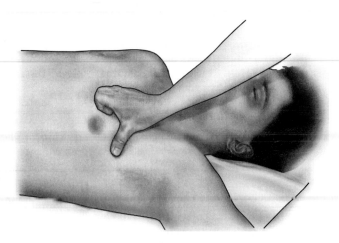

FIGURE 9–32. Direct pressure on attachments of pectoralis minor.

posture. Along with proper strengthening exercises for the back and abdominals, massage can help one maintain good upright posture.

The chest cavity expands to accommodate expansion of the lungs during inhalation. Therefore, any muscular restriction in the area can adversely affect breathing. The major muscles of respiration are the diaphragm and intercostals. Forced inhalation and exhalation also involve the abdominal muscles, and muscles that raise the rib cage such as the scalenes and levator scapulae. Massage can help maintain the muscles of respiration in optimal condition and relieve tension caused by poor posture or stress.

Rounded Shoulders. When the pectoral and anterior deltoid muscles shorten, the effect is one of rounded or forward shoulders. A program of stretching the muscles of the chest and shoulders, while strengthening the muscles of the upper back, is needed to truly correct rounded shoulders. During a massage session, rounded

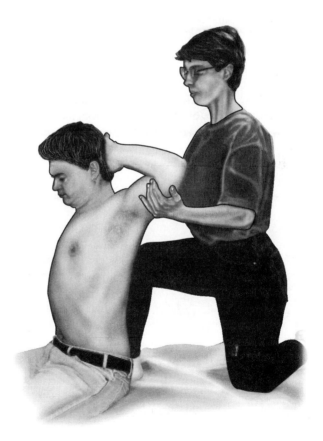

FIGURE 9–33. Stretching the pectorals with recipient in sitting position. Also used to enhance inhalation during deep breathing.

shoulders may be addressed by relaxing and stretching the pectorals and anterior deltoid.

Warm up the anterior deltoid with effleurage and petrissage. Apply compression over the anterior deltoid with a loose fist as shown in Figure 9–31. Warm up the pectorals using effleurage with the fist. Start superficially and gradually deepen the pressure. Once the muscles are warmed up, you may apply circular friction along the sternal and clavicular attachments of pectoralis major. Apply deep effleurage with the thumbs along the length of pectoralis minor, pausing to hold static pressure over the attachment on the third, fourth, and fifth ribs. See Figure 9–32.

Stretch the arm overhead to lengthen pectoral muscles. At the end of the session, have the recipient sit on the edge of the table with his hands behind his head. Get up onto the table behind the recipient and brace his back with your hip. Pull back on the elbows for a stretch of the pectorals as shown in Figure 9–33. Have the recipient inhale as you pull back and expand the chest.

Enhancing Respiration. Breathing is easier when muscles of respiration are relaxed. Muscular tension in the diaphragm, intercostals, abdominals, scalenes, and levator scapulae can inhibit proper expansion and lifting of the chest during inhalation.

During massage of the cervicals, perform effleurage specifically over the scalenes with the thumb to help relax them. When the recipient is prone, perform thumb stripping along the levator scapula to its point of attachment on the superior medial border of the scapula, lengthening the muscle. These are the muscles that elevate the shoulders and help expand the chest. They may be tense in people who are stressed and are breathing shallow from the shoulders.

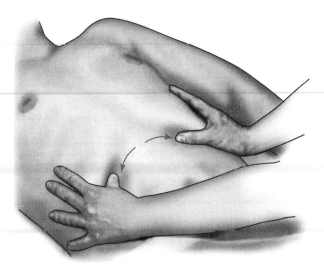

FIGURE 9–34. Sliding the thumbs along the attachment of the diaphragm.

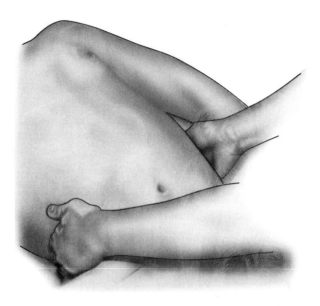

FIGURE 9–35. Sliding and lifting the abdominals around the waist.

When the recipient is supine, lengthen the pectorals as described above to create space across the chest. Then perform effleurage over the rib cage from the opposite side of the table. Reach around as far as you can and pull up and over the rib cage with spread fingers. Try to find the spaces between the ribs to massage the intercostals. Rock the rib cage to further relax the area.

Stand at the waist of the recipient facing the head. Place your thumbs just beneath the sternum and have the recipient take a deep breath in. As he exhales, press in and slide your thumbs along the attachment of the diaphragm along the outline of the rib cage as shown in Figure 9–34. Be careful to avoid pressure on the xiphoid process. Finish by lifting up and around the sides of the abdominals. See Figure 9–35.

You may want to spend some time with the recipient practicing diaphragmatic breathing, and taking a full breath beginning with the diaphragm and expanding the chest. The stretching exercise shown in Figure 9–33 can also be used to help the recipient feel the expansion of the chest during inhalation.

■ SUMMARY

Practitioners may want to focus more time and attention on a particular part of the body. This could be the result of recipient request; the judgment of the practitioner from observation, palpation, or information from a health history form; or a specific referral from a health care provider.

Even though the body is massaged in parts during a session, the interconnectedness of the body as a whole should be kept in mind. In addition, different parts of the body have different meaning for each recipient. Practitioners need to be aware that they are not just touching body parts, they are touching a person.

For purposes of discussion, the body may be thought of in sections, that is, head and face, cervical region, back, buttocks, lower extremities, upper extremities, chest and abdomen. This is generally how the body is addressed during a massage session. To benefit recipients most, practitioners should understand the meaning of the section in human terms, the applications of massage related to each section, cautions that apply, and the anatomy of the area.

Practitioners may perform additional techniques to a certain area for more specific attention with the goal of muscular relaxation and lengthening. They may also choose to focus on enhancing a specific function of the area, for example, mobility in the lower extremities or respiration.

III

Contemporary Massage and Bodywork

10

Polarity Therapy

Beverly Shoenberger

Polarity therapy is a holistic health practice involving exercises, nutrition, and love, as well as gentle bodywork techniques. Polarity techniques involve simple touching and gentle movements. The practitioner always has both hands on the receiver's body, either resting them in specific places, rocking the body, or rhythmically pressing in at various depths. These touches are designed to release obstructions to the free flow of energy through the body, so that the person is supported in returning to health.

■ HISTORY

Polarity therapy was developed in the middle 1900s by Randolph Stone (1890–1981), who was trained in the natural healing methods of chiropractic, naturopathy, and osteopathy. Stone was intrigued by the thought that there must be a basic principle underlying the effectiveness of diet change, manipulations, exercise, and other natural cures. Why did the same health problem respond positively to diet change in one person, spinal manipulation in another, and exercise in another? Why did some people seem predisposed to illness, whereas others seemed to have an innate vitality?

The search for this underlying principle led Stone to study Chinese acupuncture and herbal medicine, the Hermetic Kabalistic systems of the Middle East, and the ancient Ayurvedic medicine of India. In each of these traditions, he found two complementary elements, that is, the belief in a subtle form of life energy that permeates the body and gives it health, and the understanding that disease is a result of obstruction to that flow of energy. Stone theorized that all natural healing techniques are effective because they support the individual's innate capacity for health by stimulating the free and balanced flow of life energy. He combined his Western skills with techniques from all the Eastern traditions he had studied and explored them from the unique vantage point of their effect on the subtle life energy.

Stone then spent many years practicing methods for freeing energy flow and studying meditation in India. Indian philosophical framework permeates his writings on polarity therapy. The life energy is described in terms of longitudinal, horizontal, and diagonal lines of force, *chakras* (energy centers in the body), and the five elements (earth, water, fire, air, and ether). Foods, hands-on work, and exercises are discussed according to their effect on the balancing of these elements. This rather esoteric aspect of polarity therapy, along with the incorporation of chiropractic and osteopathic techniques, makes his writings difficult for the average reader.

After Stone's retirement in 1973, Pierre Pannetier began to spread the practice of polarity therapy across the United States through seminars. Pannetier did much to systematize the series of physical mobilizations and make the more esoteric nature of Stone's work accessible to the lay practitioner.

However, the very eclectic nature of Stone's teaching makes it difficult to actually define polarity therapy. In its truest sense, polarity therapy includes anything that promotes life. Through the years, different practitioners have tended to incorporate whatever supplemental skills they might have, and rightly so, in order to best support the health of the client. Various schools of polarity therapy that have sprung up are very different from each other in style of hands-on work, amount of pressure used, emphasis on the esoteric, and supplemental skills such as training in Gestalt therapy.

Many polarity therapists emphasize the esoteric aspect of the tradition and may use this framework to explain or develop their sessions, "I am working with your fire current, as an imbalance in it is undermining the health of your sinuses." However, acceptance of the esoteric aspects is not at all essential to the practice of polarity. Pannetier often advised his students to forget their intellects, including all thoughts based on Ayurveda. He would instruct them to sense the obstructions with their hands and work intuitively in that present moment of touching, using Stone's manipulations as springboards and developing new ones as needed. There is a vast wealth of powerful and effective techniques in the system of polarity, and this attention to intuition is in no way meant to downplay or degrade the value of learning technique. It is simply that the practitioner must learn to go beyond the intellect's limitations into the direct experience of working with the subtle energies.

Studying polarity therapy is similar to studying music where many "scales" are practiced, new "melodies" and "styles" are learned in order to stretch the student's capacity and stimulate creativity. Theory can be a valuable aid, but is not essential. The desired end result is to play from one's heart in a responsive manner that is open to the needs of the present moment.

▪ PHYSIOLOGIC EFFECTS

To date, Western science has expressed little interest in researching this so-called life energy. Although we have yet to reach scientific understanding of what happens during polarity therapy, something does happen. There are subjective as well as objective indications that some principle not yet recognized by Western medicine is involved.

- Subjectively, health is often equated with being full of energy, whereas the first sign of impending illness is often its absence.
- Subjectively, the therapist feels a definite tingling in his or her hands when doing the various mobilizations. The degree and pattern of this tingling vary with the state of health of the area being worked, and they change as the area is treated.
- Subjectively, the patient and therapist often note simultaneous changes in their sense of energy. The receiver feels freer, lighter, more relaxed; the therapist notes a balancing and strengthening of the tingling in his or her hands, and a sense of an overall increase in energy.

The polarity therapist views these changes as a response to unblocking the life energy by affecting muscular relaxation, structural change, and balancing the autonomic nervous system. Western medicine would probably say that the tingling is simply vasodilation in the hands; the talk of energy is pseudoscience; the positive health gains are a result of the placebo effect.

Yet Western science would also have to note that there are objective changes taking place. After just a few minutes of polarity therapy, signs of deep relaxation appear. Often, cheeks flush, blood pressure drops, salivation increases, the heart rate slows, the eyes may tear, and the stomach and intestines may grumble with the increase in peristalsis. These are objective signs of a relaxation response from the parasympathetic nervous system.

Closer examination reveals clear physiologic rationales for the effectiveness of many of the specific techniques. Many can be seen as stimulation to nerve centers. For example, one commonly given technique involves very light oscillating pressure over the pressure-sensitive baroreceptors in the carotid arteries along the sides of the neck. It is probable that, although the pressure is so slight as to cause no interference with the blood supply to the brain, it is sufficient to activate the neurologic reflex signal that slows the heart rate and lowers blood pressure. This same reflex is usually triggered by stretching of the baroreceptors from within when the blood pressure going to the brain is too high.

Polarity techniques often involve rocking motions of the limbs and trunk. These vary from small, gentle oscillations to large, vigorous oscillations that move the entire body. This rocking commonly induces relaxation, lowers muscle tone, reduces pain, and encourages an increase in the active range of motion afterward. Western medicine is just beginning to be aware of the tremendous benefits of this pain-free way of stimulating the joint mechanoreceptors, the nerve endings that receive messages about movements in the joints. It appears that when these receptors are gently stimulated, a reflex response will lower muscle tone, increase circulation, and stimulate endorphin release, which results in a decrease in pain sensation.

In addition, it appears that the alternating rhythmic manner with which the two hands are used and the style of touch often induce a light hypnotic trance. Recipients frequently report experiencing an unusual mind state in which they feel as though every part of their body and mind were relaxed and even asleep, except for their simple awareness of sensory stimuli. This state of deepened relaxation lays the foundation for health and well-being by returning the body and mind to a state of balanced homeostasis. Even if only temporary, the moments of peace provided by a polarity session are a much needed experience in this stressful culture. In addition, this state of quiet awareness allows people to see their problems from a broader perspective, often seeing solutions that had previously been buried by the noisiness of the conscious mind. Hidden feelings may surface, making polarity therapy an excellent adjunct to psychotherapeutic work. Thus, although Western science does not view energy as a structurally existing entity, it would seem apparent that, functionally, the human body responds to the polarity touch in a manner that supports health of the body and mind.

It is interesting to note how many of the techniques are as easily set within the framework of modern medicine as they are within Ayurvedic philosophy. It is as though the basic principle Stone sought transcends all ideas, ancient or modern, and is instead embodied in the actual experience of the hands-on work, rather than in the particular theories used to explain it. Energy is simply an abstracted metaphor—one way of looking at the results obtained through polarity therapy. Neurologic reflex is another abstracted metaphor—a way of explaining a mechanism we cannot see, except in its effects.

▪ PRINCIPLES OF POLARITY THERAPY

The basic principles of polarity therapy are related to the concepts of energy, love, working with obstructions, understanding, and nutrition and exercise. The following sections briefly explore these concepts in the context of polarity therapy and offer some experiential exercises.

Energy

Working with energy is a concept foreign to most Westerners. And yet it is not as difficult or unusual as we might expect. In this culture, not much time or value is placed on subtle awareness of changes in the hands. A simple experiment can show how these sensations can be picked up and amplified.

Rub the palms of your hands together, waking the nerve endings and bringing your awareness to your palms. Then hold them about six inches apart; relax, and center your awareness, amplifying incoming sensory input by focusing. Experiment with moving your hands closer and farther apart to see if and how the feeling changes. Then move the hands so that the palms are no longer facing, and be aware of how they feel.

Many people find that when the palms are facing each other, there is a tingling sensation of relatedness, as though the hands were "plugging into" each other. Try the same sequence with your eyes closed; from the sensation or its absence you may know whether or not your palms are directly opposite each other.

Love

The foremost principle espoused in polarity therapy is the importance of working with love. Pannetier used to say that love was the most vital element of the whole session. He would say, "If you don't know what to do, just put your hands on the person and love them."

What is this love? Obviously it is not sloppy sentimentality or an overbearing affection. Beyond that, it is difficult to put into words. Trying to act in a loving manner, or matching an idea of what we think Pannetier is talking about, misses again. To really love is a matter quite different from holding an idea about love. This love of which he spoke has no objective, not even that of healing or helping someone. It is a caring so powerful that it carries with it no agenda, no end result that must be obtained.

The practitioner does his or her work simply, always responding to the felt need, and yet without attachment to healing. This love is serving life. The practitioner who "cares enough not to care," as Dylan Thomas once said, "can truly let go and trust in the universe." The seeds of this relaxation are then watered in the recipient's own being. This fosters and extremely deep state of relaxation and trust. It is in this relaxed state that healing occurs, if it is meant to be.

Once the practitioner has begun to understand this principle, the rich wealth of polarity techniques can be explored, but always with the understanding that it is not the particular technique that heals. This attitude of surrender and openness, this simple "getting out of the way" of the body's inherent tendency to homeostasis allows healing on many levels. Muscles relax, digestion improves, circulation increases in areas where it is needed, hormone levels normalize, endorphins increase, breathing deepens, and so on.

A good place to begin exploring this quality of love is a simple "front-to-back" polarity technique. You will need a partner for this exercise.

Instruct your partner to sit on a stool or sideways in a chair so that the chest and thoracic area (upper back) are both easily accessible. Stand at the person's left side, and slowly and gently place your left palm over the person's heart and your right palm over the upper back between the shoulder blades. Move your hands slowly around until you feel a sensation of the palms "plugging into each other," as though they were connected by a flow of energy. See Figure 10–1.

Simply hold your hands in place. Check your own posture to see that it is relaxed and that your breathing is natural and uncontrolled. After a bit, your palms may begin to tingle more or less strongly, or feel unusually warm. Some practitioners do not experience these signs, but feel an inner sense of rightness, an increasing sense of peace and completion. The experience is different for everyone. The recipient may sigh, visibly relax, and show a change in his or her breathing pattern. You may feel a change in your hands or in your mind state at about the same time. After a few minutes, very slowly withdraw your hands.

Many practitioners find that their discursive intellects are quite loud during this exercise and that they are unable to tune into their hands or their subtle feelings. They are so busy watching for results or criticizing their own efforts that awareness of subtle changes in their hands is impossible. It takes practice and a continual "letting go" on the part of the giver.

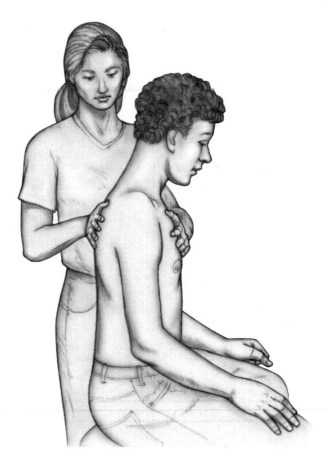

FIGURE 10–1. Feeling palms "plugging into each other."

▪ WORKING THE OBSTRUCTIONS

Another principle in polarity is that the obstructions must be released for optimal results. An obstruction is an area of the body where there seems to be a stagnation or a holding pattern that somehow interferes with a free flow of energy. In simple terms, for example, a person who is experiencing chronic anxiety may have abdominal tension, disturbed peristalsis, and nausea. Their posture may be somewhat caved in, as though they were trying to protect themselves from imminent danger. If you were to look at such a person, you might imagine that any lines of energy trying to flow vertically through that person might be really disturbed in the abdominal-diaphragmatic area. The practitioner using polarity would respond to those obstructed areas with techniques that would tend to release tension and encourage a free flow of naturally organized and balanced energy.

An alert practitioner will begin assessing clients visually as soon as they walk in the door. They will be looking for areas that seem out of alignment, do not move with the rest of the body when the person walks, seem held or protected. Further clues are found from the receiver's self-resorts, and by touch, as the bodywork session begins. The following exercise is designed to introduce you to the principle of finding and locating obstructions.

Have your partner lie supine, facing upward. Slowly and gently place your right palm on his or her abdomen between the navel and the pubic bone. You may sense tension or the opposite—flaccidly—in the musculature. You can become alert to the breathing pattern. Does it seem restricted or unusually fast or slow? Does the breathing pattern change as you touch the person? You may sense irregularities in the skin temperature, or a tightness only in a certain area as though there were a pocket of gas under your hand. Make certain that your hand, wrist, elbow, and shoulder muscles are completely relaxed, and that your own breathing is calm. The touch should be light. If you are able to relax, you can increase the pressure slightly, first with the heel of the hand and then the fingers, alternating in wavelike motion.

Leaving your right hand resting on the abdomen, place your left hand over your partner's forehead as shown in Figure 10–2. With practice, you will be able to sense whether the head is held rigidly by the neck muscles and whether the person is subtly moving toward or away from your hand. As you lightly touch, see if you can feel the sensation of your hands "plugging in" again. Feelings of warmth or tingling may begin in one or both hands. Gently rock the lower body a few minutes with the right hand, as though you were rocking a baby to sleep. The left hand should remain resting lightly on the forehead throughout, without rocking. As the

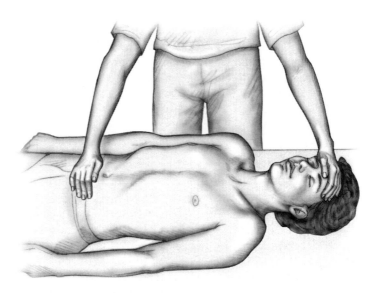

FIGURE 10–2. General position for releasing blocks in the torso and head.

sensation of connectedness or tingling increases, you may see signs of an increased energy flow. Your partner's face may show more color, muscles may relax, and the breathing may deepen and become more regular. You have helped melt areas of tension, or obstructions, in the areas under and between your two hands.

▪ UNDERSTANDING

In the above exercise, it is also quite possible that your partner experienced the opposite of the relaxation response. At times, the muscular armoring has served an important function for the person, helping him or her feel safer, for example. As these muscles release their tension, it is common for fear to arise. The person may be confused by this response, which can be of some magnitude. For this reason, many schools of polarity include basic counseling skills. Pannetier used a commonsense approach emphasizing a caring attitude, acceptance, and trust that whatever happens is from the "clearing of blocks" and is for the best.

Polarity is a gentle art. The giver invites the receiver to enter a deeply relaxed state and invites the muscles to relax. Nothing is ever forced. Pannetier would often say that no harm can come from polarity so long as the touch is gentle enough not to override the receiver's natural tendency to homeostasis. If the receiver wishes to enter into and pass through the feeling of obstruction, the practitioner will continue to work with areas of holding, deepening the relaxation, allowing the energy flow between the hands to build and balance. If the receiver wishes to pull away from the experience, reassurance can be given and alternate areas can be worked that are not threatening, perhaps building trust for work with the more tightly defended areas at a later time. It is often the case that as the receiver lets go in other areas, highly charged areas may release without his or her conscious awareness.

Thus, Pannetier would say, it is vital for the practitioner to have a proper understanding of personal responsibility. The recipient is reaping the effects of past actions and present decisions. The giver is not there to rescue the receiver, but to plant seeds of letting go and trusting, to be an accepting friend. This attitude protects the practitioner from taking on the recipient's ailments in a misguided attempt to heal.

▪ NUTRITION AND EXERCISE

Both nutrition and exercise take a prominent part in the therapeutic regimen. Commonsense stretching and toning, sometimes with the addition of sounds to stimulate the flow of energy, are suggested. Their selection is again based on the Ayurvedic concepts of freeing and balancing the life energy. The specific system of exercise is loosely derived from yoga, but it has become more eclectic as teachers have incorporated their own experiences and viewpoints. The one basic stretch is the youthful pose, or squatting posture. In this position, it is said, all the currents are stimulated and the cosmic forces are attracted for health and rejuvenation.

Dietary suggestions are primarily based on Ayurvedic theory, that is, on the energetic qualities of various foods. Clients or patients are commonly led through a period of "cleansing," during which intake of certain foods is severely limited. Daily use of a liver flush, a drink made of garlic, olive oil, and lemon juice followed by specific herbal teas, is often recommended. A simple vegetarian diet is recommended for daily fare. It should be noted that the primary emphasis in polarity is on eating with a relaxed mind state, rather than on the particulars of what is eaten. Just as in hands-on work, the subtle mental aspects of diet are far more important than the material aspects and serve as a foundation for digesting and assimilation of whatever is eaten.

The emphasis on eating nutritious foods while in a relaxed state of mind and on exercising in a balanced manner is certainly basic to a Western view of health. However, the particulars are controversial, and unless one is approaching polarity in its entirety as an offshoot of Ayurvedic medicine, they are not essential to an appreciation of the hands-on technique. For this reason, the remaining section of this chapter will deal solely with the hands-on art of polarity.

■ BASIC POLARITY MOVEMENTS

Beginning polarity students are taught a general session of 22 movements that serve to stimulate and balance the entire body. The gentle holding, rocking, and probing techniques form a generally relaxing session and also aid the practitioner in locating areas that appear to be obstructed and in need of further work.

Some of these techniques are derived from osteopathy, craniopathy, and chiropractic of the 1930s and 1940s. Some were derived by Stone from observations made by psychics, from his study of acupuncture, and from Egyptian medicine. Some were derived from theories of harmonic resonance, that is, that certain parts of the body will vibrate harmonically when other areas are worked. All in all, the techniques form a fascinating and rich array of moves that must be experienced and done in order to be appreciated.

■ ABBREVIATED GENERAL SESSION

What follows is an abbreviated version of a general session of polarity therapy. For simplicity, the receiver will be consistently referred to as "him." To begin, have the receiver lie on his back on the massage table, while you sit on a chair at his head.

1. *The tenth cranial ("the cradle").* Overlap the last three fingers of your left hand on the last three fingers of your right hand, palms up, to form a cradle as shown in Figure 10–3. Rest your hands on the table, supporting the recipient's head in your palms. Your index fingers should extend along the grooves beside the sternocleidomastoid muscle (where the carotid artery and tenth cranial nerve travel). Rest your thumbs on your index fin-

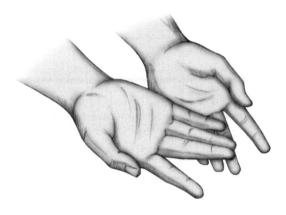

FIGURE 10-3. Hand position for the cradle.

gers rather than over the receiver's ears. Hold 1 to 2 minutes, or until the current is strongly felt. See Figure 10–4.

2. **Neck stretch.** Rest the receiver's head on the palm of your right hand, so that your first or second finger and thumb can take a firm hold on the base of his skull. Your left hand rests lightly on his forehead with your left thumb on the anterior fontanel (the "soft spot" in an infant). With firm steady pressure from the right hand only, apply gentle traction toward you. As the recipient exhales, slightly release; as he inhales, slightly increase the traction. This move is contraindicated if the receiver is know to be hypermobile or if there is any increase in pain in the arms, shoulders, neck, or head during the movement. See Figure 10–5.

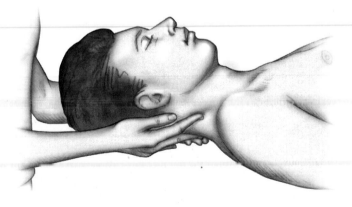

FIGURE 10-4. The cradle.

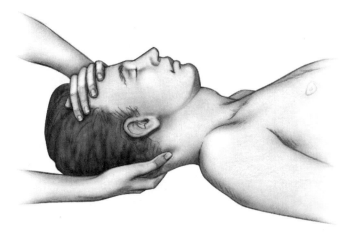

FIGURE 10–5. The neck stretch.

3. **Tummy rock.** Standing on the recipient's right side, rest your left hand on his forehead and your right hand on his abdomen halfway between the navel and the pubic bone. Rock the abdomen gently, trying to tune into the person's natural "rocking rhythm." This movement was also described earlier, as a means of releasing blocks in the torso and head. See Figure 10–6.

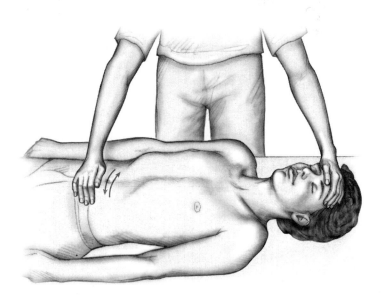

FIGURE 10–6. The tummy rock

4. **Leg pull.** Grasp both feet behind the heels and gently pull legs straight toward you several inches above the table. Rest the legs back on the table gently and place your hands over the feet for a few moments before proceeding.

5. **Inside ankle press.** You can sit on a stool at the receiver's feet if that is more comfortable for you than standing. Support the heel of his right foot with your left hand. With your right thumb, press gently in an arc under the inner ankle bone (medial malleolus). Pay special attention to any tender areas, applying rhythmic gentle compression until the points are pain free. Keeping your right hand in place, press on the ball of the foot with your left hand to flex the ankle forward (dorsiflexion). With practice, you will be able to alternate rhythmically between pressing an ankle point and flexing the ankle. See Figure 10–7.

6. **Outside ankle press.** Now, support the heel of his right foot with your left hand. (If the receiver has a markedly externally rotated hip, you may need to lift the entire leg and rest it in your palm in a more neutral position in order to have the outside of the ankle accessible for work.) With your right thumb, find any tender areas along the area under the outside ankle bone (lateral malleolus). With your right hand, press the top of the foot downward (plantarflexion) giving a good stretch. Alternate rhythmically as describe above. See Figure 10–8.

Note: Movements 7–11 are performed in sequence on the right side and are then repeated on the left side with instructions for left–right reversed, before moving on to movements 12–15.

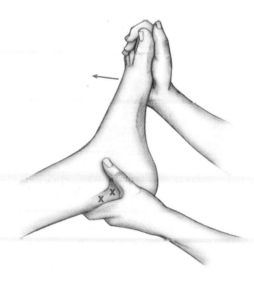

FIGURE 10–7. Inside ankle press.

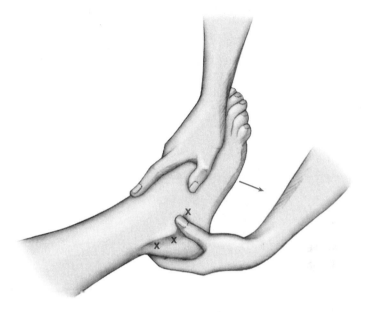

FIGURE 10–8. Outside ankle press.

7. ***Pelvis and knee rock.*** Hold the feet again for a moment, and move up to the person's right side. Place your left hand on his lower right abdomen, just above the thigh crease, with the fingers pointing down toward the feet. Place your right hand just above the knee. Very gently apply pressure with the right hand in a rhythmic fashion, gently rocking his leg. Continue for 10 to 30 seconds. Allow the leg to slow and then to be still. Continue holding for 30 seconds or so, again being aware of any sensations you feel. Carefully and slowly remove your hands. See Figure 10–9.

8. ***Arm–shoulder rotations.*** Hold the receiver's right wrist as show in Figure 10–10. Controlling movement from the wrist, gently rotate the shoulder in a small circle, alternately compressing and distracting the shoulder point. Do this about 10 times toward you and 10 times away from you.

9. ***Thumb web–forearm stimulation.*** Using the thumb and finger of your left hand, squeeze the webbing between his thumb and finger, concentrating on any tender areas. Press the pad of your right thumb into a point 1 inch below the elbow crease and ½ inch from the inside of his arm. Rhythmically alternate stimulation with each hand. See Figure 10–11.

10. ***Elbow milk–abdomen rock.*** Place your left hand under the recipient's right elbow and lay your thumb across the elbow crease. Milk upwards with your thumb. Place your right hand lightly along the bottom edge of the rib cage, and gently rock the abdomen. Alternate milking and rocking, about 10 to 12 times each for about a minute. See Figure 10–12.

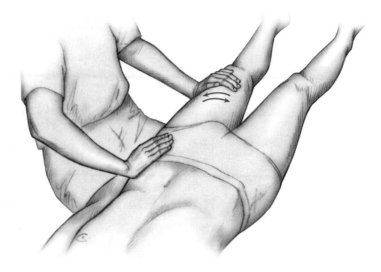

FIGURE 10–9. Left-side pelvis and knee rock.

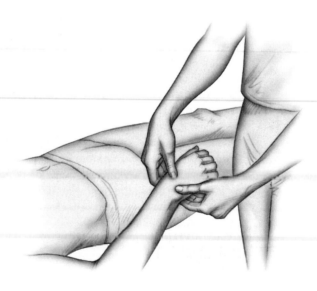

FIGURE 10–10. Arm shoulder rotation.

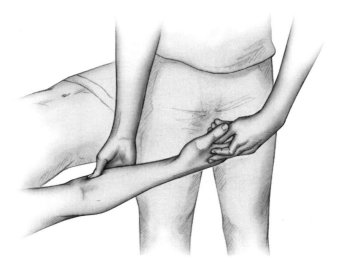

FIGURE 10–11. Forearm stimulation using the thumb.

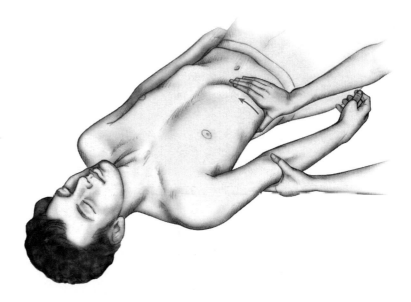

FIGURE 10–12. Elbow milk and abdomen rock.

11. **Pelvic rock.** Place your right hand over the recipient's left hip bone (anterior superior iliac spine). Place your left hand over his right shoulder. Stabilizing the shoulder girdle with your left hand, gently rock the trunk with the right. Gradually increase the rocking movement for 20 seconds, and then gradually decrease. Hold for a moment before moving on. See Figure 10–13.

12. **Occipital press.** Sitting at the recipient's head, turn his head slightly to the left. Using the second finger of your right hand, perform circular friction to the suboccipital muscles just under the base of the skull and to the right of the midline. Your left hand should be supporting his head by resting lightly on the left side of his forehead. Your index finger should rest gently on the spot known in India as the "third eye," the area between and just above the eyes. The hand on the back of the head should feel as though it were plugged into the palm of the hand on his forehead. Hold and feel for a sensation of tingling. When a steady gentle pulsation is felt in the hands, or a minute or so has passed, turn the head to the other side and repeat, switching hands. See Figure 10–14.

13. **Cranial polarization.** Lightly place both thumbs on the anterior fontanel, with both index fingers touching on the "third eye" and the remaining fingers across the forehead. If your hands are large enough, rest your little fingers on the temperomandibular joints, with the other fingers evenly spaced on the forehead. It is important that you really relax your hands,

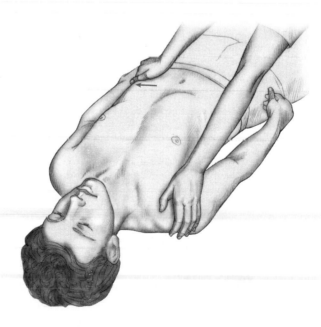

FIGURE 10–13. Pelvic rock.

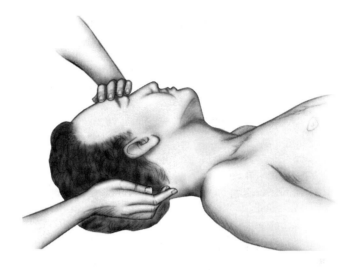

FIGURE 10–14. Occipital press.

arms, and shoulders as much as possible, and that your breathing is relaxed and your posture comfortable. Hold for about one minute, or until a steady gentle pulsation is felt. See Figure 10–15.

14. ***Navel–third eye.*** Move to the recipient's right side. Lightly place your left thumb pad between his eyebrows and your right thumb in his navel, with the thumbs pointing toward each other. Hold one minute, and then lift hands very slowly, initiating movement from the thumbs, rather than the shoulders.

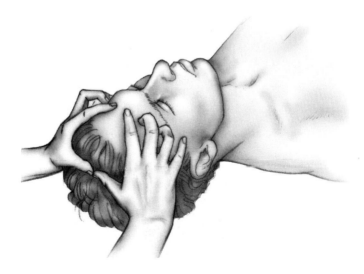

FIGURE 10–15. Cranial polarization.

15. ***Brushing off to finish.*** Wait a few moments, and then in a quiet voice ask the person to sit up with his legs off the side of the table. Standing behind him, place your hands on his shoulders. With a sweeping motion, brush your hands across the spine then down to the sacrum, and out to the crest of the hips. Repeat several times. See Figure 10–16. Standing in front of him, place his hands on his knees. Place your hands on his shoulders, and in a sweeping manner, brush down his arms to the knees and down his legs. Repeat several times. See Figure 10–17.

If you decide to explore these techniques, remember the primary principle of love. If you get confused, let yourself laugh. If you find the rhythm difficult, re- member to let your breathing relax, your shoulders down. If you are relaxed and ac- cept yourself, the receiver will benefit, regardless of your skill level. Do the best you can in a simple way, and be kind to yourself. Although you are not "the healer," you may find yourself being healed while giving polarity. You may find that in the circle of love and self-acceptance your own obstructions begin to disappear and you are no longer sure who is "giving" polarity to whom.

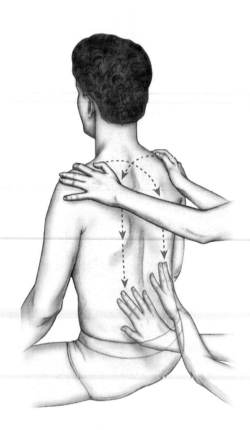

FIGURE 10–16. Brushing off the back.

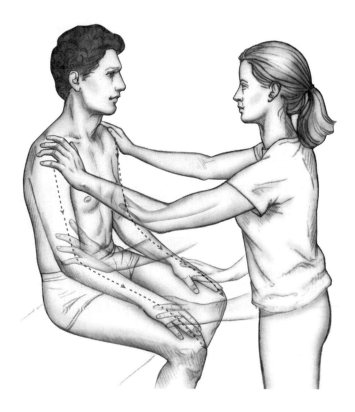

FIGURE 10–17. Brushing off the front.

You may integrate any of these movements into a classic Western full-body massage. You may find them useful for beginning or ending a session, or before the receiver turns over from prone to supine. During a full-body session, you may sense energy blockages and use one or more of these basic techniques to try to allow energy to flow freely again. Once you are familiar with them, you can insert them where it seems like the right thing to do.

▪ SOME FINAL THOUGHTS

The unique gift of polarity therapy is its simplicity. Behind the techniques and esoterica is an opening and surrendering to life and to being at home with our natural energies. The ideal supplement to this brief introduction would be to receive a session from a professional polarity therapist, as it is very difficult to convey in writing what the experience of polarity is like. Polarity therapy is truly an art form, requiring much study and dedicated practice to master the rhythm and quality of touch that are so important to the effects. In addition, the hands-on work is only a small part of the therapy, which usually includes basic nutritional guidance, exercise, and support for emotional balancing.

■ SUMMARY

Polarity therapy is a holistic bodywork approach that involves simple touching and gentle movements such as rocking and pressing. Polarity techniques are designed to release obstructions to the free flow of energy through the body, thus supporting health and healing.

Objective changes in the body observed during polarity sessions indicate deep relaxation and include flushed cheeks, drop in blood pressure, increased salivation, muscle relaxation, slower heart rate, and grumbling in the digestive system associated with the activity of peristalsis. Western science may find physiologic reasons for some of these effects such as stimulation of nerve centers and mechanoreceptors in joints.

The basic principles of polarity therapy are related to the concepts of energy, love, working with obstructions, understanding, and nutrition and exercise. The techniques involve gentle holding, rocking, and probing movements that are combined into relaxing sessions. Techniques also aid the practitioner in locating areas that appear to be obstructed and in need of further work.

Polarity techniques may be used alone or integrated into a traditional Western massage. The unique gift of polarity is its simplicity.

■ BIBLIOGRAPHY

Gordon, R. (1979) *Your healing hands: The polarity experience.* Santa Cruz, CA: Unity Press.

Siedman, M. (1982). *Like a hollow flute: A guide to polarity therapy.* Santa Cruz, CA: Elan Press.

Siegel, A. (1986). *Live energy: The power that heals.* Bridgeport, Dorset, England: Prism Press/Colin Spooner.

Myofascial Techniques

Myofascial techniques address the body's fascial system, that is, the fibrous connective tissue that holds the body together and gives it shape. The general intent of myofascial techniques is to restore mobility in the fascia and to soften connective tissue that has become rigid. These techniques remove restrictions in the fascia that cause limited mobility, postural distortion, poor cellular nutrition, pain, and a variety of other dysfunctions.

▪ HISTORY

There have been several manual techniques or systems of treatments that have focused on the fascia of the body. For example, connective tissue massage (CTM), sometimes known as Bindegewebsmassage, was developed by Elizabeth Dicke of Germany in the late 1920s and 1930s. CTM, as Dicke taught it, is the systematic application of light strokes without oil to various areas of the skin. CTM is thought to improve circulation in subcutaneous connective tissue, which may result in reflex actions to other parts of the body including the visceral organs. CTM is currently popular in Europe, although it has been slow to catch on in the United States (Cantu & Grodin, 1992).

Renewed interest in the body's fascial system appeared in the mid-twentieth century. Structural integration, or Rolfing, was developed by Ida Rolf (1896–1979) and taught at the Esalen Institute in the 1960s. Rolfing seeks to reestablish proper vertical alignment in the body by manipulating the myofascial tissue so that the fascia elongates and glides, rather than shortens and adheres. Rolf's work spawned a number of other systems of bodywork that address realignment of the structure of the body through manipulation of the deep fascia.

The term *myofascial release* is said to have been coined by osteopath Robert Ward in the 1960s to describe his system of treating the body's fascial system. In the 1980s, the term *myofascial release* (MFR) was adopted by a physical therapist named John Barnes as the designation for his method of freeing restrictions in the myofascial system. The overall intention of MFR according to Barnes is to relieve pain, resolve structural dysfunction, restore function and mobility, and release emotional trauma (Knaster, 1996).

Variations of myofascial techniques continue to be developed and are known variously as myofascial release, myofascial unwinding, myofascial manipulation, and myofascial massage. They all view a healthy fascial system as integral to good health.

■ THE NATURE OF FASCIA

Fascia is loose irregular connective tissue found just about everywhere in the body. It is described by Cantu and Grodin as sparse, with a loose arrangement of collagen fibers, and with greater amounts of elastin than the dense regular connective tissue found in ligaments and tendons (1992). Figure 11–1 illustrates the multidirectionality and low density of fibers in typical fascia.

Fascia has a greater amount of ground substance than other types of connective tissue and is the immediate environment of every cell in the body. It forms the interstitial spaces and has important functions in support, protection, separation, cellular respiration, elimination, metabolism, fluid flow, and immune-system function. Any restriction or dysfunction of the fascia can lead to a variety of problems, including poor exchange of cellular nutrients and wastes, pain, and poor mobility.

Fascia surrounds every muscle, nerve, blood vessel, and organ. It holds structures together, giving them their characteristic shapes, offers support, and connects the body as a whole. It can be thought of as winding through the body in a continuous sheet. Sheets of fascia are formed by hydrogen bonds between collagen fibers. These bonds give all connective tissue its tremendous strength.

Fascia displays an intriguing characteristic called *thixotrophy,* that is, it can change from a more solid to a more liquid gel consistency. It becomes more pliable with movement and increase in temperature (Juhan, 1987).

Three types of fascia are subcutaneous fascia, deep fascia, and subserous fascia. Subcutaneous fascia is a continuous layer of connective tissue over the entire body between the skin and the deep fascia. Deep fascia is an intricate series of connective sheets and bands that hold the muscles and other structures in place throughout the body. Subserous fascia lies between the deep fascia and the serous membranes lining the body cavities in much the same manner as the subcutaneous fascia lies between the skin and the deep fascia (Anderson & Anderson, 1990).

John Barnes defines another layer of fascia that he calls *deepest fascia,* which is within the dura mater of the craniosacral system (cranium, spine, and sacrum) (1987). It is interesting to note that one researcher reported finding cerebrospinal

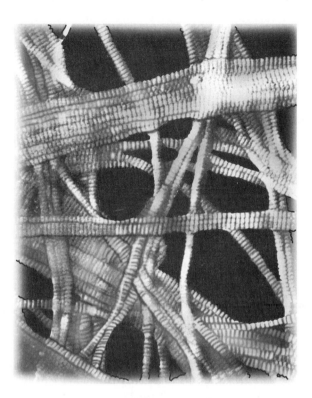

FIGURE 11–1. Illustration of multidirectionality and low density of fibers in typical fascia, that is, loose irregular connective tissue.

fluid inside collagen fibrils, which suggests that the connective tissue framework may function as a circulatory system carrying chemical messages throughout the body (Juhan, 1987). There is clearly much more to learn about this important system of the body.

The pervasiveness and interconnectedness of fascia throughout the body creates a situation in which restriction in one part of the body can affect other parts as well. A metaphor often used to describe the fascia is a knitted sweater. Because all of the threads of yarn are connected, a pull in one section of the sweater may cause a pull in a spot distant from the original, or distortion of the shape of the entire sweater.

▪ MYOFASCIAL TECHNIQUES

Myofascial techniques are generally applied using very little, if any, lubricant. Practitioners must be able to feel subtle restrictions in the movement of fascial tissues and the "letting go" or "melting" that occurs as the fascia elongates and becomes more pliable. Such palpation is hindered by sliding over the skin, which tends to happen when oil is used. Myofascial techniques also require traction on the skin as tissues are slowly and gently pushed, pulled, and stretched.

A simple technique used to free subcutaneous fascia is skin rolling, as shown in Figure 6–15. The skin is gently picked up and pulled away from underlying structures. This technique stretches the subcutaneous fascia, breaks cross-links, and makes the tissue more pliable. Increase in local circulation is evidenced by increased redness in the area.

Some myofascial techniques involve a sustained stretch. Figure 11–2 shows a horizontal stretch of the fascia of the back. While one hand anchors the skin near the sacrum, the other hand slowly pushes the skin and underlying tissue horizontally and superior, that is, toward the head. The stretch is held at the point of resistance. You may feel a subtle release of tissues after a few seconds. Then move to a different spot, working your way along the back toward the shoulders.

Restrictions in the deep fascia may be located by visual analysis of the receiver's posture, observing where fascia may be shortened. Restrictions may also be detected through palpation of tissues, finding where tissues seem to "stick together" or resist lengthening.

Once restrictions are located, they are released by applying gentle pressure into the direction of the restriction, usually with a sliding motion that stretches the tissues. Figure 11–3 shows a technique for releasing deep fascial restrictions in the upper back using the forearm. The forearm applies enough pressure to engage deeper connective tissues and slides along, slowly stretching the tissues underneath. Little if any lubricant is used to prevent the arm from sliding over the skin superfi-

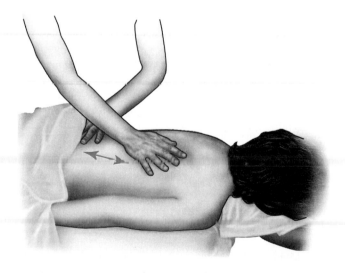

FIGURE 11–2. Horizontal stretch of the superficial fascia of the back.

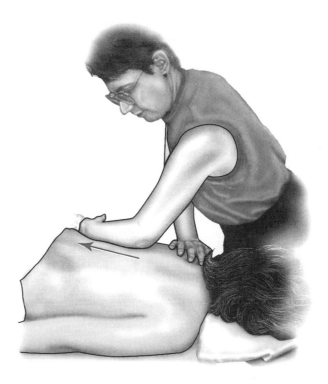

FIGURE 11-3. Using the forearm to release deep fascial restrictions in the upper back.

cially. Stretching helps elongate deep fascial tissues and frees cross-links within the tissues.

In addition to the mechanical effects of stretching the tissues, techniques applied with the practitioner's hand also impart heat to the area. The stretching and heat together help produce a softer consistency of fascial tissue and free restrictions.

In his *Myofascial Massage Therapy* training manual, Bob King (1996, p. 2) recommends that the practitioner make gentle contact, enter slowly until a point or area of resistance is felt, and wait for a feeling of *melting* (ie, softening or "giving") in tissues. He advises to shift tissues horizontally and that "pressure should be used to get you to the layer you need to work on. Once you're there, direction is what's most important." When finished, exit the tissues with as much care and awareness as when you melted into it.

Barnes describes the process as follows: "At first the elastic component of the fascia will release, and at some point in time the collagenous barrier will be engaged. This barrier cannot be forced (it is too strong). One waits with gentle pressure, and as the collagenous aspect releases, the therapist follows the motion of the tissue, barrier upon barrier until freedom is felt" (1987).

This approach has also been described as *myofascial unwinding,* referring to the unwinding of abnormal twists and turns of the fascia from a three-dimensional view of the body. The unwinding restores structural integrity and proper alignment and promotes improved functioning of tissues and organs.

Myofascial techniques may be integrated into a general full-body massage or may be used as the primary approach in a session or treatment. For best results, myofascial release techniques are often combined with soft-tissue mobilization, trigger point therapy, and craniosacral manipulation. Proper exercise, nutrition, relaxation, and psychotherapy may also be involved for a complete approach to a problem for which myofascial release is indicated.

▪ SUMMARY

Myofascial techniques are used to restore mobility in the body's fascial system and to soften connective tissue that has become rigid. These techniques remove restrictions in the fascia that cause limited mobility, postural distortion, poor cellular nutrition, pain, and a variety of other dysfunctions.

Myofascial techniques involve the slow, horizontal stretching of tissues and are generally applied using little, if any, lubricant. Practitioners must be able to feel subtle restrictions in the movement of fascial tissues and the "letting go" or "melting" that occurs as the fascia elongates and becomes more pliable.

The stretching of tissues and the heat imparted by the practitioner's hands are thought to help produce a softer consistency of fascial tissues, which allows them to elongate more easily. As the tissues stretch, cross-links within the tissues are freed. Myofascial unwinding refers to the process of freeing fascial tissues systematically over the whole body, thus restoring structural integrity and proper alignment.

▪ REFERENCES

Anderson, K. N., & Anderson, L. E. (1990). *Mosby's pocket dictionary of medicine, nursing, & allied health.* St. Louis: C.V. Mosby.

Barnes, J. F. (1987). Myofascial release. *Physical Therapy Forum,* September 16.

Cantu, R. I., & Grodin, A. J. (1992). *Myofascial manipulation: Theory and clinical application.* Gaithersburg, MD: Aspen Publishers.

Juhan, D. (1987). *Job's body.* Barrytown, NY: Station Hill Press.

King, R. K. (1996). *Myofascial massage therapy: Towards postural balance.* Self-published training manual by Bobkat Productions, Chicago.

Knaster, M. (1996). *Discovering the body's wisdom.* New York: Bantam Books.

Trigger Points

Knowledge of trigger points and skill in deactivating them are essential for any practitioner performing therapeutic massage to relieve myofascial pain. Trigger points are often present with the muscular pain caused by trauma, poor posture, repetitive injuries, and overwork of certain muscles. Practitioners who work with athletes, musicians, and others who repeatedly overload their muscles will find trigger point work invaluable.

■ HISTORY

The origins of neuromuscular technique (NMT) can be traced in Europe to a natural healer named Stanley Lief, who was born in Latvia in the 1890s. Lief studied physical culture with Bernarr Macfadden in the United States and was trained in chiropractic and naturopathy. He established a world-famous natural healing resort in 1925 in Champneys in Hertfordshire, England. There he developed soft tissue manipulative methods that closely resemble what is known in the United States today as trigger point therapy. NMT was part of a holistic approach to healing, incorporating diet, emotional health, and hydrotherapy, as well as soft tissue manipulation (Chaitow, 1996).

Janet Travell, MD, who pioneered trigger point therapy in the Unites States, published her first work on the subject in 1952. Dr. Travell is credited with relieving the debilitating pain of the young Senator John F. Kennedy, who was injured in World War II. Dr. Travell was later appointed White House physician to both Presidents Kennedy and Johnson in the 1960s. These appointments brought Dr. Travell's work to the attention of the public (Claire, 1995, p. 42). Travell, along with David

Simons, MD, has written the definitive work on trigger point therapy in two volumes (1983, 1992). They are a wise investment for any practitioner who addresses myofascial pain and dysfunction.

■ TRIGGER POINTS

Even with no complaints of pain, practitioners will often find small spots in muscles that are sore or radiate pain when pressed. In the absence of other obvious causes, for example, bruising, trigger points should be suspected. These points of tenderness may be palpated easily as tense bands of tissue in muscles and tendons and may be relieved through a variety of methods. A trigger point is defined by Travell and Simons as:

> *a focus of hyperirritability in a tissue that, when compressed, is locally tender and, if sufficiently hypersensitive, gives rise to referred pain and tenderness, and sometimes to referred autonomic phenomena and distortion of proprioception. (1983, p. 4)*

Referral Patterns

Trigger points may cause local pain and may also cause referred pain in their zone of reference. For example, tension headaches are often caused by trigger points in the trapezius and muscles of the neck. The referred pain of myofascial trigger points is described as "dull and aching, often deep, with intensity varying from low-grade discomfort to severe and incapacitating torture. It may occur at rest or only in motion" (Travell and Simons, 1983, p. 13).

Trigger points may elicit pain on being pressed or may be tender and radiate pain without pressure. Pressing on an active trigger point usually intensifies pain in the reference zone of the trigger point. The involved muscle may be stiff and weak and may be restricted in range of motion. Attempts to actively or passively stretch the muscle usually increase the pain felt. Muscles in the immediate area of a trigger point often feel tense and ropelike.

Other sensory, motor, and autonomic phenomena may be "triggered" by active trigger points. These include pain, tenderness, increased motor unit activity (spasm), vasoconstriction (blanching), coldness, sweating, pilomotor response, vasodilation, and hypersecretion. These effects often occur at a distance from the trigger point, but within the general area to which a specific trigger point refers pain (Travell and Simons, 1992, p. 5).

Figure 12-1 shows some of the common trigger point locations. While trigger point charts are useful for confirming common locations and referral patterns, you may find points and patterns unique to each receiver.

Varieties of Trigger Points

Trigger points may be described as latent or active, primary or secondary, satellite, or associated. *Latent* trigger points are painful only when pressed. *Active* trigger points are always tender, prevent full lengthening, weaken the muscle, and refer

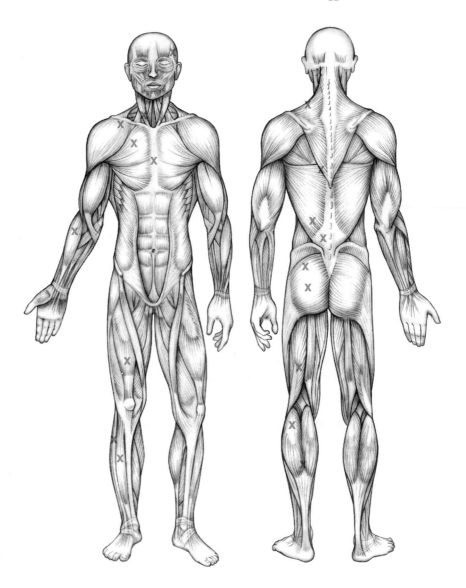

FIGURE 12–1. Common trigger point locations, anterior and posterior.

pain on direct compression. *Primary* trigger points are activated by acute or chronic overload of a muscle, while *secondary* ones become active because of their reaction to a muscle containing a primary trigger point. A *satellite* trigger point becomes active because the muscle is in a zone of reference of another trigger point. *Associated* trigger points refer to secondary or satellite points (Travell & Simons 1983, pp. 1–4).

Activation of Trigger Points

Trigger points may be activated by direct stimuli such as acute overload or over-work fatigue of a muscle, chilling, and gross trauma. Indirect stimuli may also acti-vate trigger points, for example, arthritic joints, emotional distress, certain visceral diseases, and other trigger points (Travell and Simons, 1983, p. 15).

People who perform repetitive stressful tasks such as athletes, musicians, and certain workers are prone to trigger points. Poor postural alignment, such as while sitting at a desk or driving a car, that puts undue stress on muscles may also elicit trigger points. Forward head posture, which places the upper body in a round-shouldered, slumped forward position, is known to produce trigger points in the pectoral and posterior cervical muscles (Travell & Simons, 1992, p. 20). Something as simple as carrying a heavy purse or briefcase on the same side all the time can cause the muscle overload that leads to trigger points.

Locating Trigger Points

Suspect myofascial trigger points when clients or patients complain of muscle ten-sion causing pain or localized muscle soreness and shortening, or when they de-scribe one of the common pain patterns associated with trigger points. Self-reports of when and how the pain developed may also give clues as to its origin. For exam-ple, reports of a fall or blow to a muscle, a repetitive motion, or sustained immobile posture such as in driving or sitting at a workstation all point to the possibility of trigger points.

It is useful to have recipients map out areas of pain on a blank chart, which can help the practitioner locate probable active trigger point sites. The more knowledge-able the practitioner is about trigger points and their predictable referral patterns, the more easily the exact points may be located.

Ultimately, precise trigger point locations are discovered by palpation. You may locate points from clues given from verbal reports or charts, or you may hap-pen upon latent trigger points in the course of a massage session. The taut bands of tissue characterizing trigger points can be felt. Recipients can give feedback on the exact location of the point, the degree of pain experienced, the referral pattern upon pressure, and the diminishing pain upon deactivation.

Recipients will often say something like "you're almost on it, but not quite." A slight change in location or angle of pressure is often enough to get the exact point. Often the pain reported is out of proportion to the pressure applied, and pressure elicits a "jump sign" or outcry from the recipient. With pressure directly on the trig-ger point, recipients may report increased pain in the same area or pain referral to another area.

Deactivation Techniques

It is important to locate and deactivate *primary* trigger points whether *latent* or *ac-tive*. For total relief from pain and to restore full function to a muscle, associated points (ie, secondary and satellite) must also be relieved once they are activated.

Trigger points may be deactivated by a variety of nonmanual methods, including spray and stretch, saline injection, dry needling, and anesthetics. Manual techniques found to be effective in deactivating trigger points include ischemic compression using the hands or a tool, deep stroking massage (stripping), deep friction at the trigger point site, and vibration. These techniques are typically followed by a stretch of the affected tissues.

The stretch of the affected tissues seems to be especially important to complete the deactivation of the trigger point and return the affected tissues to a normal state. Other deactivation methods that focus on stretching, and are mentioned by Travell and Simons (1992), include contract–relax, reciprocal inhibition, relaxation during exhalation, percussion and stretch, muscle energy technique, and myofascial release.

Ischemic Compression Techniques. Ischemic compression techniques are those methods in which compression of the tissues at the trigger point site causes blanching with hypoxia, followed by a reactive hyperemia (Travell and Simons 1983, p. 27). In other words, the compressed tissues become white from lack of blood and oxygen, followed by an increase in blood flow to the area once pressure is released. Ischemic compression may be created with sustained digital pressure, with a tool, or with a pincer technique.

Travell and Simons recommended application of pressure for about 20 seconds to 1 minute.

> *Pressure is gradually increased as the sensitivity of the TrP wanes and the tension in its taut band fades. Pressure is released when the clinician feels the TrP tension subside or when the TrP is no longer tender to pressure. . . . Sustained pressure should not be applied to blood vessels or a nerve; it may induce numbness and tingling. Ischemic compression should be followed by lengthening of the muscle, except when stretching is contraindicated, as in hypermobility. (1992, p. 9)*

The thumbs are commonly used to provide the sustained digital pressure in deactivating trigger points. Figure 9–14 illustrates the use of the thumb in applying direct pressure to trigger points on the suboccipital muscles.

To relieve the thumbs, other parts of the hands may be used to apply pressure, for example, the fingertips. For more heavily muscled areas, the elbow may be used. Figure 12–2 shows the use of the elbow with the recipient in the seated position to deactivate trigger points in the large trapezius muscle. The elbow is also useful when working through larger muscles to affect deeper muscles in an area, for example, to reach the deeper muscles of the gluteal area.

To protect the small joints of the hands from overuse, small hand tools may be used effectively for applying pressure. If used with sensitivity, tissues may be palpated through the tool, and the quality of touch may be indistinguishable from manual techniques. It is important to keep the wrists straight when using tools. Figure 12–3 demonstrates the use of a wooden hand tool to apply pressure to trigger points.

In all of the above examples, the tissue containing the trigger point is compressed between the practitioner's hand and tissues underneath the point. The pres-

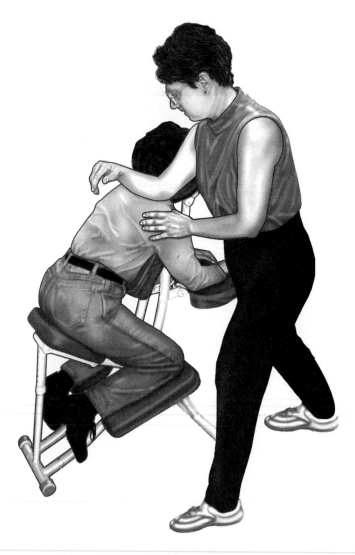

FIGURE 12–2. Use of the elbow to apply pressure to trigger points in the trapezius, sitting position.

sure is deep into the underlying soft tissue or bone. In the *pincer technique,* the tissue at the trigger point site is compressed between the fingers and thumb of the practitioner. For example, trigger points in the sternocleidomastoid may be compressed using the pincer technique as shown in Figure 12–4.

Other Manual Techniques. Deep friction, deep stroking or stripping, vibration, and stretching are other manual techniques often used in deactivating trigger points.

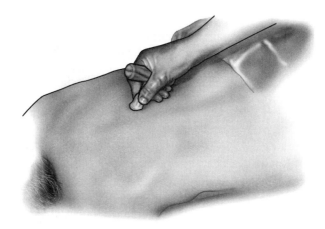

FIGURE 12–3. Use of a hand tool to apply pressure to trigger points.

These techniques are applied in conjunction with ischematic compression techniques for best results.

These techniques can be combined to help to release the actual trigger point, separate tissues that may be adhering, and improve circulation to the area to remove metabolic waste and bring nutrients for tissue maintenance and repair. Since muscle shortening is often a result of trigger points, stretching is an important finishing technique to help bring affected muscles back to full length.

A systematic approach to addressing trigger points was developed by Bonnie Prudden in the 1970–80s. Prudden's two books, *Pain Erasure* (1980) and *Myotherapy* (1984), offer practical descriptions of how to locate and relieve common trigger

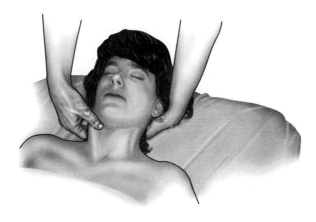

FIGURE 12–4. Squeezing the sternocleidomastoid (SCM) with a pincer technique.

points in different parts of the body. The books contain detailed descriptions of manual pressure techniques, as well as follow-up stretches and exercises.

Other systems of relieving trigger points have been promoted by their developers and have various names. A common generic designation for trigger point work is *neuromuscular therapy.*

▪ SUMMARY

Knowledge of trigger points and skill in deactivating them are essential for any practitioner performing therapeutic massage to relieve myofascial pain. Trigger points are spots of tenderness in muscles and tendons, which can be palpated as tense bands of tissue. These points often refer pain to an associated target zone when pressed. Trigger points may be classified as latent or active, primary or secondary, satellite, or associated.

Trigger points may be activated by direct stimuli such as muscle overload, trauma, or chilling. People who perform repetitive tasks, or who stress their muscles from poor postural alignment, often have active trigger points.

Trigger points may be deactivated by ischematic compression techniques. The thumbs, fingertips, elbow, or small hand tools may be used to apply direct pressure to trigger points. Other methods used include deep friction, deep stroking or stripping, fine vibration, and stretching. Since muscle shortening is often a result of trigger points, stretching is an important finishing technique to help bring affected muscles back to full length.

Trigger point therapy is also known as neuromuscular technique or neuromuscular therapy. Books by Travell (1983, 1992) and Bonnie Prudden (1980, 1984) describe trigger point theory and methods in greater detail.

▪ REFERENCES

Chaitow, L. (1996). *Modern neuromuscular techniques.* London: Churchill Livingston.

Claire, T. (1995). *Bodywork: What type of massage to get and how to make the most of it.* New York: William Morrow.

Prudden, B. (1980). *Pain erasure: The Bonnie Prudden way.* New York: M. Evans.

Prudden, B. (1984). *Myotherapy: Bonnie Prudden's complete guide to pain-free living.* New York: Ballantine Books.

Travell, J. G., & Rinzler, S. H. (1952). The myofascial genesis of pain. *Postgraduate Medicine, 11,* 425–434.

Travell, J. G., & Simons, D. G. (1983). *Myofascial pain and dysfunction: The trigger point manual.* Baltimore: Williams & Wilkins.

Travell, J. G., & Simons, D. G. (1992). *Myofascial pain and dysfunction, the trigger point manual: The lower extremities.* Vol. 2. Baltimore: Williams & Wilkins.

Manual Lymph Drainage

Manual lymph drainage (MLD) is a form of massage designed to assist the function of the lymphatic system. MLD techniques consist of slow, light, and repetitive strokes that help move lymph fluid through the system of vessels and nodes. It is a gentle and rhythmic massage used for general wellness, to remove accumulation of fluid in the tissues, to improve healing, and to treat lymphedema.

■ HISTORY

Forms of massage developed specifically to stimulate the movement of lymph fluid are found in different parts of the world, for example, Ayurvedic from India, Huna from Hawaii, and Vodder Manual Lymph Drainage (MLD) from France (Knaster, 1996). As early as 1894, massage and exercise were scientifically observed to increase the flow of lymph (Kurz et al, 1978). The most common method of manual lymph drainage used today was developed by Danish physiotherapists Emil and Astid Vodder in France in the 1930s.

■ THE LYMPHATIC SYSTEM

The lymphatic system consists of a network of vessels that function in the circulation of body fluids. Excess fluid, or lymph, is transported away from interstitial spaces and returned to the bloodstream through these lymphatic pathways. Lymph is a clear colorless fluid, which functions to remove excess fluid, bacteria, viruses, and waste products from body tissues and transports proteins back to blood circulation.

Lymph vessels are arranged in superficial and deep systems. A typical lymphatic movement may be described as follows: Tissue fluid leaves the interstitial spaces and is called lymph after it enters the lymphatic capillaries. The capillaries merge into larger vessels called afferent vessels, which take the lymph to nodes, where it is filtered. Efferent vessels then move the fluid to larger vessels called trunk vessels, which merge into collecting ducts, which empty into the subclavian vein, where lymph is added to the blood. The large lymphatic vessels have valves, similar to those in veins, which prevent backflow of lymph fluid.

The movement of the lymph is largely a passive process that requires outside forces. These forces include the contraction of skeletal muscle, the action of the diaphragm in breathing, and contraction of smooth muscles in the walls of larger lymphatic vessels. Massage may also act as an outside force to move lymph along in the vessels.

The lymphatic and circulatory systems function together to ensure the healthy circulation of fluids in the body. The uninterrupted movement of lymph is necessary for the proper functioning of the immune system, tissue repair, and maintenance of a proper fluid and chemical environment for the cells.

Abnormal accumulation of lymph fluid in tissues results in a condition called lymphedema. Lymphedema may be caused by injury, scarring, chronic infections, or surgery involving lymph nodes of the neck, axilla, pelvis, or groin. Many of the treatments for breast cancer result in lymphedema.

▪ MANUAL LYMPH DRAINAGE

Vodder's manual lymph drainage (MLD) could be regarded as one of the classical large-surface massage methods (Wittinger & Wittinger, 1986). To the casual observer, these techniques may resemble the milder manipulations of classic Western massage. However, a closer examination reveals that MLD is considerably more exact and includes techniques not found elsewhere. The effects of MLD described here presuppose that this method is applied in its original form, as taught at the Vodder School in Walchee, Austria.

MLD as developed by Vodder is a gentle method of promoting the movement of lymph into and through the lympahtic vessels. Figure 13–1 illustrates the body's superficial lymph drainage pathways. Very light pressure is used in applying MLD techniques, which directly affect the superficial vessels. Pressure on the deeper muscle layers is avoided. A general description of the process is provided by Kurz et al (1978):

The massage starts at the left supraclavicular space, draining the ductus thoracicus into the venae axillaris and subclavia. Next the stagnation created at the regional lymph nodes, either inguinal or subaxillar, is gently alleviated. Finally, the proximal, then the distal parts of the limbs are massaged. (p. 767)

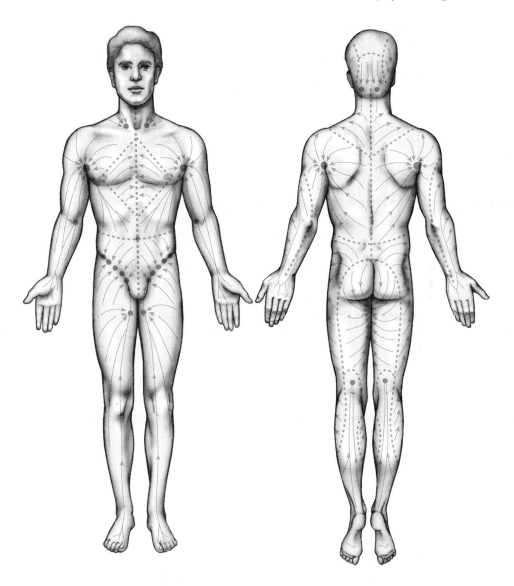

FIGURE 13–1. Schematic representation of the body's superficial lymph drainage pathways, front and rear views (From Vodder, E., *Die manuelle lymph drainage ad modum Vodder*).

The specific techniques used to effect the movement of lymph are described in more detail below. Note: Manual lymphatic drainage (MLD) should not be attempted without specific training by a qualified person, especially when used to address a medical condition such as lymphedema. Descriptions of techniques cannot teach that which must be demonstrated and practiced until the teacher is assured that the student has acquired the skill to perform the technique safely.

MLD Techniques

Vodder's Manual Lymph Drainage consists of four manual techniques used to gently move lymph fluid into and through the superficial vessels. These techniques are performed in combinations of round or oval, small or large, deep or shallow circular movements. The skin is pressed lightly during the movements. The techniques are called stationary circles and the pump, scoop, and rotary techniques.

STATIONARY CIRCLES. The fingers are placed flatly on the skin and the skin is pushed either in the same place as "stationary circles" or as expanding spirals. These manipulations are used primarily for treating the neck, face, and lymph nodes. The stationary circles are varied on the body and extremities by making circles hand on hand or with eight fingers placed next to each other. In the latter case, the fingers can press the skin circularly in one direction working together or alternately. The direction of pressure is determined by the lymph drainage. The fingers lie flat; sometimes the whole hand does. Each of these circles is executed with a smooth increase of pressure into the tissue and a smooth decrease of pressure. See Figure 13–2 for an illustration of stationary circles.

PUMP TECHNIQUE. With this technique, the palms are facing downward. The thumb and fingers move together in the same direction, pressing the skin in oblong circles. This movement of thumb and fingers is controlled by the exaggerated movements of the wrist. The fingers are outstretched; the fingertips have no function in this technique. The wrist moves like a hinge. The forward motion of the fingers is carried out under pressure, the forward motion of the wrist without pressure.

SCOOP TECHNIQUE. In contrast to the pump technique, the palm is facing upward in the scoop technique (see Figure 13–3). Vodder describes the movement as a "giving

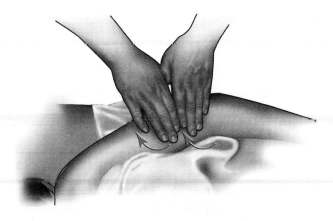

FIGURE 13–2. Stationary circles, manual lymph drainage.

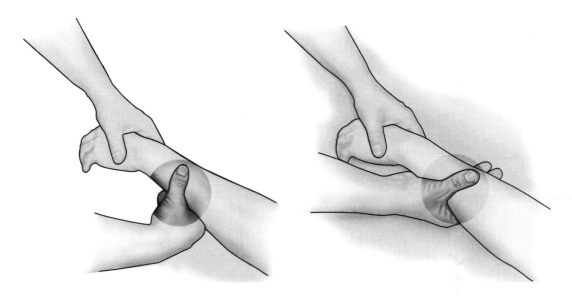

FIGURE 13–3. Scoop technique, manual lymph drainage.

motion." The rotating wrist effects a corkscrew movement of the wrist–hand unit. The fingers are outstretched and swing toward the body during the pressure phase—with pressure in and without pressure out.

ROTARY TECHNIQUE. This technique is used on relatively flat areas of the body and consists of various individual movements. The wrist moves up and down. As it moves downward, it swings from the outside toward the inside. The whole palm lies on the skin and presses it spirally inward. The thumb also makes circular movements in the direction of the lymph drainage of the skin. These motions are performed during the pressure phase. In the pressureless phase the wrist is raised, the four outstretched fingers keep on moving, and the thumb begins a new pressure cycle by completing the circular motion begun.

Basic Principles

The following are some basic principles to keep in mind when performing manual lymph drainage. They are adapted from Kurz, *Introduction to Manual Lymph Drainage* (1986, 1990).

- The proximal area is treated before the distal so that the proximal area is emptied to make room for the fluid flowing in from the distal end.
- MLD prescribes a certain pressure intensity limited to 30–40 torr.
- Each circular movement has a pressure intensity such that when the skin is released, the skin "snaps back." Think of moving only the skin with the pressure applied.

- The direction of pressure depends on the efferent lymph vessels susceptible to the massage pressure.
- The techniques and variations are repeated rhythmically, usually five to seven times, either at the same location in stationary circles or in expanding spirals. It is pointless to repeat the movements less frequently, because the inertial mass of the tissue fluid needs some time before it responds.
- The pressure phase of a circle lasts longer than the relaxation phase.
- As a rule, no reddening of the skin should appear.
- MLD should not elicit pain.

Massage Dosage

Since the effect of MLD is largely derived from the mechanical displacement of fluids and the substances they carry, it is essential that the manual techniques developed by Vodder be precisely executed. Experience shows that the more exact the technique, the better the results. The use of a certain pressure depends on the state of the tissue to be treated. One could say the softer the tissue, the softer the massage.

The length of time spent on a particular body part, the amount of pressure used, and the speed of the movements can all be explained in general terms. However, theoretical lessons are only an aid in explaining the effect of MLD and preparing the ground for an understanding of the value and use of MLD in physical therapy and health care. In practice, no two cases are identical. Ultimately, the dosage of MLD is best determined by practitioners using their knowledge, skill, experience, and intuition. Any description of MLD must be read and understood with this in mind.

▪ SUMMARY

Manual lymph drainage (MLD) is a form of massage designed to assist the function of the lymphatic system. MLD techniques consist of slow, light, and repetitive strokes that help move lymph fluid through the system of vessels and nodes.

Vodder's Manual Lymph Drainage is a systematic application of techniques using very light pressure to move the lymph fluid gently through the superficial lymph vessels. The four main techniques used are stationary circles and the pump, scoop, and rotary techniques.

When applying MLD, the proximal area is treated before the distal area to make room for the fluid flowing in from the distal end. Techniques are repeated rhythmically usually five to seven times. The amount of pressure used depends on the condition of the tissues with softer tissues requiring softer pressure. The skin does not usually redden, and there should be no pain during the application of techniques.

Vodder's MLD should be executed precisely for best results. The dosage of MLD is best determined by practitioners using their knowledge, skill, experience, and intuition.

■ REFERENCES

Knaster, M. (1996). *Discovering the body's wisdom.* New York: Bantam Books.

Kurz, W., Wittlinger, G., Litmanovitch, Y.I., et al. (1978). Effect of manual lymph drainage massage on urinary excretion of neurohormones and minerals in chronic lymphedema. *Angiology, 29,* 64–72.

Kurz, I. (1986). *Introduction to Dr. Vodder's manual lymphatic drainage.* Vol. 2, Therapy 1. Heidelberg: Haug Publishers.

Kurz, I. (1990). *Introduction to Dr. Vodder's manual lymphatic drainage.* Vol. 3, Therapy 2. Heidelberg: Haug Publishers.

Wittinger, H., & Wittinger, G. (1986). *Introduction to Dr. Vodder's manual lymphatic drainage.* Vol. 1, 3rd rev. ed. Heidelberg: Haug Publishers.

Foot Reflexology

Foot reflexology is based on the theory that pressure applied to specific spots on the feet stimulates corresponding areas in other parts of the body. For example, pressing the center of the pad of the big toe is believed to stimulate the pituitary gland. This action is thought to help normalize function and increase circulation in the part of the body affected.

Maps of the feet, like the one in Figure 14–1, help practitioners identify which part of the body is being stimulated as they press on different spots on the foot. Practitioners may use reflexology as part of a full-body or foot massage or may perform an entire session using the theory and techniques of foot reflexology.

■ HISTORY

Massaging or pressing the feet is an ancient health practice found in many parts of the world. For example, a wall painting found in an ancient Egyptian tomb depicts two seated men receiving massage of their feet. The painting is from the tomb of Ankh-ma-hor from the Sixth Dynasty, 2587–2453 B.C.E. (Knaster 1996, p. 310).

The current practice of foot reflexology has its origin in the work of Eunice Ingham (1889–1974). Ingham was a physiotherapist who lived in Rochester, New York, and spent her winters in St. Petersburg, Florida. There she worked for an eclectic natural healer named Dr. Joseph Shelby Riley. Riley introduced her to the theory of zone therapy popularized in the United States by William Fitzgerald, MD, in the early 1900s. Fitzgerald was a respected physician and senior nose and throat

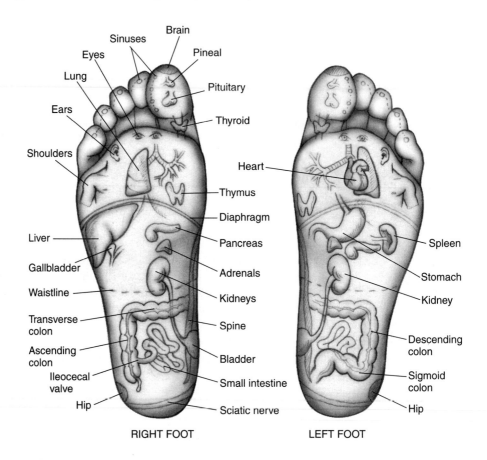

FIGURE 14–1. Reflexology map of the feet showing what area to press to stimulate the corresponding part of the body.

surgeon at St. Francis Hospital in Hartford, Connecticut. He wrote the book *Zone Therapy* in 1917 with Edwin Bowers.

Ingham is credited with taking the theory of zone therapy and combining it with compression massage of the feet, developing the prototype for reflexology systems today. Through clinical experience, she was able to make a detailed map of the feet and chart which areas of the body were affected by pressure on specific spots on the feet.

Ingham developed her method of reflexology in the years preceding World War II and, once the war was over, traveled across the United States by car teaching reflexology in workshops. Her primary audience in those early days was from the ranks of natural healers and proponents of natural health practices (Benjamin 1989a, b).

▪ THEORY

Foot reflexology was developed from the theory of *zone therapy*. According to Drs. William Fitzgerald and Edwin Bowers (1917), the body can be thought of as divided lengthwise into 10 zones, five on each side of the body. The zones have endpoints in the feet, hands, and top of the head. See Figure 14–2.

Pressure applied anywhere in the zone will affect the entire zone. Direct pressure on the endpoints will produce reflex actions along the whole length of their corresponding zones. Therefore, pressure applied to the feet can affect structures and organs in the whole body. The feet have proved an especially sensitive and easily accessed place to apply the pressure.

Charts based on zone theory have been developed that show which areas of the feet correspond to the different structures and areas of the body. These maps provide an easy reference for practitioners to know which part of the body is being affected by pressure applied to specific spots on the feet (see Figure 14–1).

Explanations of how reflexology works are still speculation. Ingham believed that with compression massage she was dissolving crystalline deposits in the feet that interfered with nerve and blood supplies (Ingham, 1938).

Kunz and Kunz view the foot as a "mirror image of the body, [which] reflects any disturbances in the body's equilibrium in the form of blockages of the zones" (1982, p. 18). They believe that the zonal blockages manifest as either internal or external blockages, for example, pooling of lymph fluid. Reflexology restores balance to the body as described below:

> *Reflexology is aimed at restoring the lost balance. This is achieved through stimulating the reflexes in the feet to cause a relaxation in the corresponding body part. Improved circulation brings in the needed elements to repair and equalize the environment. The glands and the organs in turn seek their equilibrium. The chain is completed. . . . Reflexology acts on the body to release it to do its complex job of maintaining its many operations.*
>
> *(Kunz & Kunz, 1982, p. 17)*

Some believe that the zones are more like the energy meridians of Chinese medicine, and that reflexology helps keep energy flowing freely. According to these theories, "stimulation to specific points activates the movement of energy to corresponding parts of the body to clear out congestion and restore normal functioning" (Knaster, 1996, p. 310).

▪ TECHNIQUES

The basic technique of foot reflexology is direct pressure with the thumb. A special technique called *thumb walking* is used to apply pressure quickly and systematically along the entire foot. To practice thumb walking, hold the back of the foot with one hand while the other hand performs the technique. Start at the heel of the foot and "walk" your thumb up the side of the foot by bending the thumb at the first joint,

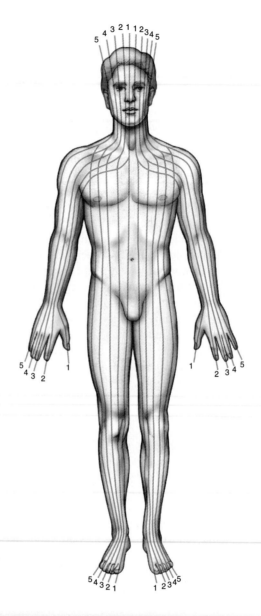

FIGURE 14–2. Zones of the body according to W. Fitzgerald and E. Bowers (1917). There are a total of 10 zones, 5 on each side.

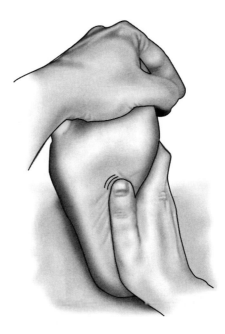

FIGURE 14–3. Bending the thumb at the first joint, "walk" the thumb from spot to spot along the foot. Pressure is applied with the outside edge of the thumb just to the side of the nail.

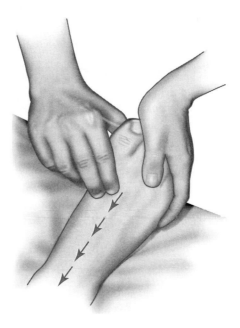

FIGURE 14–4. Finger walking along the top of the foot.

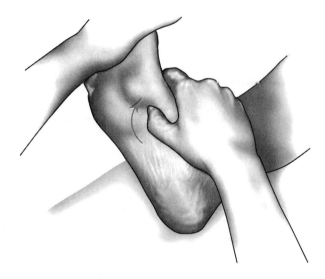

FIGURE 14–5. Hook and backup using the thumb to apply deep pressure.

pressing into the tissues, letting up pressure, and then moving to the next spot to repeat the technique. Pressure is applied with the outside edge of the thumb just to the
side of the nail. See Figure 14–3.

The thumb-walking movement should be constant and steady. The thumb always moves forward. The application of pressure is enhanced by using the four fingers of the working hand in opposition to the thumb. The holding hand can assist by
pressing the foot into the thumb as the thumb is "walking." The walking technique
may also be applied with the fingers, especially the index finger. *Finger walking* is
useful for applying pressure to the top of the foot. See Figure 14–4.

The *hook and backup* technique is used to apply deep pressure to a specific
spot. Locate the spot you wish to press, place your thumb on the spot, and bend the
first joint to begin applying pressure. Then pull back across the spot with your
thumb. This will deepen your pressure. See Figure 14–5.

These basic techniques may be combined with foot massage and joint mobilizations to stimulate the reflex points on the feet. More detailed descriptions of
how to perform a foot reflexology routine may be found in textbooks devoted to the
subject (Byers, 1991; Kunz & Kunz, 1982; Norman & Cowan, 1988).

■ SUMMARY

Foot reflexology is based on the theory that pressure applied to specific spots on the
feet stimulates corresponding areas in other parts of the body. This action is thought
to help normalize function and increase circulation in the part of the body affected.

Reflexology is based on zone therapy, which views the body as divided longitudinally into 10 zones. Pressure applied anywhere in the zone will affect the entire zone. Reflexology focuses on the endpoints of these zones in the feet. Reflexology charts of the feet show which areas of the feet correspond to different areas of the body.

Techniques used to apply pressure to the feet include thumb walking, finger walking, and hook and backup. These basic techniques may be combined with general foot massage and joint movements to stimulate reflex points on the feet.

■ REFERENCES

Benjamin, P. J. (1989a). Eunice D. Ingham and the development of foot reflexology in the United States. Part one: The early years—to 1946. *Massage Therapy Journal,* Spring, 38–44.

Benjamin, P. J. (1989b). Eunice D. Ingham and the development of foot reflexology in the United States. Part two: On the road 1946–1974. *Massage Therapy Journal,* Winter, 49–55.

Byers, D. C. (1991). *Better health with foot reflexology.* St. Petersburg, FL: Ingham Publishing.

Fitzgerald, W. H., & Bowers, E. F. (1917). *Zone therapy.* Columbus, OH: I.W. Long.

Ingham, E. D. (1938). *Stories the feet can tell: Stepping to better health.* Rochester, NY: author.

Knaster, M. (1996). *Discovering the body's wisdom.* New York, Bantam Books.

Kunz, K., & Kunz, B. (1982). *The complete guide to foot reflexology.* Englewood Cliffs, NJ: Prentice-Hall.

Norman, L., & Cowan, T. (1988). *Feet first: A guide to foot reflexology.* New York: Simon & Schuster.

IV

Asian Bodywork Traditions

Finger Pressure
to Acupuncture Points

Frances M. Tappan

■ HISTORY OF ACUPUNCTURE

Although the origin of Chinese medicine is lost in antiquity, it is assumed to have developed from folk medicine. It has many aspects in common with other Asian traditions, such as Indian herbal medicine and Persian medicine. The origin of acupuncture is, however, unique to the Chinese branch of Asian medicine.

The earliest known text on acupuncture is the *Nei Ching,* or *Classic of Internal Medicine,* traditionally ascribed to the legendary Yellow Emperor (Huang Ti, believed to have lived from 2697–2596 B.C.). The *Nei Ching* remains the basic reference on the subject and is the foundation for all development in acupuncture to the present century.

The ancient Chinese became aware of an increased sensitivity of certain skin areas (called points) when a body organ or function was impaired. It was observed that in all patients the same skin areas became hypersensitive in the presence of a specific illness or organ dysfunction. Consequently, some of the relationships between various internal organs and their functions were observed and established. These were defined and explained in terms of a complex philosophical hypothesis that attempted to relate all the observed phenomena.

Acupuncture has a known history of over 4,000 years. Over the course of centuries a long line of ancient practitioners belonging to a people noted for meticulous visual observation were able to establish the existence of a number of energy, or *chi*, meridians and their relationships with various physiologic functions. Fundamental to the concept of meridians in Chinese medicine is not only their function as imaginary lines linking a series of points on the skin that become sensitive in the presence of organic or functional disorders, but also their function as actual "energy pathways." The Chinese word for energy is *chi*.

This energy is believed to circulate throughout the body in a well-defined cycle, moving in a prescribed sequence from meridian to meridian and from organ to organ, flowing partly at the periphery and partly in the interior of the body. Like the Western concept of "nerve-energy potential" or the *prana* (life force) of Indian philosophy and medicine, *chi* is a dynamic force in constant flux.

Acupuncture was introduced to the West in the seventeenth century by Jesuit missionaries sent to Peking. Since that time, several attempts have been made to promulgate this therapy of Asia, with varying degrees of success. Not until the French sinologist and diplomat Soulié de Morant published his voluminous writings on acupuncture in the 1940s did Western physicians have a sound basis for study and application of this ancient system of healing.

Under the impetus of de Morant's work, acupuncture associations and study groups were established in many Western countries, among them France, Italy, Britain, West Germany, Argentina, and the Eastern European nations. Many countries now actively support research programs in the physiology and application of acupuncture, notably Russia, the People's Republic of China, North and South Korea, and Japan.

Acupuncture is of growing interest in the West, but it is also undergoing a resurgence of serious study in Asia. In China, acupuncture is an integral part of the nation's medical practice.

The field of acupuncture treatment is that of impaired body functions, as opposed to actual lesions. In the case of a patient with diabetes, for example, if there is no actual tissue degeneration in the islets of Langerhans, acupuncture can be extremely effective. Even if lesions have formed and are well established, the pain, discomfort, and other symptoms caused by them are greatly relieved by acupuncture. It may be impossible, however, to obtain complete and lasting relief of a functional problem that has an organic substratum by use of acupuncture.

One of the primary functions of acupuncture is to directly affect the energy level, and therefore the functioning, of the internal organs by either stimulating or depressing their actions.

▪ MERIDIANS

Chinese philosophy and medical science believe that meridians are a system of pathways, or channels. The meridian system provides for a continuous flow of vital energy to all parts of the body. Although there seem to be neither definite anatomic meridian structures throughout the body, nor a specific relationship to existing systems as we know them, Robert Tsay (1974) observes that the ". . . meridian system may differ somewhat from the nervous system, the blood circulation and the endocrine system, but it is also possible that it is intimately related to these three systems" (p. 44). The theory of the meridians is the basis for diagnosis and treatment. According to Tsay, ". . . it is impossible for the physician to differentiate symptoms, or to prescribe accurately the exact treatment for a patient without using this theory as a guide or basis. This is the reason it is necessary for the student of Chinese medicine to first study the theory of the meridian system. It is as important as the student of Western medicine having to first learn anatomy, physiology, and pathology" (p. 52).

The 12 regular meridians are listed in the order of vital energy and nutrient flow, with rare exception, as follows:

1. Lung (L)
2. Large Intestine (LI)
3. Stomach (St)
4. Spleen (Sp)
5. Heart (H)
6. Small Intestine (SI)
7. Urinary Bladder (UB)
8. Kidney (K)
9. Pericardium (P)
10. Triple Warmer (TW)
11. Gallbladder (GB)
12. Liver (Liv)

Governing Vessel (GV), and Conception Vessel (CV), the first two extra meridians, are the thirteenth and fourteenth of the most used meridians.

GV covers the total posterior midline of the body and a midline portion of the head anteriorly. CV covers the remaining anterior midline portions of the head and body.

As listed, circulation of energy starts through the Lung meridian continuing through each of the meridians in succession. From the Liver meridian the energy flows to and through the Lung meridian again. The complete cycle takes 24 hours and repeats continually throughout life. Branches of the meridians allow for the vital energy transport from one meridian to the other.

Features of the Meridians

No tangible anatomic vessels can be found by dissection. Two components of circulation go through the meridian circulatory system: *Chi,* the invisible circulation of the vital energy, and *Hseuh,* the visible circulation, including blood and lymph (Tsay, 1974, p. 40).

Meridians are named according to (1) the organ that is controlled by the energy flow, that is, lungs, stomach, spleen; (2) the function of the energy, that is, GV, Regulating Channel (RC), and Motility Channel (MC); and (3) yin or yang.

In a yin meridian, energy mainly flows upward. In a yang meridian, energy mainly flows downward. The Asian yin and yang theories compare in some ways to what Western scientists call positive and negative elements, which exist in every atom. Even when atoms are split, particles still maintain positive and negative charges. Only very recently have scientists thought that anything at all could exist without a positive and a negative particle.

The Chinese philosophy believes that the solar system is a large universe with its yin and yang. All lives are part of it, and the human body is like a smaller universe within this particular galaxy. Since an atom contains its yin and yang, a cell therefore contains its yin and yang, and an organ contains its yin and yang. Any individual body that may be deemed a unit must also contain its yin and yang.

Upon review of the literature on meridians, one will find that various authors name the system differently. For example, meridians may be called channels or pathways. The meridians may also be named in other ways, for example, lung (L) is also pulmonary (PU); large intestine (LI) is also colon (C); stomach (St) is also gastric (GA).

There are the following types and numbers of meridians: (1) 12 regular meridians; (2) 8 extra ones; (3) 12 chief branches and 12 muscle branches; (4) 15 liaison vessels; and (5) 12 cutaneous liaison vessels. The 14 meridians most often used are the 12 regular ones and the 2 extra meridians, GV and CV.

As vital energy flows during the 24-hour cycles, there are two-hour intervals when a maximum of vital energy is reached in each of the 12 regular meridians. Intervals start with 0300–0500 in the meridian. This maximum vital energy time is considered the best time to treat pathologies of that meridian. As McGarey (1974) points out,

> If asthma attacks occur, particularly at night, it is felt best to treat the problem during that two-hour period between three o'clock and five o'clock A.M. In the Western world, it does not seem likely that this would get done outside an emergency room very often, but nevertheless, this is the rule of acupuncture and should be recognized as such for whatever value it may have at some future time in one's experience. (p. 35)

Flow in the meridians follows three specific cycles within the 24-hour period. Each cycle contains 4 meridians, as grouped within the 12 meridians. Figures 15–1 through 15–8 illustrate the 4 meridians in each cycle, with the direction of the flow indicated. Figures are shown with upper extremities raised above shoulder height to better illustrate the *up* and *down* direction of the vital energy and nutrient circulation. In each figure the right side is used as the right side in both anterior and posterior views. Remember, the meridians are bilateral; therefore, the circulation is duplicated on the left.

A total of 20 enlarged dots are located on the meridians in all but one of the figures (Fig. 15–3). These indicate acupuncture points, each named according to the meridian on which it is located. The 20 points have been selected by specialists in the field and presented by Huang Min Der at a medical seminar in Taiwan in 1975. They are thought to be most effective when used, in various combinations, for treating common painful areas, that is, head, shoulder, low back, and leg. Selection was made from the 642 points found on (1) the 14 most used meridians—361; (2) special acupuncture points, also called extra points—171; and (3) new acupuncture points—110.

Each of the three cycles illustrated has the following features: each cycle is composed of four different meridians; each meridian is either a hand or a foot meridian; each is either a yin or a yang meridian; and each has a 2-hour interval

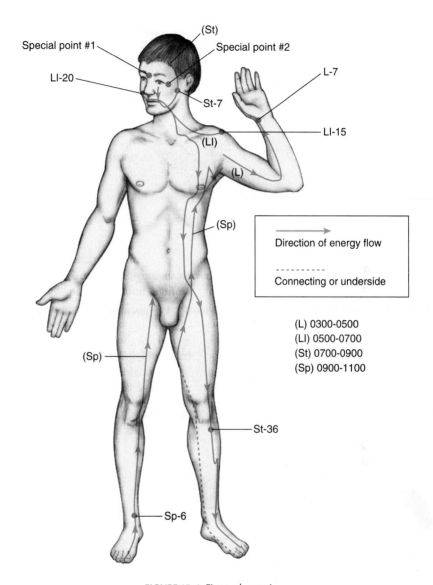

FIGURE 15–1. First cycle anterior.

when a maximum of vital energy is reached, called the maximum energy time. Each cycle also has a definite sequential direction of vital energy and nutrient flow through the four meridians of that cycle. Flow starts through a yin meridian, going *up* from the chest area to the *hand;* then from the hand, *down* toward the chest and head area via a yang meridian; from the head area *down* a yang meridian to the *foot;* and then from the foot, *up* to the chest area via a yin meridian. Then flow continues

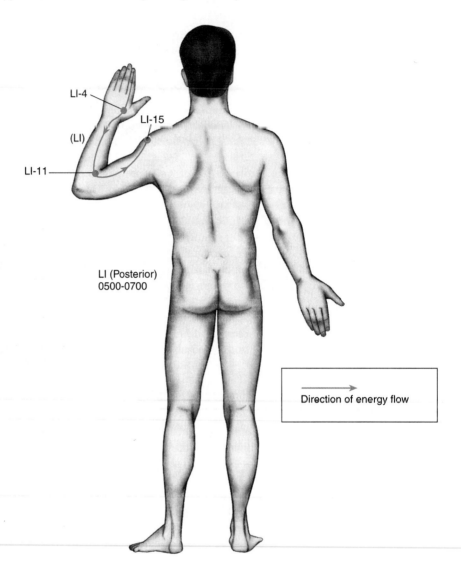

FIGURE 15–2. First cycle posterior.

to the next cycle yin meridian in the chest. Features of the three cycles are included in Table 15–1.

Governing vessel and CV, the thirteenth and fourteenth of the most used meridians, are illustrated in Figures 15–7 and 15–8. The former also shows the combined posterior acupuncture points, whereas Figure 15–8, CV, shows the combined anterior acupuncture points. For example, GV 26, one of the 20 most used acupuncture points, is seen on Figure 15–8.

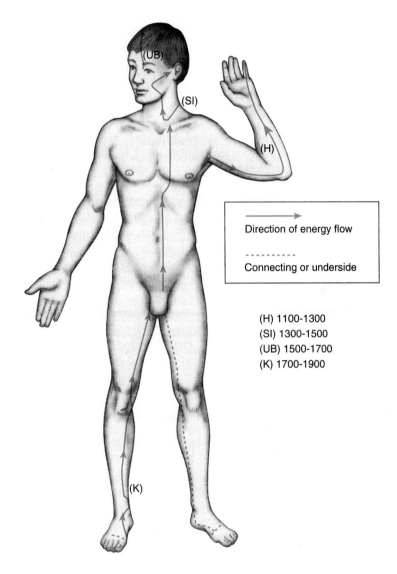

Direction of energy flow

- - - - - - - - - -
Connecting or underside

(H) 1100-1300
(SI) 1300-1500
(UB) 1500-1700
(K) 1700-1900

(UB)

(SI)

(H)

(K)

FIGURE 15–3. Second cycle anterior.

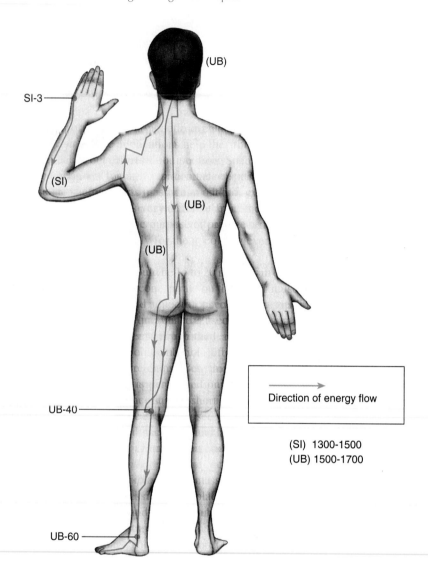

FIGURE 15–4. Second cycle posterior.

Meridians are connected, in couples, through 15 points, called Lo Meridian Points. Liaison vessels serve as links between coupled meridians. As Tsay (1974) describes them, "Coupled meridians, composed of a Yin meridian and a Yang meridian, are closely interrelated as an inseparable body. Three couples are on the hand, and three on the foot. Couples may evidence identical symptoms, and can be

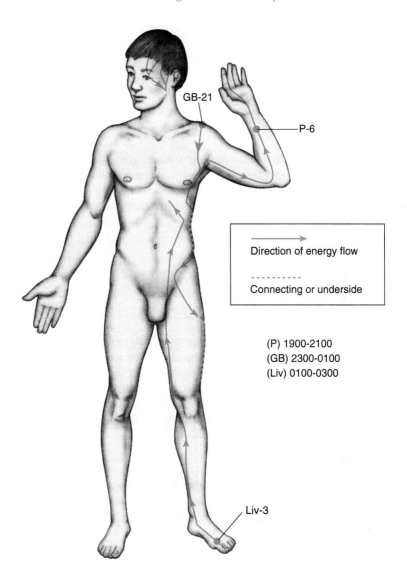

Direction of energy flow

Connecting or underside

(P) 1900-2100
(GB) 2300-0100
(Liv) 0100-0300

FIGURE 15–5. Third cycle anterior.

treated at the same meridian points" (pp. 78–79). Meridian and acupuncture points refer to the same points.

The meridian system is built anatomically in a nonspecific system functioning to balance all aspects of the human body: mental, digestive, reproductive, nerve, and circulatory processes; internal and external organs; and energy, nutrition, and consciousness. Tsay (1974) notes, "Viewing meridians as lines—it is possible to

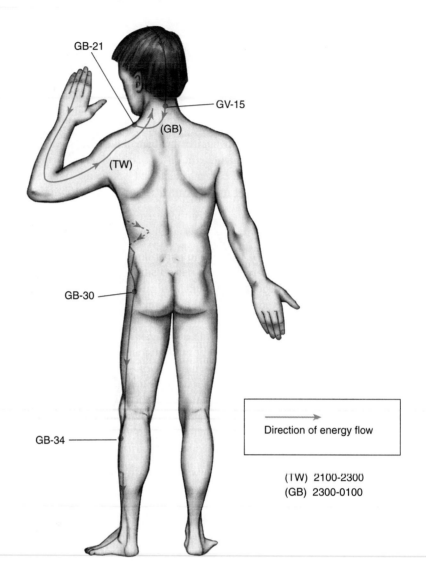

FIGURE 15–6. Third cycle posterior.

see that many meridian pathways run closely parallel to the pathway of one or more main nerve branches. The anatomical relationship of the bi-meridian points with blood vessels are [sic] also very close, but not as close as with the nerves" (p. 61). In order, then, to understand the workings of the body, to recognize symptoms of dysfunction, and to prescribe treatment, persons studying Chinese healing arts need the same basic knowledge of the meridian system as those persons studying Western healing arts need anatomy, physiology, and pathology.

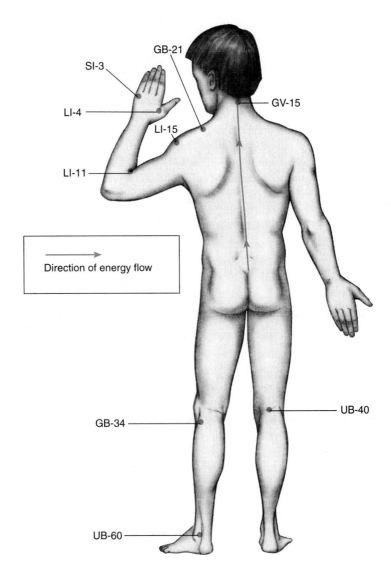

FIGURE 15–7. Combined posterior points; posterior portion of GV meridian.

■ PHYSIOLOGY OF ACUPUNCTURE

Studies showing that the electrical excitability of nerves can be reduced *solely* by acupuncture needles have been done on animals and humans (Snyder, 1977).

In 1975, Frederick Kerr, Department of Neurologic Surgery at Mayo Clinic in Rochester, MN, reported a study he conducted using rats. The first rat was given acupuncture to Ho-Ku, Large Intestine 4. This reduced its trigeminal nerve ex-

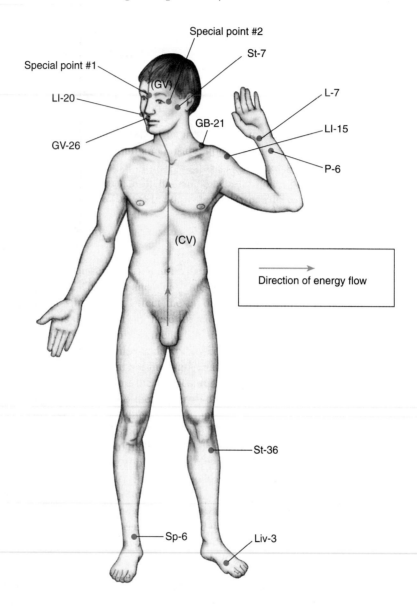

FIGURE 15–8. Combined anterior points; CV meridian; anterior portion of GV.

citability by 75%. The second rat was given no acupuncture, but was given a blood transfusion from the first rat with an acupuncture needle in his Ho-Ku. The result was that the second rat showed considerable lowering of excitability in its trigeminal nerve.

It has been shown that acupuncture points can be located with electrical apparatus, and that electrical resistance of the skin is consistently lower at acupuncture

THE THREE DAILY CYCLES OF THE MERIDIANS

TABLE
15–1

Meridian (abbr.)	Hand or Foot	Yin or Yang	Maximum Energy Time[a]	Flow: Up or Down	Points Located on Figures
First Cycle:					
(L)	Hand	Yin	0300–0500	Up	(L) 7
(LI)	Hand	Yang	0500–0700	Down	(LI) 4, 11, 15, 20
(St)	Foot	Yang	0700–0900	Down	(St) 7, 36
(Sp)	Foot	Yin	0900–1100	Up	(Sp) 6
					Special points 1, 2[b]
Second Cycle:					
(H)	Hand	Yin	1100–1300	Up	
(SI)	Hand	Yang	1300–1500	Down	(SI) 3
(UB)	Foot	Yang	1500–1700	Down	(UB) 40, 60[c]
(K)	Foot	Yin	1700–1900	Up	
Third Cycle:					
(P)	Hand	Yin	1900–2100	Up	(P) 6
(TW)	Hand	Yang	2100–2300	Down	
(GB)	Foot	Yang	2300–0100	Down	(GB) 20, 21, 30, 34
(Liv)	Foot	Yin	0100–0300	Up	(Liv) 3[d]

[a]Energy time is the time of day when the available energy is at a maximum.
[b]Points located on the anterior are shown in Figure 15–1, and on the posterior in Figure 15–2.
[c]Points located on the anterior are shown in Figure 15–3, and on the posterior in Figure 15–4.
[d]Points located on the anterior are shown in Figure 15–5, and on the posterior in Figure 15–6.

points. Acupuncture point areas often are tender, small nodules. Moreover, temperature differences in acupuncture points have been demonstrated with infrared photography (McGarey, 1974, p. 11).

Needling sites also seem to correspond with the "Head Zones" discovered by Sir Henry Head in the 1800s. Pain resulting from pathology of the viscera is often referred to clearly definable areas on the body surface known as "Head Zones." These zones closely relate to the 12 acupuncture meridians and are associated with the same organs (Armstrong, 1972, p. 1582).

Organs receive their autonomic nerve supply primarily from the homolateral part of the nervous system. Connective tissue changes can therefore be found on the corresponding part of the body surface. The liver, gallbladder, duodenum, ileum, appendix, ascending colon, and hepatic flexure receive their nerve supply mainly from the right. The heart, stomach, pancreas, spleen, jejunum, transverse and descending colon, sigmoid colon, and rectum receive their nerve supply mainly from the left.

Changes relating to the bladder, the uterus, and the head can be found in the middle of the back. Changes relating to the lungs, bronchi, kidneys, suprarenal glands, and ovaries can be found on the corresponding side of the back. Conditions affecting the nerves or vessels of either side of the body will cause changes on the corresponding side of the back.

LOCATION OF THE 20 MOST USEFUL ACUPUNCTURE POINTS

TABLE
15–2

Acupuncture Point	Chinese Name and Meaning	Location	Indications
Urinary Bladder-40 B-40	Wei-Chung "Commanding Middle"	At the center of the popliteal fossa	Low back pain Sciatica Lower extremity paralysis Leg cramp Disorders of hip joint and surrounding soft tissue Knee joint pain, arthritis Heat stroke Apoplexy Epilepsy Acute gastroenteritis Cystitis
Urinary Bladder-60 B-60	Kunlun "Mountain"	Midpoint between the posterior margin of the lateral malleolus and the Achilles tendon	Lower extremity paralysis Low back pain Sciatica Disorders of the ankle joint and surrounding soft tissue
Gallbladder-20 GB-20	Feng-chih "Wind Pond"	Midpoint of a line joining the tip of the mastoid process to the posterior midline in the groove between the trapezius and the sternocleidomastoid	Tension headache Migraine headache Stiff neck Dizziness Vertigo Common cold Hypertension Tinnitus
Gallbladder-21 GB-21	Chieng-ching "Shoulder Well"	Midway between C-7 and acromion process	Shoulder and back pain Neck pain and rigidity Upper extremity motor impairment Mastisis Hyperthyroidism Functional uterine bleeding
Gallbladder-30 GB-30	Huan-tiao "Jumping Circle"	One third of the distance from the greater trochanter to the base of the coccyx	Hip joint pain Sciatica Low back pain Lower extremity paralysis Disorders of hip joint and surrounding soft tissue

(continued)

Table 15–2 *(Continued)*

Acupuncture Point	Chinese Name and Meaning	Location	Indications
Gallbladder-34 GB-34	Yangling Chuan "Yang Mound Spring"	Anterior to the neck of the fibula	Hemiplegia Disease of the gallbladder Low back pain Dizziness Vertigo Acid regurgitation Lower extremity and knee pain
Governing Vessel-26 GV-26	Jan-chung "Middle of the Man"	One third of the distance from the inferior surface of the nose to the upper lip line	Shock Heat stroke Low back pain Epilepsy Facial paralysis
Large Intestines-4 LI-4	Ho-Ku "Meeting Valley"	Between first and second metacarpals	Foreheadache Toothache Temporomandibular joint arthritis Tonsillitis Rhinitis Oropharyngitis Facial paralysis Pain and paralysis of upper extremity Hyperhydrosis Goiter Eye disease Fever Hemiplegia Analgesia Abdominal pain Common cold—coughing Amenorrhea Delirium Induction of labor Insomnia Prostration Asthma Anesthesia for dental work—especially for lower jaw

(continued)

Table 15–2 *(Continued)*

Acupuncture Point	Chinese Name and Meaning	Location	Indications
Large Intestines-11 LI-11	Chu-chih "Crooked Pond"	Radial end of fold of fully flexed elbow	Shoulder and elbow pain Paralysis of upper extremity Hypertension Disorders of elbow joint and surrounding soft tissue Fever Common cold Chorea Eczema Neurodermatitis
Large Intestines-15 LI-15	Chien-yu "Shoulder Bone"	In the depression of the acromion in the center of the deltoid muscle when the arm is abducted to 90°	Pain and impaired movement of elbow and arm Disorders of shoulder joint and surrounding soft tissue
Large Intestines-20 LI-20	Ying-hsiang "Welcome Fragrance"	At the lower margin and lateral to the nostrils in the nasolabial fold	Facial paralysis Rhinitis Sinusitis Ascariasis of bile duct
Liver-3 Liv-3	Tai-chung "Too Rushy"	Between the first and second metatarsals, in a fossa, just distal to the heads	Headache Dizziness Epilepsy
Lung-7 Lu-7	Lieh-chueh "Listing Deficiency"	Proximal to styloid process of radius	Headache Neck pain Cough Asthma Facial paralysis
Pericardium-6 P-6	Nei-Kuan "Inner Gate"	Two cun above ventral wrist fold between the tendons of palmaris longus and the flexor carpi radialis	Vomiting Gastralgia Palpitation Angina pectoris Hiccough Chest and costal region pain Stomach pain Insomnia Epilepsy Hysteria

(continued)

Table 15–2 *(Continued)*

Acupuncture Point	Chinese Name and Meaning	Location	Indications
Small Intestines-3 SI-3	Hou-chi "Back Stream"	At the apex of the distal palmar crease on the ulnar side of a clenched fist	Neck pain and rigidity Low back pain Tinnitus Deafness Occipital headache Upper extremity paralysis Night sweating Epilepsy Malaria
Spleen-6 Sp-6	San-yin-chiao "Three Ying Crossing"	Three cun above medial malleolus, just behind the posterior edge of the tibia	Insomnia Barborymus Abdominal distention Loose stool Irregular menstruation Nocturnal emission Impotence Spermatorrhea Orchitis Enuresis Neurasthenia Frequent urination Hemiplegia Urine retention
Stomach-7 St-7	Hsia-Kuan "Lower Gate"	In the depression at the lower border of the zygomatic arch, anterior to the condyloid process of the mandible	Toothache Facial paralysis Trigeminal neuralgia Temporomandibular joint arthritis
Stomach-36 St-36	Tsu-san-li "Walk Three More Miles"	One cun distal and lateral to the tibial tuberosity	Acute and chronic gastritis Nausea and vomiting Functional gastrointestinal disturbances Digestive tract diseases Neurosis Some allergies Fever Shock Aching of hips and knees Leg edema or ache Hemiplegia Anemia Headache Epilepsy

(continued)

Table 15–2 *(Continued)*

Acupuncture Point	Chinese Name and Meaning	Location	Indications
			Lumbago Heaviness of head and frontal headache Acute and chronic enteritis Acute pancreatitis Pyloric spasm Jaundice Urogenital ailments General weakness Paralytic illness
Special Point 1	Yin-tang "Seal Palace"	At the glabella, midway between the medial margins of the eyebrows	Diseases of the nose Headache Dizziness Vertigo
Special Point 2	Tai-yang "Supreme Yang"	At the temple, one cun directly posterior to the midpoint of a line joining the lateral canthus of the eye and the lateral margin of the eyebrow	Migraine Trigeminal neuralgia Eye diseases Toothache Facial paralysis

The changes that can be observed visually may be grouped under what have for many years been called "trigger points." These include drawn-in bands of tissue, flattened drawn-in areas of tissue, elevated areas giving the impression of localized swelling, atrophy of muscles, hypertrophy of muscles and bony deformities, especially of the spinal column. Many trigger points seem to correlate with acupuncture energy points. According to this theory, pathology in muscles results in tenderness in the muscle, as well as its associated tissues and organs.

It has been evidenced that if the tissue through which a meridian runs is cut, the stimulation of an acupuncture point is not transmitted to other points of the same meridian beyond the level of the cut, and the internal organ with which the meridian is associated is not influenced by treatment with acupuncture (Armstrong, 1972, p. 1582).

The word acupuncture combines two Latin words, one being *acus* meaning needle. Therefore, those who use the term *acupressure* for finger pressure on the acupuncture energy points are in fact saying "needle pressure," which is not at all what they intend to imply. The other word is *punctura,* which means pricking. Therefore, the term *acupuncture* means needle pricking or the insertion of needles into specific points of the body known as acupuncture points. The following discussion considers how these points can also be effective in massage by applying finger pressure.

▪ TECHNIQUE OF APPLYING FINGER PRESSURE TO ACUPUNCTURE POINTS

When using finger pressure on acupuncture points, more than just the amount of pressure applied should be considered. As with all massage, the degree of pressure must be judged in relation to the tolerance of the patient. For this particular technique the more pressure the patient can tolerate, the greater the effectiveness of the treatment. However, judgment must be exercised when dealing with acute pain, swelling, local injuries to the area being treated, and systemic complications. Deeper pressure will probably be needed if the complications are chronic.

Use one finger, usually the middle finger or the thumb, to press against the acupuncture point. Small friction-like circular movements may be used to work one's way toward deeper pressure with the ultimate objective being that of deep, constant pressure on the accurate acupuncture point. Effective treatment time

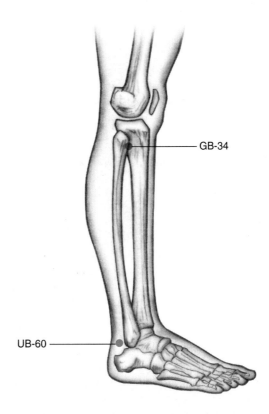

FIGURE 15–9. Acupuncture points GB-34 Yangling Chuan and UB-60 Kunlun, lateral view.

ranges from 1 to 5 minutes per point per treatment, or until the patient claims relief. The author has actually heard patients say, in reference to pain, "It's going away. . . . It's going away. . . . It's gone!"

Some contraindications exist, especially for people who are not fully trained in acupuncture. Avoid using these techniques directly over contusions, scar tissue, or infection, or if the patient has a serious cardiac condition. Discontinue treatment immediately if the patient appears aggravated or if no improvement is observable. Children under 7 years of age should not be treated with these techniques.

The 20 most useful acupuncture points will be used as examples to indicate the wide variety of disabilities that can be treated effectively using finger pressure to acupuncture points. Pressure application must be applied to the *exact point* or treatment will be useless. In traditional practice, exact point locations are found using a measurement called "cuns" based on the width of the thumb of the receiver. Table 15–2 provides information as to the location of these 20 points (see also Figs. 15–9 to 15–12 for anatomic diagrams of point locations) and the disabilities indicated that can be partially or totally relieved by pressure at these respective points.

Table 15–3 was compiled by the author using many of the sources in the references and with the assistance of Joseph Yao, Donald Courtial, and Dorothy

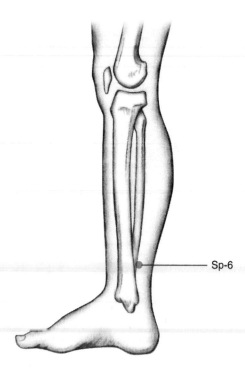

FIGURE 15–10. Acupuncture point Sp-6 San-yin-chiao, medial view.

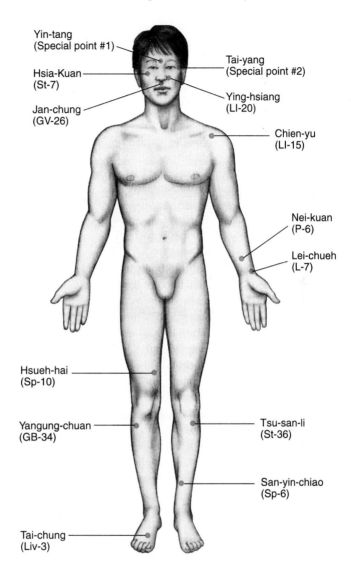

Yin-tang
(Special point #1)

Tai-yang
(Special point #2)

Hsia-Kuan
(St-7)

Ying-hsiang
(LI-20)

Jan-chung
(GV-26)

Chien-yu
(LI-15)

Nei-kuan
(P-6)

Lei-chueh
(L-7)

Hsueh-hai
(Sp-10)

Yangung-chuan
(GB-34)

Tsu-san-li
(St-36)

San-yin-chiao
(Sp-6)

Tai-chung
(Liv-3)

FIGURE 15–11. Important acupuncture points on front of body.

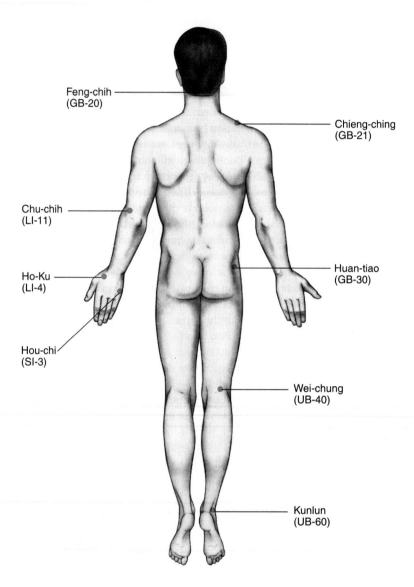

Feng-chih
(GB-20)

Chieng-ching
(GB-21)

Chu-chih
(LI-11)

Huan-tiao
(GB-30)

Ho-Ku
(LI-4)

Hou-chi
(SI-3)

Wei-chung
(UB-40)

Kunlun
(UB-60)

FIGURE 15–12. Important acupuncture points on back of body.

SOME COMBINATIONS OF THESE 20 POINTS
FOR VARIOUS DISORDERS

TABLE
15–3

Headache	

Frontal—"Heaviness of Head"
  Large Intestine 4
  Special Point 1
  Stomach 36
	Temporomandibular headache
	  Gallbladder 20
	  Special Point 2

Headache

Frontal—"Heaviness of Head"
  Large Intestine 4
  Special Point 1
  Stomach 36

Vertical headache
  Urinary Bladder 60

Tension headache
  Gallbladder 20
  Gallbladder 21
  Large Intestine 4
  Liver 3
  Special Point 1

Migraine headache
  Gallbladder 20
  Gallbladder 36
  Large Intestine 4
  Liver 3
  Special Point 2
  Stomach 36

Sinus headache—Chronic Rhinitis
  Gallbladder 20
  Large Intestine 4
  Large Intestine 20
  Lung 7
  Special Point 1

*Diseases of the head, face, trunk, and
internal organs*
  Gallbladder 34
  Large Intestine 4
  Small Intestine 3
  Stomach 36

Temporomandibular headache
  Gallbladder 20
  Special Point 2

Occipital headache
  Gallbladder 20
  Gallbladder 21
  Liver 3
  Small Intestine 3
  Urinary Bladder 60

Trigeminal nerve—Facial Paralysis
  Governing Vessel 26
  Large Intestine 4
  Large Intestine 20
  Lung 7
  Special Point 2
  Stomach 7

Generalized headache
  Large Intestine 4
  Special Point 1

From malfunction of the liver
  Large Intestine 4
  Large Intestine 11
  Urinary Bladder 40

Neck disorders
  Gallbladder 20
  Gallbladder 21
  Lung 7

Disorders of the Upper Extremity

Shoulder disorders
  Gallbladder 21
  Large Intestine 11

Elbow disorders
  Gallbladder 21
  Large Intestine 4
  Large Intestine 11
  Large Intestine 15
  Small Intestine 3

(continued)

Table 15-3 (Continued)

Disorders of the Trunk and Lower Extremity	
Low back pain	*Disorders of hip joint and*
Gallbladder 34	*surrounding soft tissue*
Governing Vessel 34	Gallbladder 30
Small Intestine 3	Gallbladder 34
Urinary Bladder 40	Urinary Bladder 40
Urinary Bladder 60	
	Knee pain
Sciatica	Gallbladder 34
Gallbladder 30	Large Intestine 4
Gallbladder 34	Stomach 36
Urinary Bladder 40	Spleen 6
Urinary Bladder 60	Urinary Bladder 40
Lower extremity involvement—pain,	*Disorders of the ankle joint and*
paralysis, fatigue	*surrounding soft tissue*
Gallbladder 30	Gallbladder 34
Gallbladder 34	Urinary Bladder 60
Stomach 36	
Urinary Bladder 40	*Muscular dysfunction of the feet*
Urinary Bladder 60	Spleen 6
	Stomach 36

Systemic Disorders	
Common cold	*Heat stroke*
Gallbladder 20	Governing Vessel 26
Large Intestine 4	Urinary Bladder 40
Large Intestine 20	
Lung 7	*Hemiplegia*
Special Point 1	Gallbladder 34
	Large Intestine 4
Cough	Spleen 6
Lung 7	
Spleen 6	*Hypertension*
	Gallbladder 20
Dizziness	Large Intestine 4
Gallbladder 20	Large Intestine 11
Gallbladder 34	Stomach 36
Liver 3	Spleen 6
Special Point 1	
	Impotence
	Stomach 36
Epilepsy	Spleen 6
Gallbladder 34	
Small Intestine 3	*Insomnia*
	Pericardium 6
Fever	Spleen 6
Large Intestine 4	
Large Intestine 11	

(continued)

Table 15–3 *(Continued)*

Systemic Disorders	
Irregular menses	*Tinnitus*
Gallbladder 21	Gallbladder 20
Large Intestine 4	Small Intestine 3
Spleen 6	
Stomach 36	*Toothache*
	Large Intestine 4
Morning sickness	Large Intestine 20
Pericardium 6	Lung 7
Stomach 36	Special Point 2
	Stomach 7
Nausea	
Pericardium 6	*Vertigo*
Stomach 36	Gallbladder 20
	Gallbladder 34
Shock	Special Point 1
Pericardium 6	
Stomach 36	

McLaughlin. It is designed to provide quick, easy reference for those using this text to enable them to incorporate finger pressure into their treatment programs.

The idea should be reinforced that any or all of the massage systems described in this text may be used alone or in combination. Any massage system used depends on the responses of individual disabilities and the particular physiologic and psychologic reactions to the treatment being given, as well as the individual's response to the person providing the treatment.

▪ SUMMARY

Since 1958, Western medicine's interest in the effectiveness of acupuncture has increased. Both Eastern and Western medicine are actively involved in research to explain physiologically or psychologically how acupuncture accomplishes anesthesia and even euphoria. The reasons for its effectiveness become clearer as research continues in the methods of pain relief and endorphins.

This chapter presents a brief history of acupuncture as well as a discussion of the Chinese medicine theories related to meridians. The discussion of 20 selected points provides the reader with general knowledge of the most commonly used points and the disabilities that can effectively benefit from finger pressure on specific points. The bibliography provides complete information related to hundreds of other acupuncture points. The reader should pursue the literature for more complete information.

■ REFERENCES

Academy of Traditional Chinese Medicine. (1975). *An outline of Chinese acupuncture.* Peking: Foreign Language Press.

Armstrong, M. E. (1972). Acupuncture. *American Journal of Nursing,* September.

Der, H. M. (1975). From a presentation at a medical seminar at Chinese acupuncture science research foundation in Taipei, Taiwan, Republic of China.

Kerr, F. W. L. (1975). Study reported at a conference at the University of Connecticut Health Center, September 29, 1975.

McGarey, W. A. (1974). *Acupuncture and body energies.* Phoenix: Gabriel Press.

Synder, S. (1977). The brain's own opiates. *Chemical and Engineering News,* September.

Tsay, R. C. (1974). *Textbook of Chinese acupuncture medicine. General introduction to acupuncture,* Vol. 1. Wappinger Falls, NY: Association of Chinese Medicine and East-West Medical Center.

Amma, Traditional Japanese Massage

Gary Bernard

The history of amma, traditional Japanese massage, dates back 5,000 years to the northern regions of China and the beginning of Chinese medical philosophy. In the United States today, amma continues to grow and evolve as a versatile and effective contemporary style of massage.

■ THE HISTORY OF AMMA

The two Chinese characters pronounced *anmo* mean "to calm by rubbing." The Japanese pronounce the same two characters *amma*, which is sometimes spelled *anma*. Japanese amma is the foundation of all forms of acupressure massage including the modern-day forms of shiatsu.

Amma originated in the tradition of Chinese medicine. It was first developed in the northern region of China in the barren lands north of the Yellow River. The inhabitants of this area used acupuncture, moxibustion and anmo, that is, manual methods, to provide cures (Serizawa, 1984). Over many years of practice and experience with massage, acupuncture, and moxa, the Chinese people came to identify the points on the body where such therapy produces maximum effects. Eventually these points, called *tsubo* or acupressure points, were documented together with the 14 major meridians or channels of energy that emerged from the patterns created by the *tsubos* (Serizawa, 1976, p. 30). Today we know this system of meridians and acupressure points as the energetic anatomy of traditional Chinese medicine.

Anmo was brought to Japan by way of the Korean peninsula at the beginning of the Asuka period in the sixth century. It was an integral part of the unified system of Chinese medicine, which the Japanese call *kampo*, "the Chinese way" (Serizawa, 1972, pp. 14–15; Serizawa, 1984). The Japanese assimilated the Chinese medical philosophy into their own culture, and amma was born as a therapeutic art form. By 701 Taiho Law referred to the new massage of Japan with the mention of "amma experts" (Joya, 1958, p. 61).

Apart from the knowledge that amma originated in ancient China, the literature that is available in English is very sketchy on the history of amma in Japan until the Edo Period in the seventeenth to nineteenth centuries. There are a few references that suggest that the perception of amma as a form of medical intervention changed from time to time. According to Yamamoto and McCarty, amma was recognized by the official medical authorities during the early part of the Nara Period (672–707 C.E.). Amma apparently lost its popularity for a time, but experienced a revival in the Edo Period (1603–1857 C.E.) (Joya, 1958, p. 61). Serizawa (1972) writes that *kampo*, of which amma was very much a part, was the main medical stream in Japan from the time it was introduced until the end of the Edo Period (p. 2).

Most of the literature agrees that during these 1,000 years, amma developed into a highly specialized style of massage involving complex techniques, which encompassed a myriad of pressing, stroking, stretching, and percussive manipulations with the thumbs, fingers, arms, elbows, and knees to stimulate points along the 14 major meridians of the body.

Amma and *kampo* reached their peak of popularity in the Edo period. During this time, students of medicine were required to study amma to understand and become familiar with the structure and function of the energetic anatomy of the body. Masunaga relates that "their training in this type of manual therapy enabled them to accurately diagnose and administer Chinese herbal medicine as well as locate the tsubos . . . easily for acupuncture treatments" (1977, p. 9).

By the end of the Edo period, two historically significant changes occurred in Japan that dramatically altered both the way amma was taught and the people's perception of *kampo* and amma. The first event occurred early in the nineteenth century when the Shogunate authorities decreed that blind persons assume the job of masseur and acupuncturist as a welfare measure (Serizawa, 1984, p. 15). As a result, many schools were created, and high-ranking amma practitioners enjoyed public respect and were honored by the court and government. However, once the schools of amma began training blind students, amma's status as a healing art gradually began to suffer because it was perceived that "blind people were at a disadvantage in receiving formal study in diagnosis and treatment" (Masunaga, 1977, p. 10). As part of its program to reserve amma as a profession for the blind, the government required that all the ammas, the name given to people who practiced amma, be licensed. The story goes that to avoid these regulations many therapists already in practice changed the name of their type of treatment. Thus, the term *shiatsu* came into use (Masunaga, 1977, p. 9).

The second change occurred during the Meiji restoration (1868 C.E.) and the modernization of Japan. Western medicine began to influence Japanese medical practices. Serizawa (1976) reports that "Western medical science as known in Germany and Holland began to influence Japanese thought, especially because of its surgical methods and its effectiveness against epidemics" (p. 30). Eventually, *kampo* was eclipsed by Western medicine, and misconceptions about amma discredited it in Japan.

Consequently, by the beginning of the 1900s *kampo* and amma had become known as "folk medicine" and amma erroneously associated only with pleasure and comfort. Amma became known as a blind person's profession, and as a result of prejudice, the word *amma* in Japan acquired some stigma as a lowly profession (Serizawa, 1984).

At the outbreak of World War II, over 90% of the people practicing amma in Japan were blind. At the end of the war, General MacArthur went into Japan and banned the traditional healing arts of *kampo* and amma. This left many hundreds of ammas out of work with no real prospects for a livelihood. The result was an epidemic of suicides among the amma practitioners. Helen Keller was informed of this tragedy and wrote to President Truman asking him to rescind the order (Ohashi, 1976). He finally did, but the damage had been done. Amma and the traditional healing arts of Japan were being further overshadowed by Western medical science.

Joya writes in her book, *Things Japanese*, "Most amma are still blind people. Formerly they used to blow a small flute as they went about, and the people used to call them in as they heard the sounds. However, except in some rural districts, this amma flute is no longer heard" (1958, p. 61).

Interestingly enough, of the many schools that teach massage in Japan today, all but two teach amma. However, most people born after World War II have never heard the word *amma* in reference to massage. In 1940, Torujiro Namikoshi opened the Japan Shiatsu School in Tokyo, which was licensed by the government in 1957. As a result Namikoshi's marketing skills in the late 1940s and '50s, "shiatsu" has become the word most commonly used to refer to massage in Japan. Shiatsu was recognized by the Japanese government as a style of massage separate from amma in 1964. The Director of the Shiatsu Massage School of California in Santa Monica, DoAnn Kaneko, told this author that many of the massage practitioners doing massage in Japan today do both the amma and shiatsu, and call it shiatsu.

■ AMMA IN THE UNITED STATES

Torujiro Namikoshi introduced Japanese massage to the United States when he brought his style of shiatsu here in the 1950s. In 1953, he brought his son, Toru, with him. Toru Namikoshi spent seven years in the United States introducing shiatsu to students at the Palmer School of Chiropractic in Davenport, Iowa. Torujiro went on to Hawaii to open a massage school. In 1969, Torujiro wrote his first book, *Health and Vitality at Your Fingertips, Shiatsu in English*, and distributed it in the United States, Great Britain, New Zealand, and Australia. This book was later translated into several other languages under the name *Japanese Finger-Pressure Therapy, Shiatsu* (1969) and distributed all over the world. Namikoshi's style of shiatsu was the primary style of Japanese massage taught in the United States until the 1960s. During the 1970s, a number of Japanese practitioners brought their styles of shiatsu to the United States, including DoAnn Kaneko, who brought a form called Amma Shiatsu; Shizuto Masunaga, who developed Zen Shiatsu; Shizuko Yamamoto, who developed Barefoot Shiatsu; and Wataru Ohashi, who developed Ohashiatsu.

Namikoshi's style of shiatsu involved the least complex of the amma techniques (finger, thumb, and palm pressure), and it did not include the traditional meridian system of amma. Sensitive to the twentieth-century enthusiasm for Western scientific medicine throughout the world, Namikoshi superimposed his points over Western structural anatomy. Toru Namikoshi details this system with diagrams in *The Complete Book of Shiatsu Therapy* (1981).

Shizuto Masunaga developed his own meridian system, which is described in his book *Zen Shiatsu* (1977). His student, Wataru Ohashi, returned to the original traditional Chinese meridian system, which he details in *Do-It-Yourself Shiatsu* (1976). Shizuko Yamamoto does not include a map of their meridian system in her book nor does she include acupressure points in her complete shiatsu treatment. She does, however, suggest a list of acupoints for treating common problems. Mr. Kaneko follows the traditional Chinese meridian system and includes many of the more complicated techniques of amma in his style of shiatsu. As you can see, when someone says, "I do shiatsu," they may be speaking about any one of a number of different forms of this ancient healing art.

Traditional amma was first formally introduced to the United States in 1971, with the opening of Kabuki Hot Springs in Japantown, San Francisco, California. Designed as a traditional Japanese spa, Kabuki Hot Springs employed sighted amma practitioners who had been trained in Japan and brought to the United States to work in the new spa. By 1977, the owners of the Hot Springs wanted to develop a local source of qualified practitioners. They asked Takashi Nakamura, a practitioner from the Kensai School of Massage, Acupuncture, Moxa, and Cautery in Osaka, Japan, to open a school in San Francisco. Although he taught amma, the school was called the Kabuki Shiatsu School of Massage.

Nakamura developed a highly choreographed one-hour, full-body table sequence using over 25 different hand and arm techniques on over 140 *tsubo*, or acupoints. He taught this sequence in the way that he had been taught in Japan. He demonstrated a small portion of the sequence on each student, they then practiced on one another, and then each student demonstrated his or her ability to repeat that segment on Nakamura. The entire sequence was taught this way, each piece building on the next. By teaching this form appropriate for a spa setting and modeling how the amma forms were taught in Japan, Takashi Nakamura helped to further an understanding of the amma tradition in the United States. Nakamura returned to Japan in 1981, after teaching his student, David Palmer, how to teach the amma spa form.

Palmer reopened the school in 1982. Recognizing the significance of the amma tradition and how it differed from the way shiatsu was being taught and practiced in the United States, he renamed the school The Amma Institute of Traditional Japanese Massage. In an attempt to make skilled touch more accessible in the United States, Palmer adapted the last few minutes of the one-hour full-body spa sequence and created a 15-minute upper-body form for clients seated in a chair. The 15-

minute chair form had made receiving amma appear safe, convenient, and affordable. Massage practitioners can once again bring their service out to the people like the blind ammas of Japan were doing over 80 years ago. In December of 1988, Palmer left The Amma Institute to develop the Skilled Touch Institute of Chair Massage. Each year his trainers introduce the techniques of Japanese massage to hundreds of professional bodyworkers. Palmer's student, the author, reopened The Amma Institute in August, 1989, and continues to carry on the tradition of teaching the original amma spa sequences.

▪ OVERVIEW OF A ONE-HOUR AMMA FORM

The one-hour amma form described here was created as a wellness or health maintenance massage. It is designed to be given on a table and includes a variety of techniques, which encompass pressing, stroking, stretching, and percussive manipulations. Techniques are performed with the thumbs, fingers, and arms to stimulate over 140 acupressure points along the 14 major energy meridians.

Amma is very rhythmic. The 60-minute form described here is characterized by a four-beat rhythm. The prescribed sequence, called a *kata*, is designed to relax and rejuvenate the body, leaving the receiver feeling refreshed and revitalized.

The intention of this amma form is to facilitate the flow of energy in the body. By improving circulation (ie, *chi* and its many manifestations such as blood, lymph, and other body fluids), the amma techniques assist the body's own healing mechanisms to operate more effectively. The practitioner's main focus is the comfort of the receiver and the precision of performance of the *kata*.

A practitioner's first consideration is to determine whether or not the receiver will benefit from the amma massage. The second is whether the service that the practitioner is providing is what the recipient is expecting to receive. Clarity of intention helps to ensure the comfort of the amma experience. To learn the receiver's expectations and determine whether or not the amma sequence will offer benefit, each session begins with a screening process.

The Screening

During the screening process, the practitioner asks five basic questions:

1. Have you ever had massage before?
2. Have you ever had a Japanese massage before?
3. Do you have any recent injuries or illnesses?
4. Are you under a doctor's care or are you taking any medication?

And we ask women of child bearing age,

5. Are you pregnant or trying to be pregnant?

Amma is contraindicated for pregnancy. Many of the points that we press are used in labor to help stimulate uterine contractions.

If the practitioner is unsure whether or not the recipient would benefit from the massage, they follow one simple rule: When in doubt, don't. The second rule they follow is: Always err on the side of caution.

And finally, before beginning the session the practitioner gives the receiver permission to give feedback regarding the comfort of the massage. The receiver decides how strong the pressure should be, not the practitioner. By following these guidelines, and by always screening, the practitioners ensure that the service they are providing is safe for the recipient and for themselves.

The Sequence

To start, the receiver lies face-down on a massage table with the arms parallel with the shoulders, and the hands by the head. The practitioner drapes the receiver with a sheet, leaving only the head exposed. All of the techniques are performed through the sheet.

The traditional one-hour form begins with the practitioner climbing onto the table and straddling the receiver by placing one knee along side of, but not touching, the hip, and the other foot near the receiver's arm pit. See Figure 16–1. This position allows the practitioner to use body leverage to apply pressure to the back.

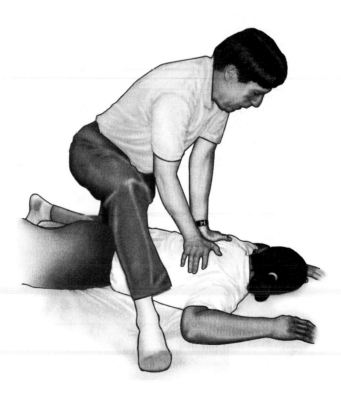

FIGURE 16–1. Amma technique called *shusho appakuho,* applying pressure with the palms.

The practitioner then presses with the palms (*shusho appakuho*) down both sides of the back on the crest of the erector spinae muscles. Start between the scapula and end just superior to the sacrum, pressing in four or five places going down the back.

The practitioner climbs off the table and moves to the shoulders. The sequence then proceeds from the shoulders to the arms all the way out to the fingertips. Once one shoulder and arm have been completed, the practitioner moves to the other shoulder and arm. This symmetry of form continues through the entire massage.

After completing the shoulders and arms, the practitioner massages the neck; from the neck to the back; from the back to the hips and legs all the way to the bottom of the feet. The practitioner completes the first side of the body by returning to the back with bilateral thumb presses and then finishes with a series of percussions. At the end of the final percussion the practitioner asks the client to "turn over, please."

After draping the receiver with a sheet and wrapping a towel across the ears and eyes, the practitioner begins with the right leg, pressing points along the top, side, and inside of the leg down to the feet and then stretching the leg. After repeating this sequence on the left leg and then stretching the toes bilaterally and shaking the legs, the practitioner moves to the head of the table. Then the practitioner massages the face, the neck, the chest, and the abdomen.

To complete the massage we sit the receiver up and work on the scalp, the neck, and the shoulders, stretch the back and arms, and finish with a closing series of percussions on the upper back and shoulders, which ends with the words "thank you very much." Palmer added "thank you very much" to all the amma sequences that are taught at The Amma Institute. He did this for three reasons: (1) to indicate to the client that the massage is over; (2) to acknowledge that a practitioner–client relationship is a peer relationship and that the practitioner would not be able to do the work they love best without the client; and (3) as a way for the practitioner to practice humility.

The Amma Techniques

Below is a list of the most commonly used techniques in the one-hour full-body sequence. Each technique would take pages of description to explain; however, there are four basic concepts pertaining to body mechanics that are common to all the techniques that are used to apply pressure.

- Weight transfer
- Perpendicularity
- Stacking the joints
- Keeping the back straight

Weight transfer allows the practitioner to find a comfortable balance, that is, pressure that is comfortable to the receiver. It also ensures that the connection that the practitioner is making comes from the whole body and not from strength. To transfer weight the practitioner must stand (or kneel) with one foot forward and the other foot (or knee) back. In a standing position the front leg must always be bent with the foot forward enough to be in front of the knee. The back leg is straight. The hips are aligned so that the back is straight. The transfer happens by taking the weight off the front leg and moving it to the heels of the hands, thumbs, or which ever part of the head or arm is being used to apply pressure.

Perpendicularity is an important part of the precision and efficiency of amma. To make sure that the pressure is sinking straight into an acupressure point, the line from the shoulders to the point of contact (heel of hand or thumb) must be 90 degrees to the plane of the surface of the point on the body. If the line isn't 90 degrees the client's skin will usually stretch in one direction or another.

Stacking the joints one on top of another is essential to the concept of perpendicularity and weight transfer. For a connection to be make with the whole body, there must be a straight line from the body, either through the shoulder, or through the elbow acting as an extension of the shoulder, to the heel of the hands or the thumbs. For example, imagine the weight moving down from the shoulder into the top third of the fingerprint part of the thumb. The shoulder is stacked over the elbow, which, in turn, is stacked over the wrist and an arched thumb. Stacking the joints in this way allows the pressure to go straight into each point effortlessly.

A *straight back* is the fourth essential part in all of the amma techniques. If the back is not straight, the practitioner often ends up pushing with the upper body instead of the more effortless feeling of transferred weight. The practitioner's weight should be held in the legs, not the back. At first, this may feel uncomfortable; however, some of the biggest muscles in the body are in the legs. They develop quickly and are much more forgiving than the small muscles of the back. If you carry the weight in the back, fatigue sets in more quickly and eventually the pain can become debilitating.

A SIMPLE EXERCISE TO FEEL THE SIGNIFICANCE OF THESE FOUR BODY MECHANIC CONCEPTS. The following is an exercise that puts all of these components together to demonstrate the sensation of transferring weight. Stand facing a wall and put both hands on the wall a shoulder's width apart and at shoulder height. Step back with both feet so that your body is at a 45 degree angle and you're leaning into the wall. Bring your hips forward so that your shoulders, back, and feet are aligned. Notice that all your weight is in your feet and in your hands. Now bring one leg forward and bend it. Make sure your foot is forward enough so that your toes are in front of your knee. The other leg stays back and straight. Keep your hips aligned with your shoulders and your back foot. Your stance should be open with your back leg centered between your hands and the front leg slightly off to the side. Keep your arms straight and relax your shoulders. Your hands are placed with your fingers out to the sides, and the heels of your hands are parallel to one another. See Figure 16–2. If you have range of motion limitations in your wrists, adjust your hands so you're comfortable. Sometimes slightly curling your fingers is enough. Now try to hold your weight in your front leg so that your hands are not supporting you at all.

Begin by slowly transferring the weight of your body from your front leg to the heels of your hands. Keep your arms straight and your hips aligned. Your hips don't need to move at all. As you feel the weight transfer to the heels of your hands,

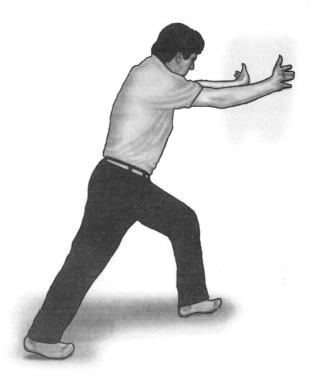

FIGURE 16–2. Wall exercise to practice transfer of weight while applying pressure for techniques like *shusho appakuho.*

you'll notice that weight is also moving to your back foot. The heel of your foot shouldn't be down. The weight is in the ball of your back foot.

To really feel this sensation, actually lift the front foot, keeping the hips quiet and the back straight. Don't bend the arms. As you lift your leg, exhale. Now lower the leg and put weight in the front leg. Remember the front foot should be far enough forward so that the toes are in front of the knee. The hands should not be holding any weight again. The hips should still be in the same place. Do not pull back with the hands. Arms can still be straight out in front. Now, transfer the weight back to the "palms" (really the heel of the hands). The above is an introduction to the first technique of amma—*shusho appakuho* as shown in Figure 16–1.

Table 16–1 contains a complete list of the amma techniques that are taught in the one-hour full-body spa sequence. Both *appakuho* (thumb pressure) and *wansho junenho* (back and forth motion with the forearms), are shown in Figures 16–3 and 16–4, respectively.

TABLE 16–1	Amma Techniques for the One-hour Full-body Spa Sequence	
	Shusho Appakuho	Palm pressure
	Boshi Appakuho	Thumb pressure
	Shusho Junenho	Back and forth movement with palm
	Boshi Junenho	Back and forth movement with thumb
	Nishi Junenho	Back and forth movement with thumb and index finger
	Shishi Junenho	Back and forth movement with four fingers
	Haaku Junenho	Back and forth movement by grasping with thumb and finger
	Rinjyo Junenho	Circular motion with thumb only
	Wansho Junenho	Back and forth motion with forearm
	Rotojyo Junenho	Waving motion with the hand
	Shusho Keisatsuho	Stroking with the palm
	Boshi Keisatsuho	Stroking with the thumb
	Shishi Keisatsuho	Stroking with the four fingers
	Shukendaho	Percussion with a loose fist
	Setsudaho	Percussion with both hands alternating
	Gasshadaho	Percussion with both hands joined
	Gankidaho	Cupped hands percussion movement
	Hakudaho	Cupped hand percussion
	Kurumade	Rolling motion from fingertips to back of hand
	Tsukide	"Finger dives"
	Tsukamide	Finger grasping in quick movements with the wrist
	Yanagide	"Willow Tree"
	Yokode	Back and fourth motion with either side of the hand

■ THE SIGNIFICANCE OF USING A *KATA* TO TEACH MASSAGE

The challenge presented to instructors in the West who are teaching Eastern styles of massage is twofold. First, the instructor needs to understand the philosophical foundation or cosmology that produced the massage form. And second, the instructor needs to be aware of his own culture's cosmology to be able to present the new information in a way that can be easily assimilated by the students.

When Takashi Nakamura began teaching amma in the Untied States in 1977, he taught a choreographed full-body sequence. The concept of *kata* is often used to help students understand the significance of the Japanese use of sequence in teaching a physical skill.

There is no exact translation of the word *kata*; however, the basic concept has to do with a form, or sequence, or system of movement that determines precisely how something is accomplished. *Katas* are studied in all of the Japanese arts; however, in our Western culture the term is most frequently used in the context of the martial arts. Students practice *katas*, or sequences of movements, over and over again until they become automatic.

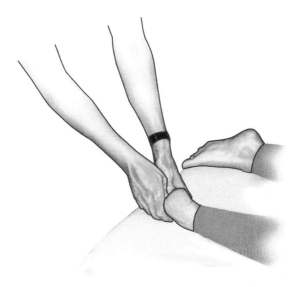

FIGURE 16–3. Amma technique called *boshi apakuho,* applying pressure with the thumbs.

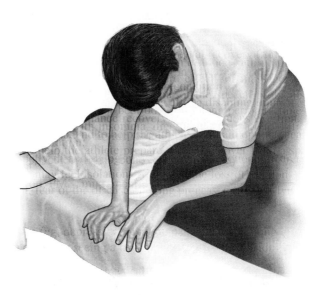

FIGURE 16–4. Amma technique called *wansho junenko,* back and forth motion with the forearms.

Practice is vital to the process involved in learning any physical skill. Teaching students a massage *kata* allows them to practice skilled touch with the confidence of knowing that the *kata* is effective in doing what it is designed to do even while the student is still integrating the sequence, the techniques and the points locations and learning how to touch someone comfortably. The student doesn't have to know Chinese medicine, for example, to give a highly effective amma massage. The *kata* "knows" Chinese medicine. The student simply has to follow the *kata*. Palmer (1995) says: "We teach a kata and it is the kata which teaches the student massage" (p. 26).

> *The Kata is like a wise elder which has the wisdom of the centuries behind it. The Kata has a long lineage that extends from teacher to teacher and is based on a theoretical foundation and philosophical world view which transcends our individual understanding.*
>
> *If you trust the Kata and develop an honest relationship with it, you will be rewarded with an unlimited stream of insights about the nature of touch, massage, service, relationships, [and] yourself . . .*
>
> *When you practice [a traditional Japanese] massage Kata it eventually becomes something like a beautiful dance or a piece of classical music. Highly structured and choreographed, it is the same each time it is performed and yet, each time, it is also different.*
>
> *(Palmer, 1995, pp. 26–27)*

■ SUMMARY

Amma is a traditional Japanese form of massage, which was brought from China during the sixth century C.E. Amma eventually became an occupation for the blind in Japan. Traditional amma was introduced to the United States in the 1970s in San Francisco.

Amma techniques include a variety of pressing, stroking, stretching, and percussive movements applied with the thumbs, fingers, forearms, elbows, and knees. These techniques are combined into sequences of movement that stimulate points along the 14 major meridians of the body.

Principles of applying amma techniques safely and effectively include weight transfer, perpendicularity, stacking the joints, and keeping the back straight. Amma is often taught in a form called a *kata*, or routine sequence of techniques designed to stimulate important acupressure points.

■ REFERENCES

Joya, M. (1958). *Mock Joya's things Japanese.* Tokyo: Tokyo News Service, Ltd.
Masunaga, S. (1977). *Zen shiatsu.* Tokyo: Japan Publications.
Namikoshi, T. (1969). *Japanese finger-pressure, shiatsu.* Tokyo: Japan Publications.
Namikoshi, T. (1981). *The complete book of shiatsu therapy.* Tokyo: Japan Publications.
Ohashi, W. (1976). *Do-it-yourself shiatsu.* New York: E. P. Dutton.

Palmer, D. (1995). What is Kata? *TouchPro massage manual.* San Francisco: Skilled Touch Institute of Chair Massage.

Serizawa, K. (1972). *Massage, the oriental method.* Tokyo: Japan Publications.

Serizawa, K. (1976). *Effective tsubo therapy.* Tokyo: Japan Publications.

Serizawa, K. (1984). *Tsubo: Vital points for oriental therapy.* Tokyo: Japan Publications.

Shiatsu: An Overview

Pauline E. Sasaki

■ SHIATSU AND ITS HISTORY

Humankind has always recognized that the hand can contribute powerfully to the healing process. No one has to be told that rubbing the eyes or the scalp helps to soothe the pain of a headache, and even in Western medicine, the role of the physical therapist has come to be widely accepted. In Japan, however, the use of the hand as a therapeutic tool has a time-honored history and a deep philosophical foundation.

The Japanese art of *shiatsu* (literally, *shi* [finger] + *atsu* [pressure]) is a system for healing and health maintenance that has evolved over the course of thousands of years. Practiced informally since at least 200 B.C., shiatsu was systematized in the early 1900s and became accepted as a form of therapy widely practiced to this day.

Shiatsu derives both from the ancient healing art of acupuncture and from the traditional form of Japanese massage, *anma.* In Japan, anma was originally considered the equivalent of Chinese acupuncture as the method one studied to treat the human body in illness. It was recognized to have bona fide therapeutic benefits up until the end of the Tokugawa period in the eighteenth century (Masunaga, 1983, p. 1). Because this was a peaceful period in Japan's history, intellectual inclinations flourished. Simultaneously, however, society became overly enamored of the pleasures and luxuries of life, with the result that anma was reduced to being merely an instrument of psychologic and sexual pleasure. Anma as it was practiced had discarded the historic foundations that had legitimized it as a therapeutic system.

Ultimately, shiatsu developed apart from anma as a therapeutic discipline based once again on its original theory. In the meantime, prior to World War II, anma became a major employer of the blind in Japan. During the American occupation of Japan when MacArthur was considering outlawing both anma and shiatsu (due to erroneous information that they had sexual connotations), the blind of Japan appealed to Helen Keller in America to intercede on their behalf. Their appeal was successful and shiatsu and anma were permitted to be practiced (Ohashi, 1976, p. 10). Eventually, this approval led to a formal school of shiatsu, the Nippon Shiatsu School, established by Tokujiro Namikoshi in the late 1940s. Since then, shiatsu has become a popular medical therapy that is recognized and licensed by the government of Japan.

■ BASIC CONCEPTS OF SHIATSU

To understand shiatsu, one must first understand some of the basic concepts shared by acupuncture, shiatsu, and the Eastern healing arts in general.

The basic tenets of Eastern medicine can be traced back to China at a time between the second and third centuries B.C., when in the Yellow Emperor's *Classic of Internal Medicine* a system of energy channels called *meridians* was described (Omura, 1982, p. 13). This perception of the body as a system of meridians formed at a time when the prevailing religion forbade any type of surgical intrusion into the human body. Denied access to procedures that would reveal the structure and functions of the human body, the Chinese developed a practical metaphor for the anatomy and physiology of the body through observation and intuition. They conceptualized the body as a living, dynamic entity subject to the influences of an underlying network of energy pathways. Thus, meridians represented the energetic, as opposed to the anatomic, structure of the body.

This emphasis on energy rather than anatomy is perhaps the fundamental difference between Eastern and Western medicine. When the body is analyzed anatomically, it appears as a collection of separate parts that exist whether the owner of the body is alive or dead. Examined energetically, however, the body appears to function as the result of a dynamic life force (referred to as chi or *ki*) that serves as the common link among all the body's tissues and organs. *Ki* ties together all bodily structures and functions so that they operate as a single entity. To the Easterner, the organs are not sufficient to sustain life unless the vital force *ki* is also present to keep the organs functional and properly interrelated. Furthermore, since *ki* represents the essence of life, this energetic structure ceases to exist once a person dies.

In its role as the life force, *ki* is always present and active within the body. Moreover, *ki* affects and even controls a person's entire life structure. To the Eastern mind, the unobstructed, balanced flow of *ki* along the meridians is both the cause and the effect of good health. Eastern medicine including the disciplines of acupuncture and shiatsu is dedicated to maintaining the balanced flow of *ki* throughout the body and to reestablishing that balance whenever it is thrown askew.

■ THE STRUCTURE OF MERIDIANS

All bodily processes are associated with various major functions, each of which is in turn associated with one or more meridians. Consequently, each meridian has been assigned the name of an organ. (Because the relationship of a meridian to an organ is metaphoric rather than anatomic, many Westerners become confused when they find, for example, that the lung meridian lies along the arm, or that the liver meridian lies along the leg. The name assigned to a meridian refers not to the meridian's external location on the body but to the functional influence of the meridian within the body.) Table 17–1 contains a list of some of the major functions and the meridians with which they are associated.

These general functions illustrate the range of roles *ki* plays in the human body and how the meridians work symbolically through the physiologic system. The theory of the life cycle of the meridians explains the sequence and the purpose of the various processes for maintaining life.

The cycle begins with the lung and large intestine meridians. As a pair, these meridians govern the intake of *ki* and elimination. The action of inhaling the *ki* from the outside world and bringing it into the body is represented by the respiratory system. The action of exhaling the extraneous *ki* is represented by the eliminative system. On a symbolic level, the breath begins life by differentiating between the *ki* from the outside world and the *ki* within the human form. An example of this is the birth of a child. A child is not acknowledged as being alive until it takes its first breath. Once the child continues to breathe, its existence as a human being is established. The *ki* from the outside world is separated from human *ki* by the existence of a border, represented by the skin. The skin acts in two ways: (1) it absorbs *ki* from

FUNCTIONS ASSOCIATED WITH MAJOR MERIDIANS

TABLE
17–1

Function	Meridians
Intake of *ki*	Lung
Process of elimination	Large Intestine
Intake of food	Stomach
Digestion	Spleen
Interpretation of the emotional environment	Heart
Assimilation	Small Intestine
Purification	Bladder
Impetus to move	Kidney
Circulation	Heart Constrictor
Protection	Triple Heater
Storage, distribution,	Liver
and detoxification of *ki*	Gallbladder

Modified from S. Masunaga & W. Ohashi. (1977). *Zen Shiatsu.* Tokyo: Japan Publications, pp. 42–47.

the outside; and (2) it excretes waste material from the inside of the body via the pores. If both activities are in balance, the human form remains an entity.

Once this is established, two requirements are necessary for survival: (1) nourishment from an outside source and (2) emotional stimuli to satisfy the spirit.

Outside Nourishment

The primary external source of nourishment is food. Therefore, the intake of food and its breakdown for human consumption as represented in the process of digestion is an important function that is necessary to replenish expended *ki*. The stomach and spleen meridians initiate these functions via the actual stomach, esophagus, and duodenum as well as via the digestive enzymes necessary for the breakdown of food.

Emotional Stimuli

The second requirement is nourishment of the psyche by giving meaning to all human actions. The heart and small intestine meridians act as the interpreter and assimilator of stimuli that affect the emotions and feelings. A person's interaction with others is dependent on these functions; if a person cannot understand and absorb stimuli from the environment, life has no meaning beyond pure existence, and the reason for relationships and experiences ceases to exist. Of all the meridians, the heart and small intestine are most associated with the spiritual aspect of *ki,* primarily compassion. They are the connecting links between the physical and heavenly bodies (ie, our relation to the universe). On a physiologic level, the qualities of the heart are symbolized by the color red in our blood. Therefore, the heart and small intestine meridians are said to influence the quality of the blood.

These three pairs of meridians all deal with extracting *ki* from the environment. When that function is completed, the *ki* is then processed internally so it can be utilized. The first step is to filter out the impurities in the *ki* taken in from the outside world and move it to the meridians that circulate it throughout the body. The bladder and kidney meridians govern the purification and movement process via urination, the autonomic nervous system, and the endocrine gland system.

When the *ki* is refined, it is sent to the central distributors for circulation and protection. The heart constrictor and triple heater meridians are the central distributors that make *ki* available to all parts of the body regardless of whether the body is active or inactive. For circulation to occur, a specific temperature must be maintained. The heart constrictor and triple heater meridians carry out these functions via the vascular system, the lymphatic system, and the metabolic processes that regulate body temperature.

When the *ki* is available for use, the liver and gallbladder meridians control how the *ki* is distributed to accomplish a specific action. For example, in the action of walking, more *ki* would be channeled into the moving leg than other parts of the body that are still. However, not all the *ki* is distributed and used. Much of it is stored for future use so that it does not have to be constantly replenished. The quality of *ki* is constantly maintained through the process of detoxification. This function of allocating *ki* for specific actions over a period of time parallels the birth and growth cycle whereby specific actions at different time periods contribute to a pattern of development. This function is represented on the physiologic level in the reproductive system. The liver and gallbladder meridians thus govern the reproductive system. Since life is a process, this cycle is ongoing until life ends.

The meaning of these functions can be interpreted on a variety of different levels including the physical, the emotional, the intellectual, and the spiritual. For example, an imbalance exhibited in the small intestine meridian indicates that the process of assimilation may not be working properly. On the physical plane, this imbalance may indicate faulty absorption of nutrients from the food in the intestines. This imbalance may express itself through physical symptoms such as acne, flatulence, migraine headaches, and intestinal problems. If the remedy addresses the problem of assimilation, the physical symptoms will automatically subside.

On an emotional plane, an assimilation problem might occur if there is an overload of emotional stimuli coming from the environment. Having to process and cope with the reactions to such stimuli disrupts the assimilation mechanism that normally adds meaning to our emotional environment. In cases such as trauma when the person cannot cope with the amount of stimuli derived from the experience, the body halts the assimilation process by going into a state of shock. This imbalance might manifest itself in symptoms such as hypersensitivity, the inability to cope with emotional situations, or the inability to recall traumatic experiences (in cases of shock).

On an intellectual plane, a small intestine meridian imbalance may indicate an inability to fully understand abstract concepts and an inability to follow through on details. Symptoms could include excessive worrying, anxiety, or too much concentration on unimportant details.

On a spiritual plane, an assimilation problem may exhibit itself by a person's being overwhelmed with emotion during religious experiences or by a lack of compassion due to an inability to react emotionally.

We can see from this analysis that a variety of symptoms can manifest themselves from one single cause—in this case, poor assimilation. If the imbalance in a particular meridian is rectified, it will have positive repercussions on all of the different planes.

■ HOMEOSTASIS

Homeostasis is a modern scientific term that happens to describe quite suitably the flow of *ki* within and among the meridians. The idea behind homeostasis is that dynamic systems (in this case the human body) naturally seek and maintain a condition of overall balance. Whenever an external force is applied to the system, at least one change must occur in the system in order to establish a new condition of balance.

With regard to the balance of *ki,* external forces resulting from physical, mental, and spiritual stresses produce internal obstructions that are released at points along the meridians, termed *tsubos.* The character of these obstructions depends not only on the meridian or meridians affected but also on the quality and quantity of the *ki* involved in the imbalance. The study of the quality and quantity of *ki* and how it influences homeostasis in the body involves the concepts of vibration quality and of Kyo-Jitsu.

Vibration Quality

Ki can be thought of as a form of vibration that ranges in frequency from low to high. *Ki* with a low vibrational quality seems heavy and slow, whereas *ki* with a high vibrational quality seems light and fast. These qualities are additionally influenced by the quantity of *ki* present, which can be either deficient or excessive. The most common sensations of vibration felt are temperature differences, ie, high vibration is sensed in heat and low vibration is sensed in the feeling of coldness. However, these are not the only barometers for measuring the quality of vibration. Trained shiatsu practitioners spend years developing sensitivity to the flow of *ki* within the body and are able to feel subtle vibrational qualities of energy imbalances associated with illness, disease, and pain.

Kyo-Jitsu

The terms *kyo* and *jitsu* refer to the quantity as well as quality of *ki*. The concept of Kyo-Jitsu is explained by Masunaga and Ohashi in the book *Zen Shiatsu* (1977). *Kyo* is defined as an area of deficient and weak *ki,* whereas *jitsu* is defined as an area of excessively strong *ki.* Imbalances generally stem from an absence of *ki* (*kyo*) because this absence retards a meridian's function. When this occurs, the life process is threatened and the remainder of the network becomes distorted as energy is redistributed in order to compensate for the weak area that is malfunctioning. As a consequence of this dynamic redistribution of energy, areas of excess *ki* (*jitsu*) appear and are necessary to sustain the distorted state. This condition persists as long as the malfunctioning area remains weak. Once the weakness is alleviated, the meridian initially affected regains its normal function, the remainder of the body is able to disperse the areas of *jitsu,* and the normal pattern of energy flow becomes reestablished.

■ TYPES OF SHIATSU

Presently, there are three major types of shiatsu being practiced, each of which approaches the goal of balancing energy flow differently: shiatsu massage, acupressure, and *zen* shiatsu.

As explained earlier, shiatsu massage is based largely on anma techniques and views the body purely from an anatomic or physiologic perspective. In conjunction with the use of massage techniques and manipulations, hard pressure is applied to the body at certain points to elicit the relief of specific symptoms. The most widely known form of shiatsu massage is the Namikoshi method, developed by Tokujiro Namikoshi (1969), and his son Toru Namikoshi (1981).

Acupressure is similar to shiatsu massage, the difference being that acupressure incorporates the same theory of meridians and *tsubos* used by acupuncture. Acupressure is advocated in books by Katsusuke Serizawa (1976, 1984) and is discussed in Chapter 15 of this book.

Zen shiatsu recognizes a broader set of meridians and *tsubos* than does acupuncture (Fig. 17–1). The level of pressure applied to the *tsubos* and meridians is significantly lighter than that in other types of shiatsu. Also, unlike shiatsu mas-

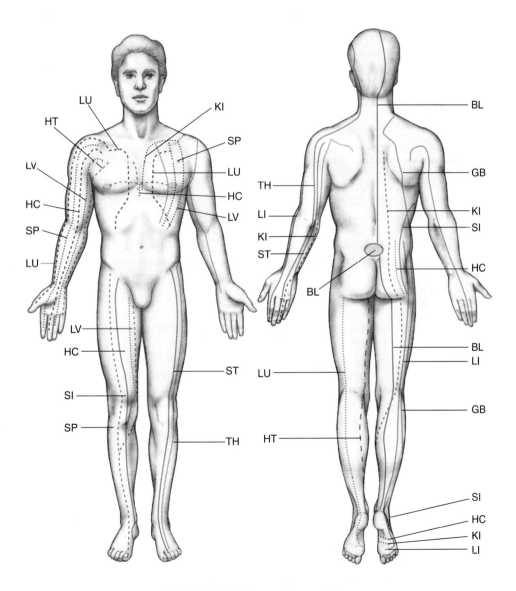

FIGURE 17–1. Meridians used in zen shiatsu.

sage and acupressure, zen shiatsu incorporates the diagnostic theory of *kyo-jitsu*. This style of shiatsu was developed by the late Shizuto Masunaga, founder and director of the Iokai Shiatsu Center in Japan (Masunaga & Ohashi, 1977). Because this style of shiatsu is unique, its basic concepts will be discussed in detail. (Hereafter, the term *shiatsu* will be used to mean zen shiatsu.)

■ THE ROLE OF THE SHIATSU PRACTITIONER

The shiatsu practitioner has three primary goals: diagnosis (to identify the nature and extent of energy imbalances in a patient), treatment (to penetrate meridians in such a way as to alleviate the imbalances that exist), and maintenance (to apply manual pressure in such a way as to sustain and strengthen the existing energy balance).

■ DIAGNOSIS

The underlying purpose of diagnosis in shiatsu is to identify the cause-and-effect relationship between a *kyo* meridian and a *jitsu* meridian, with the goal of altering the cause of the condition so that the effect will take care of itself. (In any cause-and-effect relationship, the effect will persist until the cause is dealt with. For instance, a person lacking adequate food will feel continuously hungry. Once he or she eats, however, the hunger disappears.) Specifically, a *jitsu* condition (the effect) disperses automatically once the weak *kyo* condition (the cause) is altered. Because diagnostic areas for each of the 12 meridians are located in the abdomen (Fig. 17–2), the primary means of evaluating the state of a person's energy is to palpate the abdominal area. The intent is to use findings of *kyo* and *jitsu* areas to identify those meridians in which energy levels and flow are out of balance. (Additional sites on the back can be used for visual diagnosis. When there is an imbalance in a meridian, the area where it pools in the back may appear distorted or out of proportion to the whole [Fig. 17–3].)

Skill in diagnosis is a function of the practitioner's ability to sense *kyo* and *jitsu* relationships within the abdomen. Once those relationships have been correctly identified, a talented practitioner can usually draw meaningful conclusions as to how and why the imbalance developed. Typically, a shiatsu session begins with palpation of the patient's abdomen; pressure is then applied to *tsubos* along the *kyo* and *jitsu* meridians; finally, the abdomen is once again palpated. If the practitioner has been effective, the final palpation will indicate that both the *kyo* and *jitsu* conditions have been altered and even alleviated entirely.

■ SHIATSU TECHNIQUES

Four primary principles govern shiatsu techniques:

1. The giver maintains the attitude of an observer.
2. Penetration is perpendicular to the surface of the meridian being treated.

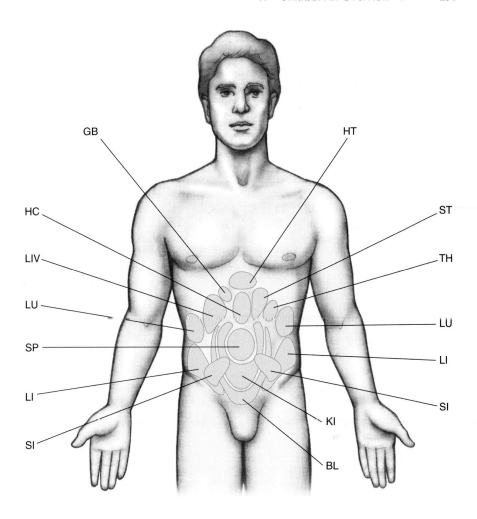

FIGURE 17–2. Diagnostic areas in the abdomen for the 12 meridians.

3. Body weight rather than strength is used to allow the hand to penetrate into the meridian that is being worked on.
4. Pressure is applied rhythmically.

The Practitioner as Observer

To tap into the body's natural source of healing energy so that it can remedy an imbalance, the shiatsu practitioner must become attuned to the internal dynamics of the *ki* structure of the body by the simple device of observation. Maintaining a relaxed hand and an attitude devoid of any intention to interfere with the receiver's *ki,* the practitioner ensures that the focus remains on using the receiver's own energy as the source of healing. The practitioner acts as a catalyst for the healing process.

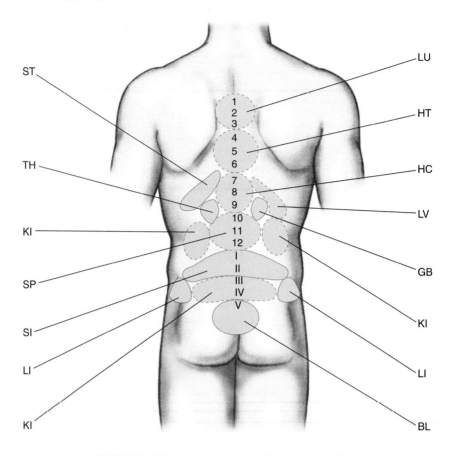

FIGURE 17–3. Diagnostic areas in the back for the 12 meridians.

Perpendicular Penetration

The purpose of shiatsu is to effect changes in the flow of energy in a meridian by manipulating the energy vortices called *tsubos*. However, contacting the flow of *ki* in a meridian is analogous to pouring water into a vase. (The word *tsubo* in Japanese means *vase*. The metaphor is of a vessel with a narrow neck.) Unless water is poured into the vase from directly overhead, much will be lost. Similarly, in shiatsu, penetration into the *tsubo* must occur at a 90 degree angle to the *tsubo* in order to have the optimum impact on the flow of *ki* within the meridian. At any other angle, the effects will remain on the surface and will not penetrate deeply enough to influence the meridian.

Shiatsu techniques that employ perpendicular penetration produce significant changes in the meridian structure that go beyond superficial stimulation.

Body Weight Versus Muscle Strength

The type of pressure applied directly affects the nature of the impact a shiatsu session has on the receiver. To apply hard pressure to a meridian, the practitioner would have to tense the upper-body muscles forcefully; to endure such hard pressure, the receiver would have to remain totally passive and would be unable to participate at all in the healing process. Since tension decreases a practitioner's sensitivity, no communication bond between giver and receiver could be established. The practitioner would dominate the process, and the receiver would remain a passive recipient. Techniques that use hard pressure require more upper-body strength than do more gentle techniques, and they can produce physical problems in the shoulders and arms of the giver.

In contrast, when penetration of *tsubos* is achieved through the use of body weight, the practitioner's hand and upper body remain relaxed rather than tense. Pressure is applied by transferring the body's weight into the hand. The receiver senses this type of pressure as firm but gentle, with the result that a communication line of energy is established between giver and receiver. This relaxed form of penetration draws the receiver's own energy into the area being touched. The receiver participates by using that energy to rectify the imbalance in the meridian. The communication bond enables the practitioner to detect changes as they take place in the meridian and thereby monitor the receiver's response and progress. Because giver and receiver are providing each other feedback, this type of shiatsu is beneficial to both.

Rhythm

The receiver's response to shiatsu is contingent on the quality of the pressure being used on the meridians and *tsubos*. The intervals at which pressure is felt constitute the rhythmic pattern of the technique. The response to rhythm can be seen in a person's response to music. If a piece of music has a slow rhythm, the common reaction to it is one of relaxation or of feeling soothed. A slow rhythm also allows the listener to focus on the composition of the music and how each note is played in relation to the others. If the rhythm is fast, the listener reacts excitedly, responding by moving the body or dancing. Instead of tuning in to the notes being played, the person is carried away with the active response to the beat.

The rhythms of shiatsu technique elicit similar responses. A slow rhythm is produced when perpendicular pressure is held on a *tsubo* for a short length of time (usually the time needed to create a vibrational change in the area being touched). This is the principal technique used when working along the *kyo* meridian because it brings the cause of the imbalance to the attention of the receiver. This results in more permanent changes in the energy pattern. When the pressure is held, it allows the receiver's energy to tune in to the area of weakness and remedy it. At the same time, the slow rhythm relaxes and soothes, making it easier for the receiver to participate in the healing process.

A fast rhythm, on the other hand, causes the *ki* in the *tsubo* being touched to disperse. Fast-moving, perpendicular pressure produces a rapid rhythm that distracts the receiver's attention from the cause of an imbalance. Because of this, sole use of this type of pressure throughout an entire shiatsu session produces very temporary results. This technique is used primarily on the *jitsu* meridian to assist in the redistribution of excess *ki* in an area that is exceptionally obstructed, as in cases of injury.

If these four primary guidelines are adhered to, *shiatsu* becomes a highly effective method for correcting *ki* imbalances quickly with the least amount of effort exerted by the giver. When this is accomplished, the healing power of both the giver and receiver is strengthened.

■ BENEFITS OF SHIATSU

In Chinese medicine, a therapeutic approach was considered valid if it produced consistently positive results over a long period of time with little or no ill effect. This contrasts with Western medicine, in which the focus is on fast relief of the present symptoms in the shortest period of time, often without regard for the long-range effects. Although Western science still does not recognize the existence of the meridian structure of the body, there is no doubt that the practical application of the basic principles of shiatsu work.

■ SUMMARY

Humankind may have changed through the years, but the relationship of the human species to natural law has remained the same. Shiatsu is based on that law, and its tool, the hand, is imbued with the sensitive qualities necessary to evaluate the impact those laws are having on an individual. Just as the ancient system of meridians and *tsubos* is as effective today as it was thousands of years ago, shiatsu continues to unify body, mind, and spirit and contribute to a life lived to its highest potential through healthful and fulfilling experiences.

■ REFERENCES

Masunaga, S. (1983). *Keiraku to shiatsu.* Yokosuka: Ido-No-Nihonsha.
Masunaga, S., & Ohashi, W. (1977). *Zen shiatsu.* Tokyo: Japan Publications.
Namikoshi, T. (1969). *Shiatsu.* San Francisco: Japan Publications.
Namikoshi, T. (1981). *The complete book of shiatsu therapy.* Tokyo: Japan Publications.
Ohashi, W. (1976). *Do-it-yourself shiatsu.* New York: Dutton.
Omura, Y. (1982). *Acupuncture medicine.* Tokyo: Japan Publications.
Serizawa, K. (1976). *Tsubo.* Tokyo: Japan Publications.
Serizawa, K. (1984). *Effective tsubo therapy.* Japan Publications.

18

Jin Shin Do

Jasmine Ellen Wolf, Iona Marsaa Teeguarden

Jin Shin Do® is a relatively new method of releasing muscular tension and stress by applying deepening finger pressure to combinations of specific points on the body. These points, called *acupoints,* are highly energized spots along the meridians—pathways of energy associated with body organs.

Jin Shin Do, which may be translated as *the way of the compassionate spirit,* is a modern synthesis of traditional Asian acupressure–acupuncture theory and techniques, breathing exercises, Taoist philosophy, and modern psychology. Iona Marsaa Teeguarden researched various acupressure techniques and wrote *Acupressure Way of Health* in 1978. This book describes the basic principles behind her synthesis, which she calls *Jin Shin Do.* In the ensuing years, she added psychology to this synthesis, as described in *The Joy of Feeling: Bodymind Acupressure™* (1987). In 1982, Teeguarden founded the Jin Shin Do Foundation to train and network authorized teachers of this method.

▪ ARMORED ACUPOINTS

Applying simple, direct finger pressure to acupoints helps to release tension and reduce physical and emotional stress. In Chinese medicine terms, these acupoints are places along the meridians where the life force energy comes close to the surface of the body. In Western terms, they are places of high electrical conductivity or low electrical resistance, compared to the surrounding area.

When a person experiences stress due to environmental, social, emotional, or physical stimuli, tension (and energy) tends to collect at some of these points. If the tension is not released, the tension acts like a record of the stressful experience or situation. Future incidents may remind the person unconsciously of the original stress or trauma. For instance, a child who is physically or emotionally abused may tighten certain body parts to numb the pain or to suppress tears or shouts in order to avoid further punishment. Stress may be induced years later by the replication of smells, sights, or sounds experienced during these early traumatic events, but the person may not be aware of why she or he is feeling more stressed in these situations. Meanwhile, the points of tension (eg, in the neck, shoulders, or back) become tighter and tighter and feel increasingly hard to the touch. This chronic tension, called *armoring,* is often located on the acupoints.

Because armored points contain a psychologic history, sometimes suppressed emotions or old defensive attitudes will surface to conscious awareness during the release of these points. Jin Shin Do practitioners are trained to empathize with and help people go through such emotional releases as well as to help release physical stress and refer people to psychotherapists and doctors when necessary. Jin Shin Do is not a medical treatment. It is a transformational process, involving consciousness in restoring balance to body, mind, emotions, and spirit.

Jin Shin Do is a gentle way to release muscular tension and armoring. The practitioner starts with light pressure and penetrates deeper when "invited in" by the client. The practitioner stays on the point for a relatively long time and is, therefore, able to work deeply. While one hand is holding a tense place, the other hand holds a series of other points, which helps release the tension and balance the body energy, enabling the release to be more pleasurable and more effective. Even so, it is rarely possible or advisable to release all the tension from an armored area in a single session. People are usually not able to handle too revolutionary a change at once, just as they are not prepared to confront their entire psychologic history too quickly.

Trained practitioners help people pay attention to the sensations and feelings that accompany release or armoring, and to learn and grow from the emotions and imagery that arise. Release is often accompanied by deep relaxation, or occasionally by tingling and trembling, crying or shouting. Sometimes, the process is peaceful and internal, perhaps with the recipient falling asleep during the session. Often the release is followed by a new resolution, on a conscious or unconscious level, and a renewed ability to live joyfully.

▪ STRANGE FLOWS

Ancient Chinese philosophers believed that the body is a microcosm of what is on earth and in the universe. These philosophers observed that when rivers overflow, the excess water forms channels and flows to a river that lacks water. Therefore, these philosophers postulated that when a meridian becomes excessively filled with energy, the excess collects in channels and is redistributed to deficient meridians. These channels are called *strange flows* or *wondrous channels.*

Unlike the flow through the meridians, energy does not flow continuously through the strange flows, but only when the energy is unevenly distributed among the meridians. The strange flows have no acupoints of their own—all their points are on major meridians. An exception is the great central channel (GCC) formed by the conception vessel (CV) and the governing vessel (GV) combined.

If the strange flows were free from blockage, the body would maintain harmony and balance through the meridians. However, the strange flows are also subject to armoring and blockages. A Jin Shin Do practitioner can balance the meridians without assessing them by releasing the strange flows.

There are four pairs of strange flows—the yin and yang great regulator channels (GRC), the yin and yang great bridge channel (GBC), the belt channel (BC) and penetrating channel (PC), and the conception vessel (CV) and governing vessel (GV). The CV and GV combined are the GCC. Release of the GCC (which is shown in a simplified form in Figs. 18–1 and 18–2) is good for people with minor

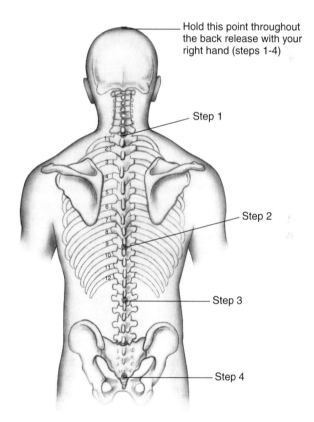

Hold this point throughout the back release with your right hand (steps 1-4)

Step 1

Step 2

Step 3

Step 4

FIGURE 18–1. Location of points for the back release. The back release for the Great Central Channel is performed with the receiver face up. The practitioner sits on the receiver's left side, and places a finger or the palm of the right hand on top of the receiver's head. The right hand remains in place for the entire release. The left hand reaches under the receiver's back, and *gently* presses straight up into each point on the back. Step 1 is between the seventh cervical and first thoracic vertebrae. Step 2 is between the ninth and tenth thoracic vertebrae. Step 3 is between the second and third lumbar vertebrae. Step 4 is placement of the palm of the left hand against the receiver's coccyx.

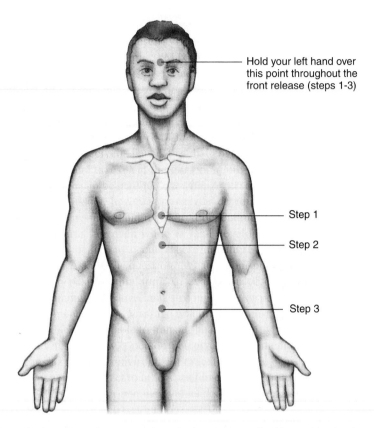

Hold your left hand over this point throughout the front release (steps 1-3)

Step 1

Step 2

Step 3

FIGURE 18–2. The front release (the conception vessel). The practitioner should sit on the right. The receiver lies face up. Step 1. Place the palm of your left hand over the receiver's "third eye" (just above and between the eyes). Your left hand will stay on the third eye throughout the next three steps. Place either one finger or the palm of your right hand over the midpoint between the receiver's nipples and press. Step 2. Place your right palm over the receiver's solar plexus and press. Step 3. Place your right palm over the receiver's lower abdomen (hara).

spinal or constitutional disorders (check with their doctor or chiropractor first) and it is used to balance the reproductive system, particularly in women. It is also effective for helping psychic energy flow. The yin and yang GRCs are used for people who are suffering from shoulder or neck tension or from nervous tension. The yin and yang GBCs are chosen for people with back tension. They also help increase a person's energy and are the channels that are traditionally released on athletes. The PC and BC help release the abdominal and low back areas and strengthen the sexual energy and organs. Detailed instructions for releasing all the strange flows can be found in Teeguarden (1978) *The Acupressure Way of Health,* and (1996) *A Complete Guide to Acupressure.*

■ ASSESSMENT OF MERIDIANS

Although the strange flows can be released without assessment, more accurate meridian balancing requires assessment of the energy flow. Theoretically, if the energy were flowing freely, our bodies would be working perfectly, and we would not experience physical, mental, emotional, or spiritual tension or dis-ease. In Jin Shin Do, releasing tension and enhancing bodymind well-being involves the assessment of which meridians and flows are imbalanced, as well as of which parts of the body are most tense or armored.

The emphasis is on energetic imbalance and muscular relaxation, not on symptoms. For example, in the case of the common cold, there may be imbalance of the lung meridian, which would be the most obvious possibility. Nevertheless, assessment of the meridians may indicate that the problem is imbalance of the triple-warmer meridian (which pertains to the maintenance of homeostasis of body temperature and energy production). Or the problem may have begun with a liver meridian imbalance; perhaps the patient is having a problem with toxicity (perhaps toxic anger). Or there may be a kidney meridian imbalance, indicating that the patient's reserve energy is drained (perhaps due to chronic stress). People with imbalanced gallbladder meridians may be so tortured by decision making that they make themselves sick. Wherever the imbalance starts, if it is not corrected, other meridians may gradually be affected in a domino-like fashion. According to the traditional theory behind Jin Shin Do, the bodymind is one whole, and problems in one part of the system will affect other parts.

It is important to note that we are assessing meridians, *not* organs. A meridian can be out of balance, and yet the person can be physically healthy. For instance, a heart meridian imbalance is much more likely to indicate heartache or difficulty with intimate relationships than physical heart problems. Meridians are symbols, and as such they have many meanings. In Chinese medicine theory, the meridians are associated not only with body organs, but also with specific senses, colors, expressions, emotions, tastes, and activities. An imbalance in a meridian may be reflected as either an excess or a deficiency in these areas. There are seasons and times of day when the energy is strongest in each meridian. During a meridian's associated "time" or "season" strengths and weaknesses of the meridian are accented.

The 12 "organ meridians" fall within the five categories of metal, earth, fire, water, and wood. These elements are symbols for five energic tendencies, or for five aspects of the bodymind whole.

Some key associations for each meridian are listed in Table 18–1. This is not a definitive list, but these functional relationships will give the reader some idea of the essentially holistic concepts of acupressure theory.

There are several ways to assess the related meridians, including pulse reading and assessing the abdomen (*hara*) and back. Another method is to observe and ask questions, designing the questions to find out information such as that given in Table 18–1. Let us consider some examples.

Which sense is most important or works best for the recipient? Which sense is weak? If a recipient has a problem with a sense organ, weakness in the correspond-

QUALITIES OF THE FIVE ELEMENTS

TABLE
18–1

Element	Metal	Earth	Fire	Water	Wood
Yin	Lung	Spleen	Heart & pericardium	Kidney	Liver
Yang	Large intestine	Stomach	Triple warmer & small intestine	Bladder	Gallbladder
Sense	Smell	Taste	Speech	Hearing	Sight
Sense organ	Nose	Mouth, lips	Tongue	Ears	Eyes
Liquid	Mucus	Saliva	Sweat	Urine	Tears
Color	White	Yellow	Red	Blue, black	Green
Expression	Weeping	Singing	Laughing	Groaning	Shouting
Extreme emotion	Grief, anxiety	Worry, reminiscence	Shock, overjoy	Fear	Anger
Balanced emotion	Openness, receptivity	Sympathy, empathy	Joy, compassion	Resolution, trust, motivation	Assertion
Taste	Pungent, spicy	Sweet	Bitter, burned	Salty	Sour
Season	Fall	Indian summer	Summer	Winter	Spring
Related activity	Letting go	Mental activity	Inspiration & intimacy	Willpower & vitality	Planning & decision making
Times	Lung, 3–5 AM	Stomach, 7–9 AM	Heart, 11 AM–1 PM	Bladder, 3–5 PM	Gallbladder 11 PM– 1 AM
	Large intestine, 5–7 AM	Spleen, 9–11 AM	Small intestine, 1–3 PM	Kidney, 5–7 PM	Pericardium, 7–9 PM
					Triple warmer 9–11 PM

ing meridian may be indicated. For example, depending extensively on the sense of sight and not being able to smell very well may indicate both metal and wood imbalance. Similarly, too much or too little of a body liquid could indicate an imbalance. For instance, if a person creates too much mucus or too little there may be an imbalance in the metal element—either the lung or large intestine meridian.

Look at the colors a person wears and the hue of the person's face. For instance, asthmatics are often very white, indicating a lung meridian imbalance. People with metal imbalances may love white or hate it. Listen to the patient. Some people have voices that sing (earth) and others are always shouting (wood imbalance). Some people giggle at inappropriate times, for example, when they talk about having been hurt (fire imbalance).

Which emotions cause problems? Some people are so sympathetic that they are swallowed by other people's sorrows, whereas others are unable to feel or express their sympathy. In both cases there is likely to be an earth imbalance.

Times of day when a person feels tired or uncomfortable can help point out imbalances. A person who feels tired at 2 PM probably has a small intestine meridian imbalance since the small intestine "time" is from 1 to 3 PM.

The way people express themselves also reveals imbalances. For example, intellectuals tend to have earth imbalances as do people who scorn the intellect, whereas a fear of intimacy suggests a fire imbalance.

Assessment is nonjudgmental. In the Chinese philosophy frame of mind, nothing is good or bad. In Western society, anger is often considered "bad." Notice that anger is a wood element quality along with spring and green. When it flows smoothly, anger is an honest, spontaneous emotion from the heart, and such anger is often felt toward a loved one or someone considered important. Healthy anger can be a renewal because it can clear away the debris in a relationship. On the other hand, stifled anger festers and becomes toxic, and like explosive anger it suggests a wood imbalance.

Another way to assess meridians in the body is to touch the *associated points* and determine whether they are tense or sore. These points are located on the back along the two bladder meridian lines that are on the edges of the erector spinae. On these lines, the points parallel to the spaces between the vertebrae correspond to specific meridians (Fig. 18–3). If the tension is mostly on the medial edge of the erector spinae, then the problem is short term or in the early stages of development, and if the tension is on the outer edge of the muscle then the imbalance is chronic. For instance, the points on these lines that are next to the discs between the third and fourth thoracic vertebrae are associated with the lung meridian. If the lung meridian is weak, then the third or fourth thoracic vertebrae may be out of alignment or the area around one or both of the lung-associated points may be tense or lifeless, colorless or excessively colored, hot or cold, or may have some other unusual quality. These points may be sore when touched or may be so armored that they are numb. There may also be muscle spasms in this area.

In Jin Shin Do, the practitioner first chooses a meridian to work with and then chooses a point on that meridian needing to be released. For instance, in working with the lung meridian, a point called #30 is a good choice for a *local point,* that is, a point that is the site of the problem or of excessive tension. This point is held for about two minutes while at least two other points on the lung meridian are pressed, one after the other. These points are called *distal points* because they are distant from the site of the problem, but they facilitate deeper release of the local point. Because of the connection created between the two stimulated points, both points are released more efficiently than they would be if only one point were held at a time. It is necessary to study Jin Shin Do with a trained practitioner in order to know how to

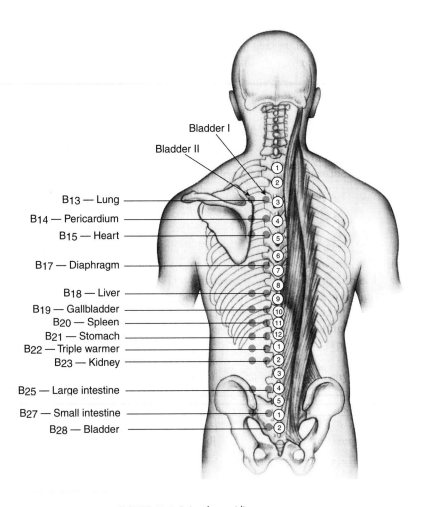

FIGURE 18–3. Points for meridian assessment.

effectively release the meridians, but Figure 18–4 provides an example of how you might work with the lung meridian.

■ BODY SEGMENTS

Jin Shin Do practitioners also work in terms of *body segments*. These are groups of muscles that are functionally related and that work together to make expressive movements and gestures. For example, if you grit your teeth you can feel the back of your neck tensing. Therefore, these areas are part of the same segment. For this

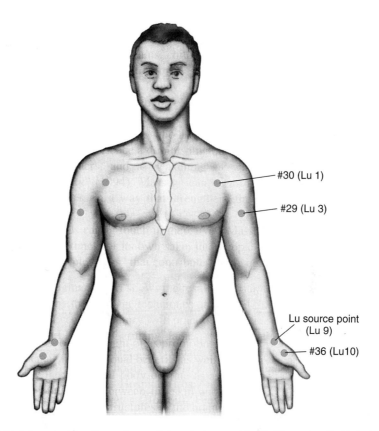

#30 (Lu 1)

#29 (Lu 3)

Lu source point
(Lu 9)

#36 (Lu10)

FIGURE 18–4. Lung meridian. Some release points on the lung meridian. While one hand holds the local point known as #30 in Jin Shin Do numbering (called Lung 1 in acupuncture), the other could hold several distal points along the lung meridian, such as point #36 (Lung 10 in acupuncture) at the base of the thumb.

reason it is impossible to fully release the neck until tension is released from the jaw. The major body segments are shown in Figure 18–5.

Determining which segments are tense also helps the practitioner understand a patient's emotional conflicts. The chest, for instance, reveals how we do or do not let our feelings flow. People with inflated chests are likely to have a macho facade and to act stronger than they really are. One way to correlate the segments and emotions is to think of clichés associated with the tight segments, such as "carrying the weight of the world on my shoulders," or "I can't stomach the situation." Table 18–2 provides examples of emotional correlations with the major body segments.

Usually, all the segments need some release. In Jin Shin Do, the usual procedure is to release the segments from the top down, first freeing the areas related to

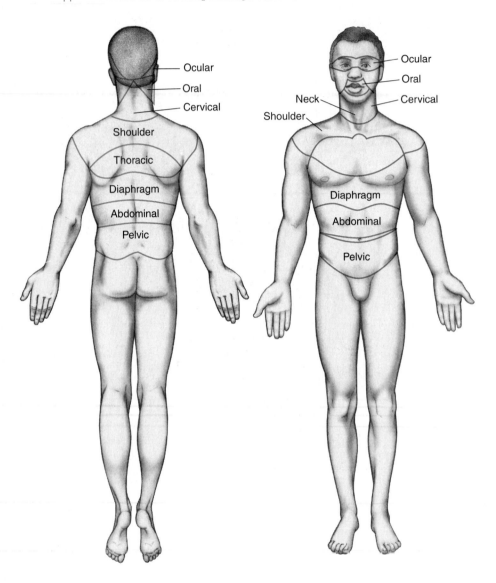

FIGURE 18–5. Major body segments, posterior and anterior.

self-expression. Then, when energy is released in the lower segments, it does not get stuck when it flows up the back along the strange flows. When the upper segments are free, the person is more able to release stagnated energy through vocal expression. All Jin Shin Do sessions end with a neck release to be sure that this often tense area is relaxed—and because the neck release is very pleasurable (Fig. 18–6).

EMOTIONAL ASSOCIATIONS WITH THE BODY SEGMENTS

TABLE 18–2

Body Segment	Emotional Association
Ocular and oral	Expression of feelings Rational thinking
Neck	Division between rational and feeling parts of the body Choking down feelings Difficulty in expression
Shoulder	Responsibility Judgment (including self-judgment)
Chest	Restricting the flow of our emotions Restricting breathing is the way to restrict feelings In the heart segment we experience appreciation and love as well as the loss of love (heartache or heartbreak)
Diaphragm and abdominal	Emotional and intrapersonal power Fear of losing oneself to one's feelings In this society we are told to hold our stomachs in, an area related to our personal power and gut feelings. In the Orient, by contrast, the ideal is a relaxed belly
Pelvic	This is the segment we cannot talk about in social settings—sex and elimination Fear of our primary survival needs or of losing control to our primal self

More information on the segments is found in Iona Marsaa Teeguarden (1987) *The joy of feeling: Bodymind acupressure™*, and (1996) *A complete guide to acupressure*.

▪ HOW TO GIVE JIN SHIN DO SESSIONS

It is very simple to learn to use Jin Shin Do at a basic level for self-help and to help family and friends. After studying the 40-hour basic course, students are able to give many types of full sessions by following various release examples, or by creating their own combination of points. The only motion in a Jin Shin Do session is pressing points and holding them. The point most requiring release is called the local point. The local point is held continuously while at least two distal points are held, one after the other. The distal points are chosen by their relationship to the local point. Usually, the two points are in the same segment, on the same meridian, or on the same strange flow.

A pressure point is held by pressing a finger against the point firmly, but not so deeply that the recipient cannot relax. As the point releases, the practitioner's finger will automatically sink deeper into the point. The points are held for an average of one to two minutes or until the following occurs:

1. The practitioner feels the muscle relax to a significant degree.
2. The practitioner feels a pulsation or an increase in pulsation. (It might take practice to be able to feel this.)
3. The recipient feels a decrease (or sometimes, first, an increase) in sensitivity.

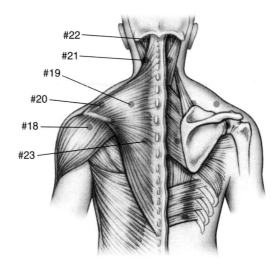

FIGURE 18–6. Neck and shoulder release. The recipient lies on his or her back; the operator sits at the head. Place hands under the shoulders and use one finger of each hand to hold both 23s until they release. Then hold both 18s until they release. Then with the fingers over the shoulders, press the thumbs into the 19s until they release, followed by thumb pressure to the 20s until they release. Next press the 21s with the fingers. The operator finishes by pulling the occipital ridge toward him or her, pressing the 22s until they release. Adapted from JSD Neck Release (Teeguarden, 1978).

■ BENEFITS OF JIN SHIN DO

Psychologic Benefits

Much disease is associated with destructive thought patterns often created in early childhood as an adaptive mechanism.

Now a woman in her 30s, Andrea was taught by her father not to be an "over-emotional wimp." When Andrea first came to the author for treatment, she had severe asthma and had taken medication nightly for the past 12 years. The medication was no longer of value. Andrea told the author that she never cried and that she held her anger inside until she exploded uncontrollably. When she was angry she would grit her teeth, sometimes to the point of breaking them. Andrea had a very white complexion and assessment indicated that the energy in her lung meridian was excessive. The author used the lung meridian release in the *Jin Shin Do Handbook* (1981, p. 8), which includes #30 (lung 1), several other lung meridian points, and other points on the chest segment.

During the sessions, Andrea explained that her asthma had been very severe for the past month. Asked if anything significant had happened in her life a month ago, Andrea explained that her aunt had died, but true to her training, she had not cried. When the author explained that Andrea might be choking on her own emotions, Andrea agreed to let herself cry rather than suffocate herself. By the end of the session, her complexion was red. She did not need to use her medication once for as long as the author kept in contact with her, which was nine months. Although hiding her emotions was destructive, this behavior was originally adaptive, for it had helped Andrea to win her father's love.

One purpose of Jin Shin Do is to help people become aware of the bodymind connection. Very often, people believe their body is "doing it to them." Our bodies are not separate entities that are giving us pain. When we learn to look for the cause of our pain within ourselves, we can accept it and then be ready to use our minds to transform our health. It is important to learn from our tensions rather than judge them. The Chinese word for crisis is composed of two characters—"danger" and "opportunity." It is the practitioner's job to help the client become aware of the opportunity for growth that is contained in tensions, pains, or other health crises. Patients can use this knowledge as they wish. Some people need their dis-eases.

Jin Shin Do practitioners are not magical healers. They are more like midwives to a client's self-healing. They assist the self-healing process by holding acupoints and by making suggestions to facilitate release. People can only heal themselves. (As noted earlier, they occasionally need the help of doctors, physical therapists, or psychotherapists to do so.)

In Jin Shin Do practice, health is seen as a balance of the vital energies and of the bodymind–spirit. Health is not an achievement to be maintained, but a continual process that includes growth and knowledge of ourselves and the world.

Physical Benefits

Because both the length and depth of pressure are paced to the receiver's needs, Jin Shin Do helps provide gentle and deep release of tensions, as well as reduction of stress. As Jin Shin Do involves no movement, it is excellent for people who cannot be moved or who must be worked in a specific position. Although only a small area is touched, muscles and meridians are affected all over the body. Jin Shin Do is, therefore, effective in conditions that cannot be touched. For example, a practitioner could not work directly on an injured disc, but could help the surrounding muscles to relax. In such cases, the practitioner must always work with the permission of a chiropractor or a doctor.

Jin Shin Do is excellent to use just before a chiropractic adjustment because the adjustment is likely to be easier and to last.

Project PRES (Physical Response Education System) conducted research in California on effects of weekly Jin Shin Do sessions on handicapped children. More recently, Steve Schumacher in Kentucky has conducted similar studies as described in Chapter 20 of A Complete Guide to Acupressure (Teeguarden, 1996). The research has demonstrated many benefits to these children including improvement in learning and decrease in allergies, seizures, bedwetting, constipation, night coughing, lung congestion, ear infections, runny noses, nosebleeds, skin conditions, and weight problems. The researchers reported that children were less hyperactive, less angry, and happier. One child who had never talked began to talk in three-word sentences. Another child made a gain of almost two grade levels in language development. This study suggests that the use of Jin Shin Do with normal children might be of great benefit (Teeguarden, 1985, p. 22).

■ SUMMARY

Jin Shin Do is a form of acupressure that works by releasing two points simultaneously. Practitioners release body segments, meridians, or strange flows (channels which balance the organ meridians). Because the entire body is connected, the effects of Jin Shin Do are often felt in areas that the practitioner has not touched. The practitioner paces the depth and length of pressure to the receiver's needs. Jin Shin Do practitioners also help their clients understand how their thoughts and attitudes may be related to their physical imbalances. Occasionally, the effects of Jin Shin Do are not felt for the first one or two sessions. However, they often last a lifetime. To find a registered practitioner or authorized teacher, contact the Jin Shin Do Foundation for Bodymind Acupressure (see Appendix B).

■ REFERENCES

Teeguarden, I. M. (1978). *Acupressure way of health: Jin Shin Do.* New York/Tokyo: Japan Publications (distributed by Putnam).

Teeguarden, I. M. (1985). Acupressure in the classroom. *East West Journal, 15* (August), 22.

Teeguarden, I. M. (1981). *Jin Shin Do handbook,* 2nd ed. Felton, CA: Jin Shin Do Foundation.

Teeguarden, I. M. (1987). *Joy of feeling: Bodymind acupressure.* New York/Tokyo: Japan Publications (distributed by Putnam). Harper & Row.

Teeguarden, I. M. (1996). *A complete guide to acupressure.* New York/Tokyo: Japan Publications (distributed by Putnam).

V

Applications
of Massage

Sports and Fitness

Massage has been used since ancient times in the training of athletes. This tradition from ancient Greece and Rome is carried on today in a specialization called *sports massage*. Chapter 2 contains a brief historical survey of sports massage in ancient and modern times.

Sports massage is defined as "the science and art of applying massage and related techniques to ensure the health and well-being of the athlete and to enhance athletic performance" (Benjamin & Lamp, 1996). Most of the principles of sports massage are also applicable to those engaged in physical fitness activities. Many fitness participants train just as hard as athletes and have similar needs, even though they may not enter competitions. Massage helps care for the wear and tear and minor injuries sustained in the performance of any strenuous physical activity.

There are five major applications of massage in sports as described by Benjamin and Lamp (1996). The first four applications may also apply to fitness participants.

- Recovery. To enhance physical and mental recovery from strenuous physical activity
- Remedial. To improve a debilitating condition
- Rehabilitation. To facilitate healing after a disabling injury
- Maintenance. To enhance recovery from strenuous exertion, to treat debilitating conditions, and to help the athlete maintain optimal health
- Event. To help the athlete prepare for and recover from a specific competitive event

▪ TECHNIQUES AND KNOWLEDGE

Sports massage as practiced in the United States today is based in classic Western massage. Some techniques are used more than others, depending on the situation and the desired results. For example, compression is often used to increase circulation in pre-event and post-event situations when athletes are clothed (see Fig. 19–1), while effleurage (sliding) and petrissage (kneading) are more often performed in maintenance and recovery sessions where athletes are unclothed and draped, and oil is used.

Because of the recurring stress, overload, and trauma to the body, athletes often need specific remedial work in their maintenance sessions. Sports massage practitioners should be skilled in locating and relieving trigger points as described in Chapter 12. Myofascial techniques are useful for freeing the fascia and restoring optimal mobility (see Chapter 11).

Techniques are often applied very specifically to certain muscles and tendons; therefore, sports massage specialists should have well-developed palpation skills and knowledge of musculoskeletal anatomy. Understanding of the biomechanics of specific sports and fitness activities is useful in planning sessions and locating areas of stress. Practitioners working with athletes and fitness participants should be well versed in their special needs and be able to adapt their massage sessions accordingly.

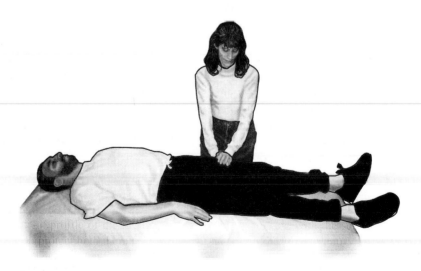

FIGURE 19–1. Compression used to increase circulation in pre-event and post-event situations when athletes are clothed.

■ RECOVERY

Recovery from strenuous exertion is a major application of sports massage. It addresses the tight, stiff, and sore muscles that often accompany exercise and helps the body heal minor tissue damage. Recovery is also a major component in maintenance sports massage. For recovery, the practitioner spends more time on body areas most stressed during an athlete's performance in a specific sport or in a fitness participant's exercise routine.

Recovery massage generally includes techniques to improve circulation, promote both muscular and general relaxation, and enhance flexibility. Effleurage and petissage may be used to improve circulation and, thereby, bring nutrients to an area and flush out metabolic waste products. When the recipient is clothed, compression is often the technique of choice to create hyperemia in a muscle group.

Joint mobilizations and stretching help muscles relax and lengthen. Jostling and rocking are good techniques to encourage "letting go" of tension held unconsciously in muscles. Broadening techniques help separate muscle fibers, which may be adhering due to the stress endured during exercise.

An important component of recovery is general relaxation. Stress interferes with the body's capacity to heal itself, and relaxation promotes the healing process. The relaxation response may be evoked with long flowing effleurage techniques or light rhythmic compressions. The environment should be as relaxing as possible with low light and little distracting noise. A hot shower, whirlpool, sauna, or steam before the recovery massage will enhance its effects.

■ REMEDIAL MASSAGE AND REHABILITATION

Remedial and *rehabilitation* applications of massage with athletes are the same as with other populations. The most common situations involve muscle tension and inflexibility, muscle soreness, trigger points, edema, tendinitis, tenosynovitis, strains, sprains, and general stress. Deep friction massage is especially useful in the development of healthy mobile scar tissue and freeing adhesions in tissues after trauma. Massage techniques used to address these situations are described elsewhere throughout the text.

■ MAINTENANCE

Maintenance is a term used to describe an all-purpose massage session received regularly that addresses the unique needs of the recipient. In maintenance sessions, extra attention is given to areas commonly stressed in the recipient's sport or fitness activity. The goal of the session is to keep the recipients in optimal condition as they are training. Maintenance sessions last from ½ to 1½ hours. Its foundation is massage designed for recovery and also includes remedial massage for problem conditions as needed.

▪ EVENTS

Applications of massage at athletic events include *pre-event, inter- or intra-event,* and *post-event.* These applications help the athlete prepare for and recover from the effects of the all-out effort of competition. Special areas are often set aside at organized competitions for athletes to receive sports massage, for example, tents are often used to shelter sports massage at outdoor events.

Pre-event massage is very different from the other applications of sports massage described thus far. The purpose of pre-event massage is to help the athlete prepare physically and mentally for the upcoming event. It may be part of the athlete's warm-up routine.

Pre-event massage should be 15 to 20 minutes in duration, have an upbeat tempo, avoid causing discomfort, concentrate on the major muscle groups to be used in the upcoming performance, and adjust for psychological readiness. If the athlete is anxious, more soothing techniques may be used, but most athletes benefit from a stimulating session. Athletes are usually clothed, and techniques used include compression, direct pressure on stress points, friction, lifting and broadening, percussion, jostling, joint mobilizations, and stretching (Benjamin & Lamp, 1996, p. 68).

Inter-event massage is performed on athletes between events at competitions such as track and swim meets. It is short (10–15 minutes), avoids discomfort, and focuses on recovery of the muscles used most in the preceding event. It must give attention to psychological recovery and also readiness for the upcoming performance. Techniques used are a combination of those used for pre-event and post-event situations.

The primary goal of *post-event* massage is physical and psychological recovery of the athlete. If the session takes place close to the time of the event, the practitioner may also identify and assess injuries received during the competition. These may be treated, given first aid, and/or referred to other health care practitioners.

Post-event massage should be short (10–15 minutes) if close to event time, or may be longer (30–90 minutes) if 1 hour or more after an event. The athlete should be cooled down, have taken adequate fluids, and be breathing normally before getting massage. Pressure used is generally lighter, pace is moderate to slow, and special attention is given to muscles used in the event. Techniques known to increase circulation and promote muscular and general relaxation are emphasized. These include compression, sliding strokes, kneading, jostling, postional release, joint mobilizations, and stretching.

▪ SUMMARY

Sports massage is the science and art of applying massage and related techniques to promote the health and well-being of athletes, fitness participants, and others engaged in strenuous physical activity. It may also be used to enhance athletic performance.

Sports massage, as practiced today in the United States, is based on classic Western massage with other techniques combined as appropriate. Trigger point therapy, myofascial techniques, and deep transverse friction are especially useful to address the physical stresses of athletes. Compressions are used frequently when working at competitive events, since athletes there receive massage fully clothed and, typically, no oil is used.

There are five major applications of sports massage: recovery, remedial, rehabilitation, maintenance, and event. The intent of recovery sports massage is to help the athlete heal from the regular stresses and strains of training and competition; remedial sports massage helps alleviate problem conditions before they worsen; rehabilitation applications address injury healing; maintenance sessions focus on recovery and remedial applications; and sports massage at events helps athletes prepare for and recover from the rigors of competition.

■ REFERENCES

Benjamin, P. J., & Lamp S. P. (1996). *Understanding sports massage.* Champaign, IL: Human Kinetics.

■ RECOMMENDED FOR FURTHER STUDY OF SPORTS MASSAGE

Benjamin, P. J., & Lamp S. P. (1996). *Understanding sports massage.* Champaign, IL: Human Kinetics.
Coseo, M. (1992). *The acupressure warm-up.* Brookline, MA: Paradigm Publications.
Johnson, J. (1995). *The healing art of sports massage.* Emmaus, PA: Rodale Press.
King, R.K. (1993). *Performance massage.* Champaign, IL: Human Kinetics.
Meagher, J. (1990). *Sportmassage.* Barrytown, NY: Station Hill Press.

Mother and Child

Massage can help relieve some of the physical and emotional stresses women experience during pregnancy. Many women find relief with massage from the strain put on the spine and lower extremities by the extra weight they gain while carrying a child. Women confined to bed during pregnancy can benefit from the improved circulation, joint movements, and social contact during massage.

▪ PREGNANCY AND THE BENEFITS OF MASSAGE

Pregnancy is a special time in which a woman's body undergoes significant changes as it nurtures, carries, and prepares to deliver the growing baby. These changes include hormonal, structural, and postural deviations from the nonpregnant state. Some of the changes can cause discomfort or distress that may be relieved with massage.

Women may experience mood swings and greater emotional reactions as hormone activity increases. Insomnia may be a problem for some.

Structural changes include enlarged breasts and additional weight anteriorly as the fetus grows. This shifting weight distribution causes postural distortion that puts pressure on the lower back, and often results in neck strain. A typical posture may be described as head forward, chest back, belly out, and hips tilted forward, locked knees, and feet turned out. Figure 20–1 shows the typical posture of a pregnant woman and major areas of stress. Pressure from the additional weight being carried and decreased physical activity as the pregnancy progresses may cause swelling of the hands, legs, and feet.

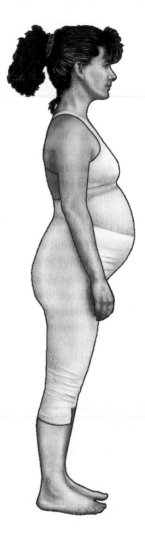

FIGURE 20–1. Typical posture of pregnant woman; head forward, chest back, belly out and hips tilted forward, locked knees.

During pregnancy, there is a softening of the connective tissue of the body, including cartilage and ligaments. This facilitates normal delivery of the baby. It may also cause some instability and pain in the joints.

The objectives of a massage session during pregnancy include helping the mother relax and release some of the emotional stress and addressing the strain felt in the lower back, neck, legs, and feet. Massage may also help reduce edema in upper and lower extremities.

Because each woman is unique, and with the many complications possible during pregnancy, it is best to get permission from the primary health care provider before giving massage. Massage may be contraindicated totally in a very few cases, or there may be cautions or restrictions to take into consideration. It is important for practitioners working with pregnant women to understand what is happening in a woman's body during that time in order to give massage safely.

Abdominal massage is contraindicated during pregnancy. A few nerve strokes, passive touch, and some forms of energy work may be performed safely. It is best to use extreme caution in the area of the belly.

Elaine Stillerman, in her book *Mother-Massage* (1992), lists the following general contraindications for massage of pregnant women: morning sickness, nausea, or vomiting; any vaginal bleeding or discharge; fever; a decrease in fetal movement over a 24-hour period; diarrhea; pain in the abdomen or anywhere else in your body; excessive swelling in arms or legs; immediately after eating (wait two hours); over a bruise or skin irritation (local contraindication).

■ THE MASSAGE SESSION

There are some things about the general environment and your equipment to keep in mind when preparing to give massage to pregnant women. They are often warm, and so the room should generally be kept 5–10 degrees cooler than usual for massage. Good air flow and fresh air are desirable. The massage space should be near a bathroom if possible, because pregnant women feel the need to urinate frequently. The atmosphere should be relaxing, including any music played.

Your table should be lower than usual, especially when the woman is further along in the pregnancy. As she gets larger, and especially in the side-lying position, you will be better able to use good body mechanics with a lower table. Have several bolsters or pillows to use as props for comfortable positioning of the pregnant recipient. A glass of water should be in reach for the recipient, and tissues handy.

A stepping stool may be useful for the woman to use to get up onto the table. You may also want to be present to assist the recipient and help her get into a comfortable position. This is especially true in the later stages of pregnancy.

Positioning

It is important for the recipient to be in a safe and comfortable position while receiving massage. The prone, supine, reclining, and side-lying positions each have their place in giving massage to pregnant women.

In the first few months, women may be comfortably prone or supine as usual for massage. Once the fetus has grown and the mother's belly starts to get larger, other positions may be more comfortable. Later in the pregnancy, the mother may not be able to lie supine without the fetus putting pressure on the decending aorta, impeding the flow of blood to the placenta and causing shortness of breath. Lying on the back may also put pressure on the inferior vena cava, resulting in feelings of lightheadedness, nausea, and backache. Lying prone may be difficult, although with proper bolstering, it may be quite comfortable.

Reclining, or half-sitting, may be a good alternative to lying supine. Bolsters may be used to prop the recipient into a half-sitting position. Some stationary massage tables have an adjustment to convert the flat tabletop into one with a back support.

Side-lying is perhaps the most common position for pregnant women receiving massage. Some doctors caution against pregnant women lying on their left side while sleeping. This may not be a problem for the short duration of massage, but it doesn't hurt to check with the woman's physician for his advice on positioning, especially if there is any complicating health factor.

A general rule of thumb for positioning and propping pregnant women is to fill in any spaces you find with bolsters, pillows, or rolled-up towels. In the supine and reclining positions, a bolster under the knees is often useful to take pressure off of the lower back. In the prone position, props may be placed under the shoulders, under the ankles, and as needed around the belly. In the side-lying position, pillows are placed around the belly for support, under the top arm, and under the top leg or between the legs. A pillow may also be needed under the head. Figure 20–2 shows the props for the side-lying position.

Techniques

The massage should generally be gentle and relaxing. Classic Western massage and its variations, various forms of acupressure and other energy work, reflexology, and other forms of massage and bodywork may be used to address the wellness of pregnant women.

While there are no special techniques for massage during pregnancy, there are some places on the body that need special attention, for example, neck, chest, lower back, hips, legs, and feet. Suggestions for massaging specific areas are described below.

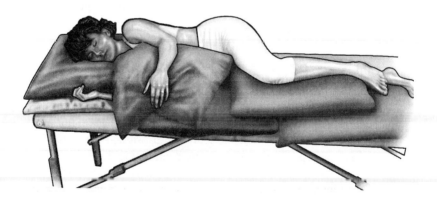

FIGURE 20–2. Props for side-lying position for pregnant woman; pillows under and around the belly, under the head, and under the top arm and leg.

Because of the forward head posture, the neck and upper back may feel strained. This may also result in tension headache. The neck is most easily accessed in the supine or side-lying positions. Effleurage, deep friction, and compression are effective in reducing tension in the muscles of the neck and upper back. There may be trigger points to be relieved. Direct pressure to certain acupressure points can also relax neck tension.

The chest may become sunken or depressed as the pregnancy progresses. The enlarged uterus also takes up a lot of room in the abdomen making it hard for pregnant women to breathe. Therefore, massage that frees up the rib cage and diaphragm can be important. Massage of the intercostal muscles and along the diaphragm promote easier breathing.

An exaggerated lordosis, which puts pressure on the lower back, often results from pregnancy. This can be addressed effectively in the side-lying position, which in itself relieves pressure in the lower back. A simple technique to help tilt the hips back into a more normal position is a firm effleurage with the palm of the hand from the upper back to the sacrum. When over the sacrum, apply a little more pressure to help reduce the lordotic curve.

Childbearing puts strain on the entire lower body. The muscles of the hips and legs have to work harder to carry the added weight accumulated during pregnancy. The lower extremities are massaged as usual, ending with distal to proximal effleurage to help accumulated fluid move out of the area.

When massaging the feet, you may want to apply some reflexology. Areas to stimulate include along the medial border, which corresponds to the hips and spine, and on the inside of the foot below the ankle bone, which corresponds to the uterus. It is now considered a myth that reflexology can cause miscarriage. Kunz and Kunz believe that reflexology is safe for pregnant women and that it has never been shown to have caused the body to do something it didn't want to do. It merely helps the body seek its own equilibrium (1980).

▪ LABOR, DELIVERY, AND RECOVERY

Midwives, childbirth assistants, and others in the delivery room may use massage as desired by the mother during labor and delivery. This may be as simple as gentle stroking to reduce anxiety.

There are also certain acupressure points which may be pressed to relieve labor pain. These include the Shoulder Well (GB21) on the trapezius; Sacral Points (GB 27–34); Hoku or Joining the Valley (LI4) in the web of the thumb; Bigger Stream (K3) near the Achilles tendon; and Reaching Inside (B67) on the little toe (Gach, 1990).

Massage may be used during recovery from labor and delivery. Classic Western techniques can help relax stressed and sore muscles and soothe nerves. Acupressure points to press for postpartum recovery include Sea of Energy (CV6) just below the naval; Inner Gate (P6) inside of the forearm just above the wrist; Sea of Vitality (B23 and B47) across the back at waist level; Womb and Vitals (B48) lateral to the sacrum; Three Mile Point (St36) just below the kneecap lateral to the shin bone; and Bigger Rushing (Lv3) on top of the foot between the big toe and the second toe (Gach, 1990).

After an appropriate amount of healing has taken place, women who had delivered their babies by C-sections may benefit from abdominal massage and massage around and on the scar itself. Deep transverse friction can help prevent adhesions and promote mobile scar tissue as in any wound healing situation.

■ WOMEN WITH INFANTS AND TODDLERS

Women with infants and toddlers have a new set of stresses from the demands of motherhood. Massage affords an opportunity to take time out and relax. It may also address the stress on the upper back and arms from picking up, holding, and nursing the growing babies.

■ INFANT MASSAGE

Massage given by parents and other caregivers is an excellent way to provide the tactile stimulation and movement essential for the healthy growth and development of infants. Massage has other benefits for infants, including releasing tension and learning to relax, bonding with parents, aiding digestion and elimination, improving sleep, easing growing pains, and helping calm colicky babies. In addition, touching and handling her baby promotes milk production in the mother by stimulating the secretion of prolactin. Massage can also provide fathers with an opportunity to touch and interact with their babies in a way that is satisfying and also builds confidence in handling the child (Schneider, 1982).

Infant massage is a simple, gentle, yet firm application of stroking, pressing, squeezing, and movement of the limbs. Examples of techniques include soft circular motions with fingertips all over the baby's head, gentle but firm squeezing and twisting the muscles of the legs, strokes with the thumbs on the bottom of the feet, circular massage of the abdomen, broad strokes on the chest, milking the arms, and small circles all around the back with the fingertips. Figure 20–3 shows the squeeze and twist technique used on the legs and arms. Grasp the limb like holding a baseball bat, then gently squeeze and twist the hands in opposite directions. Continue the motion while traveling up the leg from buttocks to feet.

Caregivers should maintain eye contact and talk or sing to the child throughout the massage. It can be a time of connecting and playful interaction that helps in the infant's emotional and social development, as well as the physical.

Massage practitioners may include training in infant massage in their services to pregnant clients before or after delivery. Dolls may be used to introduce massage techniques before the baby is delivered.

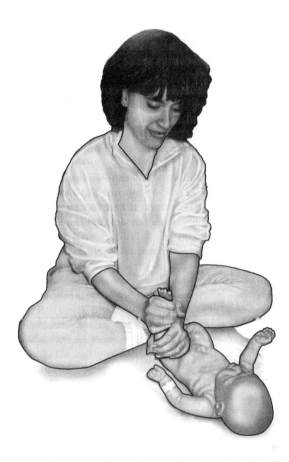

FIGURE 20–3. Gentle squeeze and twist of the muscles of the leg during infant massage.

■ SUMMARY

Massage can help relieve some of the stresses women experience during pregnancy, including strain on the spine and lower extremities. It can also be a time of relaxation and emotional relief. Massage is safe in most cases of pregnancy, but it is best to check with the mother's physician for any special cautions or directions. Abdominal massage is contraindicated, and massage should be avoided if the mother is experiencing nausea, vomiting, diarrhea, or any unusual pain, swelling or bleeding.

In the first few weeks of pregnancy, women may lie supine or prone. As the belly gets larger, switch to the reclining or side-lying positions. Use pillows and other props to support the body properly. The room temperature may be kept a little cooler than usual for massage; air should be fresh and flowing, and music relaxing. A bathroom should be accessible. A stepping stool may be useful for the recipient to get onto the table.

Techniques should be gentle and relaxing. Classic Western massage, acupressure, and reflexology have been found to address pregnant women's needs well. Focus of the sessions is on the neck, lower back, legs, and feet, and general relaxation. Massage may be performed during delivery to help reduce anxiety and ease labor pain.

Massage may be received during the weeks after birth to help recondition areas stressed during delivery. Women who receive cesarean sections may also benefit from massage during recovery and from techniques that help form healthy scar tissue. Women with infants and small children may benefit from taking time for themselves and receiving relaxing massage as part of their regular self-care.

Massage given to newborns by parents, grandparents, and other caregivers can be a playful, healthy, and bonding experience. Touch and movement have been proven to be important for proper physical, mental, emotional, and social growth and development of infants and small children. Massage techniques for infants are gentle stroking, pressing, squeezing, and movement of the limbs.

■ REFERENCES

Gach, M. R. (1990). *Acupressure's potent points: A guide to self-care for common ailments.* New York: Bantam Books.

Kunz, K., & Kunz, B. (1980). *The complete guide to foot reflexology.* Englewood Cliffs, NJ: Prentice-Hall.

Schneider, Vimala. (1982). *Infant massage: A handbook for loving parents.* New York: Bantam Books.

Stillerman, E. (1992). *Mother-massage: A handbook for relieving the discomforts of pregnancy.* New York: Delta/Delcorte.

Workplace Wellness

Massage is an increasingly popular offering of wellness programs in the workplace. Many businesses recognize the benefits of massage to their employees and are making massage available at the work-site itself. Chair massage, in particular, is becoming more popular as businesses explore ways to reduce stress on the job and to prevent job-related injuries.

■ HISTORY

In the late nineteenth and early twentieth centuries, massage was sometimes available at businesses such as large factories and retail stores as part of in-house employee services. Industrial recreation programs might provide fitness and sport activities that include massage. Large businesses often had on-site medical departments, including physiotherapy. These in-house programs largely disappeared in the mid-twentieth century.

In the 1980s, businesses began to rediscover the benefits of healthy employees and to implement programs to encourage healthy life habits. These include programs such as exercise, weight loss, smoking cessation, and stress reduction. Healthy employees tend to be more productive and lose less time due to illness or injury. Workplace wellness programs have been found to reduce workers compensation claims and absenteeism.

The invention of a specially designed chair that allows people to receive massage in a seated position has had a dramatic impact on the availability of massage in offices and other work settings. The first modern massage chair was designed in the 1980s by David Palmer of San Francisco, CA, and promoted as the foundation for "on-site massage." One of the first large corporations to provide on-site massage for their employees in 1985 was Apple Computer Corporation (Palmer, 1995).

The idea of the special chair was to make receiving massage more available. It can be transported easily, takes up less room than a massage table, and allows recipients to receive massage sitting up and with their clothes on. Massage techniques that do not need oil are used.

▪ BENEFITS OF MASSAGE IN THE WORKPLACE

Many of the tasks performed by factory workers in the past are now done by sophisticated machines run by computers. However, there are still workers who sit at workstations for long periods of time performing repetitive tasks. For example, many office workers today sit at computers for long hours, and overuse injuries from using computer keyboards are common.

Attention to ergonomics in the work environment has alleviated some potentially damaging situations. For example, care may be taken to ensure that computer keyboards and monitors are in the right relationship to the user to reduce physical injury, and phone headsets help prevent neck strain. While these practices can lessen the negative impact on employees, they do not eliminate problems altogether. The stress level of employees is also a major wellness factor. The dizzying pace of modern times, at work and in everyday life, adds to the stress of employees. A high level of chronic stress is known to have a negative effect on health.

Massage can help address many of the potentially harmful conditions mentioned above, and it has also been found to increase mental clarity and alertness (Field et al, 1993; Massage, 1996). This can only enhance worker productivity. Practitioners can adapt massage sessions to address the needs of workers, and chair massage makes offering this service in the workplace convenient.

Some of the benefits of massage, especially chair massage, in the workplace are listed below. The list was adapted from the information brochure, *On-Site Therapeutic Massage: Investment for a Healthy Business* (Benjamin, 1994):

- Reduces the physical and mental effects of stress, thus helps prevent burnout and stress-related diseases.
- Reduces the adverse effects of sitting for long periods of time in the same position, such as at a desk or other workstation.
- Relieves physical problems associated with repetitive tasks such as computer keyboard use, sorting, filing, and assembly-line tasks.
- Improves alertness and ability to focus, an antidote for work slumps.
- Helps relieve common problem conditions such as tension headaches and stiff and sore muscles.
- Is thought to improve immune system functioning for better general health and resistance to colds and other illnesses.
- Leaves employees feeling revitalized and ready to return to work.

▪ CHAIR MASSAGE FOR OFFICE WORKERS

Chair massage does not require a special space. It may be given at a workstation, in an empty office or cubicle, or in any small space such as the corner of a conference or work room. Chair massage sessions for office workers typically last from 10 to 20 minutes. Recipients may be seated at their workstations or may be in portable massage chairs. Figure 21–1 shows a tabletop unit that offers recipients support when receiving massage at desks.

The recipient is clothed, but may remove jacket, tie, large jewelry, or other things that might interfere with the massage. Practitioners should ask permission to work on the face if the recipient is wearing makeup, and on the scalp if it would disturb the hair.

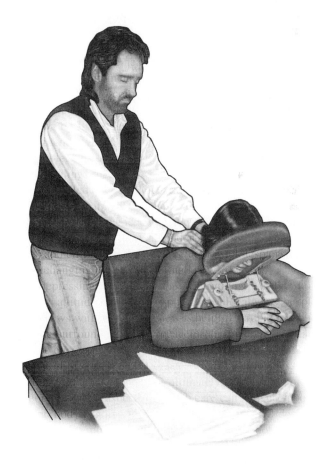

FIGURE 21–1. Portable table-top equipment that provides support for recipients receiving massage at their workstations.

Sessions focus mainly on the upper body. Areas of concern for office workers might be the neck and shoulders, head and scalp, upper back, and forearms, wrists, and hands. Techniques that are effective without the use of oil are used; for example, forms of petrissage, friction, tapotement, light stroking, and joint movements. Forms of energy balancing such as polarity may be incorporated into a session.

Shiatsu, acupressure, and amma are particularly adaptable for chair massage since they are given without lubricant and include techniques such as direct pressure, compressions, and percussion. Figure 21–2 shows the practitioner applying direct pressure to the muscles along the spine.

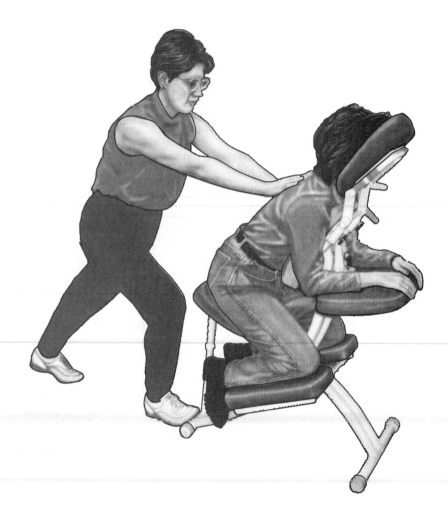

FIGURE 21–2. Application of direct pressure to muscles along the spine during upper body massage in special massage chair.

■ POPULARITY OF WORKPLACE MASSAGE

Massage is popular with employers and employees for a number of reasons. It has immediate positive effects since recipients usually feel better right away. It may alleviate some of the physical aches and pains developed from sitting long hours doing deskwork. In contrast to other wellness practices, massage requires no practice or effort on the part of the recipient. It complements other health practices such as exercise and stress-reduction programs.

Massage programs help increase good feelings about the workplace and loyalty to businesses that show caring for their employees' well-being. They may boost productivity, and may be taken advantage of by all workers (Benjamin, 1994).

■ SUMMARY

Massage is becoming an increasingly popular part of workplace wellness programs. Employers are recognizing the benefits of massage for helping workers stay healthy and productive. Massage can help relieve muscular tension in those who sit at workstations for long periods of time or perform repetitive tasks, and help reduce the effects of work environment stresses.

The invention of a special massage chair in the 1980s has helped make massage more accessible. Massage may be given in small spaces, and recipients are sitting up and receive massage through their clothes. Massage techniques that do not require oil are used; for example, the classic Western massage techniques of petrissage, friction, tapotement, and other approaches such as amma, shiatsu, and polarity therapy. Massage leaves employees feeling revitalized, alert, and ready to return to work.

■ REFERENCES

No author. (1996). Massage helps lower stress of working, taking final exams. In *Massage, 62* (July/August), 148.

Benjamin, P. J. (1994). *On-site therapeutic massage: Investment for a healthy business.* Information brochure. Rockford, IL: Hemingway Publications.

Field, T. M., Fox, N., Pickens, J., Ironsong, G., & Scafidi, F. (1993). Job stress survey. Unpublished manuscript, Touch Research Institute, University of Miami School of Medicine. Reported in *Touchpoints: Touch Research Abstracts, 1*(1).

Palmer, D. (1995). The death of on-site massage? *Massage Therapy Journal, 34*(3), 119–120.

Mental and Emotional Wellness

Although massage is most often thought of as promoting physical well-being, there are many mental and emotional benefits as well. Relaxation, anxiety reduction, release of emotional tension, increased mental clarity, and the experience of caring touch are all possible effects of massage.

Theories about how the body, mind, and emotions are interrelated are discussed below. Some of the practical applications are also presented. Research on the mental and emotional aspects of massage are reviewed in Chapters 3 and 25, while some of the major theories and findings are summarized in this chapter.

▪ THE INDIVISIBLE BODY AND MIND

The body and mind function as a single unit. For example, emotions are felt in and expressed through the body. Love is felt deeply in the physical self, as is hate. Facial expressions are a window to our emotions. Mental and physical pain can be indistinguishable.

Physical manifestations of emotions include the blush of embarrassment, sweaty palms in nervousness, the clenched fist of anger, wide-eyed fear, and the quickened heartbeat of those in love. Some believe that body posture may be read for its emotional sources. For example, raised shoulders indicating fear; rounded shoulders carrying the weight of the world; or forward, hunched shoulders for self-protection and fear of being hurt (Dychtwald, 1977).

Skin as the Outer Surface of the Brain

The connectedness of body and mind can be traced to our beginnings as an embryo. In the third week of life, there are three layers of cells. The outer layer, or ectoderm, eventually develops into the skin, brain, and nervous system. Thus the physical structures that allow us to feel physical sensations are from the same source as those through which we experience emotions. Juhan observes that "depending on how you look at it, the skin is the outer surface of the brain, or the brain is the deepest layer of the skin" (Juhan, 1987, p. 35).

This connection between the skin and the nervous system has profound implications when studying the effects of massage on the mind and emotions. In touching the outermost part of the physical body, we are able to touch the innermost parts of our patients and clients.

Research on touch has borne out this connection. For example, babies deprived of touch fail to develop properly and suffer retarded bone growth, failure to gain weight, poor muscular coordination, immunologic weakness, and general apathy (Montagu, 1978). Massage, as a form of structured touch, has been used successfully to help premature infants, and infants from mothers who used cocaine, gain weight and thrive (Field et al, 1986).

The Limbic System

The concept of the *limbic system* helps shed light on how the physical and emotional components of a person are related and how body memories are created. From a physiologic perspective, the lymbic system is defined as follows:

> *Limbic system—a group of structures within the rhinencephalon of the brain that are associated with various emotions and feelings such as anger, fear, sexual arousal, pleasure and sadness. The structures of the limbic system are the cingulate gyrus, the isthmus, the hippocampal gyrus, the uncus, and the hippocampus. The structures connect with various other parts of the brain.*
>
> *(Anderson & Anderson, 1990)*

Memory researchers have been able to trace the flow of information from touch receptors in the skin through the spinal cord and brain stem into different parts of the brain. This activates the limbic system to experience emotions related to the touch and to create memories or images of tactile experiences (Knaster, 1996, pp. 123–124).

There is the possibility, therefore, that memories may be activated, as well as created, by touch. This has a variety of important implications for practitioners. For example, if the recipient of massage has experienced caring touch primarily in a sexual context, the touch of the practitioner might bring up feelings and memories that would be confusing and inappropriate during a session. Or a recipient who has been physically or sexually abused may have difficulty accepting healing touch without hardening against it. Touch may similarly be used to help in the healing and recovery process.

Character Armor

Wilhelm Reich (1897–1957) introduced the concept of *character armor,* or muscular tension caused by supression of emotions. For example, unexpressed anger may cause tension in the muscles of the back and arms that would have been used to strike out. Or unexpressed grief may result in shallow breathing and stiffening of muscles used in crying. In the process of relaxing the affected muscles, the supressed emotions may be felt by the recipient. Massage practitioners may encounter such armoring and should be prepared to help the patient or client understand the release of emotions that sometimes happens.

The above discussion merely touches lightly on the complexity of the body, mind, and emotion relationship. Many of the concepts are in the theoretical stages of development. Research into the holistic nature of human beings is continuing to confirm and clarify ideas that have been little understood before in the context of Western medicine. In her book *Discovering the Body's Wisdom,* Mirka Knaster explores these ideas in more detail and offers a comprehensive introduction to the subject (1996).

■ APPLICATIONS FOR MENTAL AND EMOTIONAL WELL-BEING

Massage has been called a *body-centered therapy* since it works primarily through touch and movement of the body to enhance the overall well-being of the recipient. This concept may include the energetic aspect of the person as well, as, for example, in polarity therapy and Asian forms of bodywork.

Explained in Western scientific terms, massage may produce effects on the parasympathetic nervous system, release endorphins, stimulate sensory receptors, relax muscles, or give pleasure. Any of these effects may, in turn, enhance the mental and emotional well-being of the recipient. The following sections briefly discuss some of the more common benefits of massage involving the mind and emotions.

Stress and Relaxation

One of the most recognized effects of massage on the body and mind is relaxation. Certain types of massage (eg, a gentle back rub) are known to stimulate the parasympathetic nervous system, eliciting the relaxation response. This has a soothing emotional effect, reduces anxiety, calms the mind, and promotes feelings of well-being.

Massage has been used in medical settings for this very effect. It has been shown to be beneficial for patients hospitalized for serious medical conditions, the institutionalized elderly, people with conditions worsened by stress, and psychiatric patients. The relaxation elicited by massage has contributed to healing and sense of well-being. Some of these studies are described in more detail in Chapter 25.

Anxiety Reduction

Massage has been found to be useful in reducing anxiety in a variety of situations. Many studies that have observed physiologic indications of relaxation after massage also noted a reduction in anxiety. This may be connected to the release of endorphins thought to occur with certain types of massage, as well as the effects of the relaxation response. They are no doubt intimately related.

Anxiety reduction may be beneficial in situations such as relieving everyday tensions at home and at work, worry due to disease or injury to self or a loved one, or a sense of grief caused by the death of someone close. Massage has been used with hospital and psychiatric patients to help reduce their uneasiness of mind, improve their mental states, and facilitate their recovery.

Release of Tension

Muscle tension is often the result of coping with the stressors of everyday life. The tension caused by chronic stress may manifest in such common ailments as backache, tension headaches, grinding the teeth, and TMJ. Because massage promotes relaxation and anxiety reduction, it may help prevent this buildup of tension.

A phenomenon called emotional release may happen during massage as suppressed emotions are allowed to surface. The release may be expressed in simple ways such as the eyes tearing or in crying and shaking.

Trauma, such as from an automobile accident or from physical or sexual abuse, may also lead to muscle tension. Memories of these events may be stored in the body and manifest as chronic aches and pains or more serious disease. Clyde Ford, a chiropractor and psychotherapist, specializes in using touch, movement, and awareness to help adult survivors of childhood sexual abuse recover and heal from their traumatic experiences (Ford, 1993).

Some forms of bodywork help recipients become aware of the sources of their muscular tension and then release it. The Rosen Method, developed by physical therapist Marion Rosen, is one such form. The Rosen Method uses gentle touch, awareness of breath, and verbal interaction to help clients unlock old memories that have settled in their bodies in unhealthy ways. In the process of letting go of suppressed emotions, recipients often report a release of chronic muscular tension and an improvement in overall well-being (Claire, 1995).

Mental Clarity

Massage can be relaxing without making recipients drowsy or sleepy. By using a varied rhythm, faster pace, shorter sessions (10–15 minutes), and incorporating techniques that are stimulating, the results may be mental clarity and alertness. Pre-event sports massage and massage given in special chairs at the workplace or in other public places are examples where this type of massage would be appropriate. The mental effects of alertness and clarity are the result of increased sensory stimulation and circulation.

Need for Caring Touch

People in all stages of life—infants, children, adults, elders—need caring touch to thrive. Massage is a form of structured, safe touch available to those who would otherwise be deprived of the touch they need. This is especially true for infants and elders, who are the most dependent on caregivers for meeting their needs.

In the preface to her book *Compassionate Touch,* Dawn Nelson says: "I believe that those in later life stages who are similarly deprived of tender and nurturing physical contact experience a diminishing quality of life, a lessening of their desire to relate to others, and a weakening of what may already be a fragile relationship to reality" (1994). Massage can be a time for elders to connect with themselves and others in a way that strengthens their social and emotional well-being.

Everyone needs caring touch in their lives. Massage can be a vehicle to bring caring touch, sometimes for its own sake, into people's lives in healthy ways. It is one of the "healthy pleasures" that contributes to the quality of life.

▪ SUMMARY

Massage is most often thought of as promoting physical well-being; however, there are many mental and emotional benefits as well. Modern science is beginning to understand how the mind and body operate as a unit and to recognize the profound physiologic connections between the skin and nervous system. For example, the limbic system, a group of structures in the brain, is activated as we experience emotions related to touch. It creates memories or images of tactile experiences. "Character armor" is another important concept that describes how muscle tension is created by the suppression of emotions. These ideas help explain how massage may impact the whole person and why it may elicit certain reactions from the recipient.

The potential effects of massage related to the mind and emotions include relaxation and stress reduction, anxiety reduction, release of tension, and increased mental clarity. Massage can provide healthy caring touch necessary for well-being and may be one of the "healthy pleasures" that contributes to the quality of life.

▪ REFERENCES

Anderson, K. N., & Anderson, L. E. (1990). *Mosby's pocket dictionary of medicine, nursing, & allied health.* St. Louis: C. V. Mosby.

Claire, T. (1995). *Bodywork: What type of massage to get and how to make the most of it.* New York: William Morrow.

Dychtwald, K. (1977). *Body-mind.* New York: Jove Publications.

Field, T. M., Schanberg, S. M., Scafidi, F., et al. (1986). Tactile/kinesthetic stimulation effects on preterm neonates. *Pediatrics, 77*(5), 654–658.

Ford, C. W. (1993). *Compassionate touch: The role of human touch in healing and recovery.* New York: Simon & Schuster.

Juhan, D. (1987). *Job's body: A handbook for bodywork.* Barrytown, NY: Station Hill Press.

Knaster, M. (1996) *Discovering the body's wisdom.* New York: Bantam Books.

Montagu, A. (1978). *Touching: The human significance of the skin,* 2nd ed. New York: Harper & Row.

Nelson, D. (1994). *Compassionate touch: Hands-on caregiving for the elderly, the ill, and the dying.* Barrytown, NY: Station Hill Press.

Healthy Aging

Massage can be an important component of a life-long personal wellness program. It promotes general physical and emotional well-being, addresses conditions commonly associated with aging, and enhances the quality of life. It can help slow the aging process and maintain youthful characteristics longer.

Massage works best if received regularly and over a period of years. Who we are as we grow older is an accumulation of a lifetime of both good and poor health practices. Along with good eating and exercise habits, regular massage can help prevent or retard some of the decreases in condition and function experienced as we age. It can help improve an already deteriorated condition, but works best as a measure of prevention.

■ THE EFFECTS OF AGING AND BENEFITS OF MASSAGE

The physical effects of aging are perhaps the most visible and begin noticeably for most around age 30. These include decrease in general mobility and muscular strength, slower nerve conduction, less efficient circulation, less tissue elasticity, thinner and drier skin, loss of bone mass, decreased function of the senses, and a less efficient immune system. This is often experienced as general aches and pains, slower movement, and less stamina. Research has found that many of these "biomarkers" can be slowed considerably with a healthy lifestyle, including good nutrition and exercise (Evans & Rosenberg, 1991).

Massage may directly address the effects of aging. For example, it promotes well-nourished skin by increasing superficial circulation and may help moisturize skin through the use of oils and lotions. Massage improves general blood circulation, especially in the extremities. Immune system function is strengthened with improved lymph flow and general relaxation.

It has been found that chronic stress and inactivity accelerate the aging process (Evans & Rosenberg, 1991). Massage helps reduce the physical and mental effects of stress and anxiety. It is known to trigger the relaxation response, relieve muscular tension, reduce anxiety, improve sleep, and increase feelings of well-being.

Older adults find massage useful for reducing the muscular tension and the aches and stiffness that often accompany an exercise program. By keeping muscles more pliable and increasing flexibility, massage can reduce the potential for injury during workouts. Chapters 3 and 25 review the research on the effects of massage discussed in this section.

■ BENEFITS FOR ELDERS

Massage has special benefits for elders in addition to those mentioned above. For example, it helps people 65 years and older maintain mobility and independence longer by improving tissue elasticity and joint flexibility. Along with exercise, it helps elders keep the flexibility and strength needed to do simple things like get up out of a chair, dress and undress, climb stairs, and get in and out of a bath tub.

The later years of life are often a time of loss, frustration, and fear about the future. There could be loss of work, home, spouse, family, friends, independence, or financial security. Some elders will have better coping skills than others. The caring touch and relaxing benefits of massage help ease these emotional pains.

Massage also provides an avenue for social interaction, especially for elders in nursing homes or homebound. The personal interaction with the practitioner helps reduce feelings of social isolation, and the touch inherent in massage provides a special connection to others.

In her book *Compassionate Touch,* Dawn Nelson lists some of the common conditions that the elderly experience and that massage can help alleviate. These include insomnia, loss of appetite, constipation, immobility, poor circulation, decreased immune system functioning, skin problems such as loss of elasticity and dryness, bedsores, physical discomfort and pain, chronic stress, chronic depression, feeling alone and useless (1994).

Chapter 25 reviews some of the research that has been done on massage in medical settings. They have shown massage to be beneficial to those hospitalized for a number of conditions, including heart disease, cancer, and psychiatric problems. The benefits of back massage to institutionalized elderly included relaxation, improved communication, and reducing the common dehumanizing effects of institutional care (Frazer & Kerr, 1993). These results were confirmed by another study of slow stroke back rub for the elderly by nurses (Fakouri & Jones, 1987).

■ WORKING WITH THE ELDERLY

Elders are perhaps the most distinctive population to work with. Individuals in this age group are generally more different from each other than those in other age groups. By the time people have reached 65+ years of age, they exhibit the accumulated effects of a lifetime of good and poor health habits, diseases and injuries, and life experiences. They are more likely to have chronic health problems and to be on medications. Care should be taken in learning about them and planning their massage sessions.

It is useful to think about older adults in terms of *physiologic age,* rather than *chronologic* age. People age at different rates depending on their genetic makeup, life-long health habits, and unusual life events such as car accidents or sports injuries. Diseases experienced earlier in life may have an effect later, such as the incidences of post-polio syndrome affecting people 40–50 years after the fact.

Elders may be thought of as falling into one of three categories, that is, robust, age appropriate, and frail. *Robust* elders show few outward signs of impaired health, look younger than their chronologic age, are mentally sharp and physically active. People who show some of the typical signs of aging are considered *age appropriate. Frail* elders look and feel fragile to touch (Meisler, 1990).

Robust elders can generally be treated like the typical middle-aged recipient of massage. Information obtained on a health questionnaire can help you identify any areas of caution that are not obvious. Age appropriate elders will have some problems associated with aging. Information from a health questionnaire may be useful to identify areas of caution. Use pillows and bolsters to ensure maximum comfort and the least stress on joints. Limit the prone position to 15–20 minutes. After the session, help the recipient sit up, or at least stay until he or she is sitting up. Leave the room only when you are sure that the recipient is not lightheaded and can get off the table safely.

Frail elders need special care. Check with their physicians before massaging the very frail. Frail elders will probably need assistance getting onto and off of the table. You might find it necessary to massage them in a regular chair or on their beds. Limit the session to 15–20 minutes until you know that they can handle longer sessions. Watch them carefully in the prone position on the table to be sure that they can lie there comfortably. Be extra gentle in lifting frail elders, avoiding pulling on their arms to help them up. Cradle their bodies to help them change position (Meisler, 1990).

■ MASSAGE TECHNIQUES

There are no special massage "techniques" that slow the aging process. However, there are certain points to keep in mind in working with adults, and especially with the elderly.

Do include the following in your massage session:

- Techniques to improve circulation in the extremities. Effleurage moving distal to proximal enhances venous return, and relaxing the muscles with kneading and jostling improves local circulation.
- Kneading and other petrissage movements that help keep muscle and connective tissue pliable and elastic.
- Joint mobilizations and stretches of the lower extremities for improved mobility and flexibility. Spend time on the feet to relieve soreness, improve cir-

culation, and mobilize joints. Mobilizing the legs and feet can help increase kinesthetic awareness, and thereby improve movements such as walking and climbing stairs.

- Mobilizations and stretches for the shoulders to help maintain some important daily living functions such as getting dressed and undressed and reaching for things overhead. The hands may benefit from special attention to help them to stay mobile and sensitive.
- Passive motion and stretches for the cervicals to help maintain normal range of motion in the head and neck. With declining peripheral vision, the ability to turn the head to see things in the environment is important. This is essential for the safety of elders who drive motor vehicles.
- Techniques that focus on lengthening the front of the body, especially abdominals and pectorals, to help maintain an erect posture. Exercises are also needed to keep postural muscles strong and to avoid a bent-over or collapsed condition later in life.
- Abdominal massage for the viscera, which may be important for sedentary elders to improve digestion and elimination. Use gentle but firm pressure, always going clockwise during circular movements.

Cautions

Some problem conditions are more common in older adults and warrant special attention. Massage is rarely contraindicated totally, but certain cautions apply with the conditions mentioned below. It is important to take a thorough health history to identify the conditions that are contraindicated or for which cautions are important. Always consult the recipient's physician when in doubt about a condition or disease mentioned by a recipient of massage.

- Massage may be contraindicated with certain medications. If you work regularly with older adults and elders, it would be wise to have a reference book that explains the effects and possible side effects of common medications. Check with the recipient's physician if in doubt about the advisability of receiving massage with a certain medication.
- Elders usually have thin and delicate skin and may bruise more easily than younger people. Pressure used in massage should be gentle to moderate depending on the recipient's general condition.
- Watch for varicose veins, which tend to appear in the legs, and do not perform deep effleurage or strong kneading over them. Light effleurage and jostling movements are better for circulation in this case. Elevating the legs slightly when the recipient is supine will help venous return during the massage.
- Older adults and elders may have diagnosed or undiagnosed atherosclerosis, or hardening of the arteries. This is especially dangerous in the cerebral arteries, which pass through the neck. Avoid deep work in the lateral neck area. Avoid movements that put the neck in hyperextension or increase the cervical curve. This position may further occlude blood vessels to the head and cause fainting.

- Use great care in performing joint movements and stretches involving the hip joint for those who have had hip replacements. Avoid movements involving abduction and circumduction. Consult the recipient's health care provider for instructions. Extreme care should be taken in the case of any joint replacement because of the potential instability of the joint.
- In the case of cancer patients, always check with the physician before performing massage. Some types of cancer may spread with massage, while some will not be affected. It may be possible to perform massage away from the site of the cancer and do no harm.
- Older adults and elders tend to have problems in their joints, including osteo- and rheumatoid arthritis. Massage of the area should be avoided if the joint is inflamed. When there is no inflammation, massage of the surrounding muscles is indicated to help relieve stress on the joint.
- Because massage is commonly done directly on the skin, practitioners may detect skin cancers of which recipients of massage are unaware. Basal and squamous cell carcinoma and malignant melanoma usually appear on sun-exposed areas of the body, including the face, arms, and chest. Malignant melanoma may develop at the site of a mole. Report any lesion or suspicious-looking skin condition to the recipient, or to the caregiver in the case of frail elders, and suggest that it be checked out by a physician or dermatologist. Do not massage directly over the site.

▪ SUMMARY

Regular massage can help retard some of the decreases in function and condition that are part of the normal aging process. Massage promotes well-nourished skin, improves general blood circulation and lymph flow, helps keep fascia and muscles more pliable, improves joint flexibility, and strengthens immune system function. It helps reduce the physical and mental effects of stress that may accelerate the aging process.

Massage is especially beneficial for elders of 65 years old or more. It helps them maintain mobility and independence longer and helps ease the pain of loss and frustration often experienced in later years. It may alleviate some common problems such as insomnia, constipation, and depression. Massage offers regular caring touch, relaxation, and social interaction to homebound elders and those in institutions.

It is useful to think of older adults in terms of physiologic, rather than chronologic, age. Elders may be thought of as either robust, age appropriate, or frail. Frail elders need special care. Common conditions that may be contraindications, or for which special cautions apply, include certain medications, thinning skin, skin growths, circulatory problems, joint disease, and joint replacements.

There are no special massage techniques that slow the aging process. However, massage sessions may be tailored to meet the needs and concerns of older adults related to maintaining healthy tissues, mobility, and independence, good posture, and physiologic functions such as digestion. Massage can be an important part of a life-long personal wellness program and an aid to caring for elders in institutional settings.

▪ REFERENCES

Evans, W., & Rosenberg, E. H. (1991). *Biomarkers.* New York: Simon & Schuster.

Fakouri, C., & Jones, P. (1987). Relaxation RX: Slow stroke back rub. *Journal of Gerontological Nursing, 13*(2), 32–35.

Fraser, J., & Kerr, J. R. (1993). Psychophysiological effects of back massage on elderly institutionalized patients. *Journal of Advanced Nursing, 18,* 238–245.

Miesler, D. W. (1990). *Geriatric massage techniques: Topics for bodyworkers no. 2.* Guerneville, CA: Day-Break Productions.

Nelson, D. (1994). *Compassionate touch: Hands-on caregiving for the elderly, the ill, and the dying.* Barrytown, NY: Station Hill Press.

Terminally Ill and Dying

Massage may be used in hospital, hospice, and home care to bring comfort and caring touch to the terminally ill and dying. Simple massage techniques may be used by health practitioners and taught to nonprofessional caregivers to aid those seriously ill or approaching the end of their lives.

▪ THE CARING TOUCH OF MASSAGE

In the wellness model, even those with terminal illnesses or nearing death continue to strive for optimal well-being in their life circumstances. Although massage may not "cure" or save someone from imminent death, it can help improve physical function and ease some of the pain and anxiety felt. As Dawn Nelson points out in her book *Compassionate Touch*, "attentive nurturing touch can be a significant therapeutic factor in treating despondency in the aging and/or the ill because of its multiple psycho-social, mental, emotional, and physical benefits" (1994, p. 12).

General relaxation, improved circulation of blood and lymph, reduced muscular tension, and stimulation of the skin are effects of massage with benefits for everyone. These effects may address some of the special problems of those who have been physically inactive or bedridden for a long period of time. Massage may help alleviate problems with insomnia, digestion, constipation, difficulty in breathing, and skin degeneration.

The terminally ill and dying may experience emotional distress for a number of reasons. They may feel isolation, grief from the loss of freedom and friends, fear of abandonment, fear of the disease or aging process, or fear of dying. Depression is common among the seriously ill and elderly and may be caused or deepened by touch deprivation.

Gentle relaxation massage is known to reduce anxiety, provide a sense of connection, and generate feelings of general well-being. Massage may also facilitate a release of pent-up feelings, frustrations, sadness, and emotional energy. Pain that is aggravated by stress may be lessened with relaxing massage.

■ FOR THE DYING

Near the end of life, massage can provide comforting touch and communicate caring and love in a nonverbal way. It is important that the quality of touch be gentle, and the techniques simple such as stroking and holding.

In his book *Touching is Healing* (1982), Jules Older describes a program in New Zealand for the seriously ill and dying called the TLP Programme. TLP stands for Tender Loving Physiotherapy. The function of TLP is short-term rehabilitation and clearing the chest, and if appropriate, easing the transition from life to death. When death is near, smooth, soothing touch is used as a form of comfort and a means of communication. Some technical skills are needed to avoid causing pain or damaging delicate tissues.

Cathleen Farnslow, R N, describes how she uses Therapeutic Touch with the dying in *The Many Facets of Touch* (1984):

> *When treating people near the end of the life continuum, I am drawn to place my hands on or near the heart, since this is the area of relationship and fear and requires life energy so that the dying can make amends and say good-bye, I'm sorry, or I love you before death occurs. As I hold my hands on or near the heart I am consciously sending thoughts of peace, love, and wholeness, which makes energy available for patients to finish their business with those who remain here and decreases pre-death anxiety. The elders feel a deep warmth penetrating the heart area and report a sense of peace and deep calm. (p. 187)*

In hospice and home-care situations, family members and other caregivers can be taught simple ways of giving massage to the dying person. This has benefits for both parties since it offers caregivers something active to do with their loved one and provides a means of connection even for those who may not be able to speak.

■ KNOWLEDGE AND SKILLS

A medical profile of the recipient is essential in working with the seriously ill and dying to protect both them and you. As in any other massage, identify contraindications and areas of caution before proceeding with a session. It may also be useful to understand the symptoms expected as a specific disease or condition progresses.

Specific technique is less important than other essential skills when working with the terminally ill and dying. Dawn Nelson points out that:

If you develop the ability to "see" an individual rather than just looking at a body, and if you reach out to that individual with a caring and open heart, your touch is likely to be far more effective than that of a highly trained professional who may be simply going through the mechanics of manipulating a physical body. Out of your real and pure contact with the individual, you will intuitively know what to do and how to proceed. (1994, p. 43)

Intuition and sensitivity to others are important qualities for those giving massage to the terminally ill and dying. Other characteristics and abilities recommended by Nelson (1994) include being touch oriented, able to adapt, open-hearted, able to focus energy, willing to face death, and able to focus on the individual. The skills she identifies as important include sensitive massage, active holding, listening and feedback, visualization and guided fantasy, guided meditation, shared breathing, and communicating with the dying. While some of these skills may seem outside the scope of a massage practitioner, they may be useful in working with certain populations.

In planning massage sessions for the terminally ill or dying, there are no specific procedures to follow or ironclad rules to memorize. Each individual will be different in how he or she experiences dying and in how massage might be of benefit. However, there are some general guidelines to keep in mind.

In general, massage sessions with the dying should be softer, gentler, and shorter. A person may only be able to benefit from 10–20 minutes of contact. Techniques may vary from simple hand holding to full-body massage. Massage may be given with the receiver lying on a standard massage table, sitting in a chair or wheel chair, or lying in bed. Patients may be in hospital beds with tubes or IVs in their bodies. Massage practitioners in these situations need to be versatile and able to adapt to the circumstances. Listening and feedback skills are important since communication may be a great need among those facing death. The key here is to be caring, supportive, and accepting.

Hand and arm massage is a useful approach for getting to know a new patient or client and for nursing home and hospice volunteers to perform. The hands are easily accessible, relatively safe to massage, benefit from the application of lotion, and are a familiar place of contact with other people. Having the hands touched is comforting in itself and affords the opportunity for eye contact while talking.

▪ SELF-CARE

Working with the terminally ill and dying can be physically and emotionally challenging. It is important to practice conscious self-care to help maintain your own well-being.

The actual massage techniques used with the seriously ill or elderly tend to be simple and light and easy on the practitioner's hands. However, maintaining good body mechanics may be difficult when working with people in chairs or in bed. The general principles of good mechanics apply here also, and you need to find creative ways to keep your back straight and spine and neck in good alignment.

If the recipient has a communicable disease, proper precautions and hygiene should be observed. Latex gloves, although awkward, should be worn if necessary for protection.

Maintaining emotional well-being involves a variety of factors. It helps to have confronted your own issues and fears around illness and death to a point of acceptance. Conscious awareness of how you feel when with someone seriously ill or nearing death can help you work through those feelings with a friend, co-worker, or supervisor.

Eventual loss is expected in working with the dying. It is natural to develop caring relationships with your patients or clients. When one of them dies, be sensitive to your own process of grieving and letting go. Ongoing professional supervision or peer counseling may be of benefit when working with this special population.

▪ SUMMARY

Massage may be used to bring comfort and caring touch to the terminally ill and dying. Simple massage techniques may be used by health practitioners and taught to nonprofessional caregivers to help improve the physical and emotional well-being of those approaching the end of life. Gentle, soothing stroking and holding are the main techniques used to relieve anxiety and produce a sense of calm. Massage may have benefits related to improved circulation, healthy skin, and general relaxation. Touching in itself may communicate caring and love and help those suffering depression from touch deprivation.

In general, massage sessions with the dying are softer, gentler, and shorter. Practitioners need to use their intuition and sensitivity in determining how to approach each person. Knowledge of the recipients' medical profiles can help practitioners plan massage sessions better and provide a safe environment for both giver and receiver. Physical and emotional self-care practices help practitioners maintain their own well-being while working under unusual circumstances and in facing loss and grief encountered when working with the terminally ill and dying.

▪ REFERENCES

Fanslow, C. (1984). Touch and the elderly. In *The many facets of touch* edited by C. C. Brown. Skillman, NJ: Johnson & Johnson Baby Products Company.

Nelson, D. (1994). *Compassionate touch: Hands-on caregiving for the elderly, the ill and the dying.* New York: Station Hill Press.

Older, J. (1982). *Touching is healing.* New York: Stein & Day.

Massage in Medical Settings

Massage has been used to treat medical conditions since ancient times. The earliest known record of medical massage is found in ancient Sumeria (2100 B.C.E.) in a prescription written on clay tablets. It calls for an herbal mixture to be rubbed on a diseased part, followed by frictions and more rubbing with oil (Time-Life Books, 1987, p. 41).

Massage has been used throughout history within the established medical professions, as well as among natural and traditional healers. Its acceptance within the medical establishment has hit high and low points at different times in the past. Manual therapies are currently enjoying a resurgence of interest within medical professions. See Chapter 2 for further information on the history of massage in medical settings.

Massage has been found to be beneficial in the overall healing process, as well as for specific local effects. In this chapter, we will review some of the ways massage is used as treatment, or as an adjunct to treatment, within the professions of nursing, physical therapy, massage therapy, and chiropractic.

■ MASSAGE AS INDICATED FOR TREATMENT

The success of the use of massage as a medical treatment is determined by how much it contributes directly and measurably to the alleviation of the targeted condition. It is in this sense that massage can be said to be *indicated* for treating a certain disease or injury. Massage may be *contraindicated,* or not advisable, if its use as a form of treatment would be detrimental to the patient.

Massage is sometimes indicated as an *adjunct* to treatment to create an environment or state of being in which the effects of more targeted treatment are enhanced. This is especially true in the uses of massage to help patients relax and reduce their anxiety, thus enhancing and removing blocks to the body's own capacity to heal.

Massage is used in different health care professions to varying degrees and within their various scopes of practice. Some of the uses of massage in medical settings and the research addressing its efficacy in various situations will be reviewed in this chapter.

Physical Rehabilitation

In Ontario, Canada, where massage therapy is part of the health care system provided by the government, massage is used in the treatment of a wide range of conditions. In her book *Massage Therapy: An Approach to Treatments* (1994), Fiona Rattray, a Canadian Registered Massage Therapist, describes how massage is applied in conditions as varied as burns, "frozen shoulder," fibromyalgia, cerebral palsy, Parkinson's disease, Bell's palsy, and whiplash. This is similar to what physical therapists typically see in the United States. It is beyond the scope of this book to describe all of the applications of massage in physical medicine, but the following paragraphs mention some of the common uses for musculoskeletal conditions.

Massage or manual therapy is routinely incorporated into the rehabilitation of musculoskeletal injuries by physical therapists, athletic trainers, and massage therapists. It is particularly effective in relieving muscle tension, increasing range of motion, promoting healthy scar tissue, and reducing pain. See Chapter 3, "Effects, Benefits, and Indications."

Deep transverse friction applied to a painful site is known to result in a high degree of analgesia, which in turn allows the patient to move more normally, thereby preventing the formation of adhesions (de Bruijin, 1984). When treating tendinitis and tenosynovitis, deep transverse friction is used to relieve pain and to promote healthy scar formation. Massage is also used to reduce edema in the area and reduce hypertonicity, spasm, and trigger points in the surrounding muscles. Massage increases circulation to the area, facilitating healing, and helps maintain normal range of motion in affected joints (Rattray, 1994, pp. 256–257).

Tapotement or percussion is used in treatment of respiratory conditions (eg, bronchitis) to loosen mucus in the system. Mobilization of the chest is important in conditions such as bronchitis, emphysema, and asthma (Rattray, 1994). Trager Psychophysical Integration, a form of loose mobilizations, appears to have a positive effect on the restrictive component of chronic lung disease (Witt & MacKinnon, 1986).

Relaxation and Anxiety Reduction

The ability of certain applications of massage to elicit the relaxation response accounts for much of its value as an adjunct to regular medical treatment. Nurses in particular have found massage useful in caring for patients hospitalized for a variety of conditions. Two nurses, Frazer and Kerr (1993), found back massage to be an effective, noninvasive technique for promoting relaxation and improving communication with elderly, institutionalized patients. They noted its promise for reducing the common dehumanizing effects of institutional care. The results were confirmed by another study of slow stroke back rub for the elderly by two other nurses, Fakouri and Jones (1987).

An interesting study by nurses Bauer and Dracup (1987) found that back massage consisting of effleurage had no detrimental cardiovascular hemodynamic effects on patients with acute myocardial infarction. Although they could not confirm certain physiologic benefits from back massage, they noted its usefulness in the perception of relaxation and comfort reported by patients.

In a study of patients hospitalized in a cardiovascular unit of a large medical center in New York City, it was found that patients who received Therapeutic Touch had a significantly greater reduction in posttest anxiety scores than those who received casual touch or no touch (Heidt, 1981). See below for a description of Therapeutic Touch.

A study by nurse Ferrell-Torry and Glick (1993) examined the effects of therapeutic massage consisting of effleurage, petrissage, and myofascial trigger point therapy on hospitalized cancer patients. They found that massage therapy significantly reduced the patients' perceived level of pain and anxiety, while enhancing their feelings of relaxation. Objective physiologic measures (heart rate, respiratory rate, and blood pressure) tended to decrease from baseline, providing further indication of relaxation.

Massage for Cancer Patients

Massage is often listed as a general contraindication for cancer patients. However, this conventional wisdom is being challenged on several fronts. An article appeared in the Summer 1995 issue of *Massage Therapy Journal* called "Massage for Cancer Patients" A Review of Nursing Research" (MacDonald). Five studies were reviewed (Ferrell-Torry & Glick, 1993; Rhiner, Ferrell, Ferrell, & Grant, 1993; Sims, 1986; Tope, Hann, & Pinkson, 1994; Weinrich & Weinrich, 1990).

MacDonald (1995) reports three general findings from the research to date. First, massage often helps alleviate symptoms related to cancer or side effects from treatment procedures (eg, nausea, fatigue, insomnia, and pain). Second, massage increases relaxation and decreases muscle tension. Third, patients report an increased sense of well-being and reduced anxiety and sense of isolation. MacDonald concludes that "no evidence exists that comfort-oriented massage is deleterious, and what research there is indicates that it is often beneficial" (1995, p. 56).

Current thought is divided on whether massage will spread a cancer that metastasizes (Curties, 1994). Rattray recommends contacting the recipient's physician for information on the type of cancer the person has and, when obtaining consent from the recipient, informing him or her that it is unclear whether massage would promote the spread of the disease. If the cancer is terminal, the recipient may desire massage for palliative reasons (1994, p. 461).

After cancer surgery, patients may benefit from massage for stress reduction and relaxation, relieving pain and insomnia, promoting healthy scar tissue, treating edema, and lymph drainage. Rattray also mentions the role that positive touch can have after cancer surgery in regaining self-image and body awareness (1994, p. 462). Chamness (1996) identifies three common goals for the breast cancer patient receiving massage: stress reduction and relaxation; reclamation of her body as an ally; and maintenance of range of motion following surgery and physical therapy.

Edema and Lymphedema

Edema, or excess interstitial fluid in the tissues, is not a disease, but rather a manifestation of altered physiologic function. Edema may occur when an increase in capillary pressure causes excess movement of fluid from the capillary bed into the interstitial spaces. It may also occur when plasma protein levels become inadequate to exert the osmotic force necessary to move fluid back into the capillaries from the tissue spaces (eg, in early stages of a burn). Edema may also result from increased capillary permeability or obstruction of lymph flow.

Massage in general and manual lymph drainage in particular are useful methods of reducing edema in the extremities. The beneficial effects of manual lymph drainage for patients with chronic and postmastectomy lymphedema continues to be confirmed. It has been noted that permanent and regular treatment is necessary for these conditions (Kurtz et al, 1978; Zanolla, Monzeglio, Balzarini, & Martino, 1984). Manual lymph drainage is discussed further in Chapter 13.

Therapeutic Touch

Therapeutic Touch is a form of manual therapy (ie, performed using the practitioner's hands) in which the energy field of the recipient is rebalanced, thus promoting health and healing. Although it does not fall directly into the category of soft tissue massage, it is performed by many massage practitioners and integrated into their work. It has found special acceptance by nurses, who find it useful in caring for patients.

Therapeutic Touch as developed by Dolores Krieger, PhD, RN, in the 1970s. She explains the technique as one of centering; then placing the hands in the recipient's energy field to detect a break in energy flow, pressure, or dysrhythmias; then rebalancing or repatterning the energy field by sweeping hand movements a few inches above the skin. She explains what happens as a profound relaxation response that has a positive effect on the immune system, which allows self-healing to reassert itself (Karpen, 1995).

Kreiger explains that Therapeutic Touch has been found to have more effect on some conditions than others. For example, it seems to have a positive effect in working with fluid and electrolyte imbalances, dysfunctions of the autonomic nervous system, lymphatic and circulatory dysfunctions, and musculoskeletal problems. She further explains that:

Some collagen dysfunctions respond, such as rheumatoid arthritis, but lupus is resistant. Within the endocrine system, the thyroid, adrenals, and ovaries respond, but there is little success with the pituitary and variable success with the pancreas in treating diabetes. In psychiatric disorders, manic depressives and catatonics respond, but there has been little success with schizophrenics.

(Karpen, 1995)

It was found that Therapeutic Touch may have potential in the treatment of tension headache pain (Keller & Bzdek, 1986). Therapeutic Touch has also been used successfully to help reduce the stress of hospitalized children (Kramer, 1990). More research on the use of touch and massage with children is presented below.

Research and articles about Therapeutic Touch can be found in nursing journals such as the *American Journal of Nursing* and *Nursing Research.* Further information about Therapeutic Touch research is available from the Nurse Healers–Professional Associates, which was established in 1977 under the leadership of Dolores Kreiger (see Appendix A). The NH-PA is a voluntary, nonprofit cooperative whose international exchange network facilitates the exchange of research findings, teaching strategies, and developments in the clinical practice of Therapeutic Touch.

Pediatric Care

Massage is being used increasingly in the care of hospitalized children from infants to adolescents. Many of the uses of massage in pediatric care are similar to uses for adults, eg, rehabilitation and anxiety reduction. A unique benefit for infants is the tactile stimulation provided by massage, which is essential for proper growth and development.

Much of the recent interest in massage for children has been generated by the work of Tiffany Field, PhD, who in 1991 founded the Touch Research Institute (TRI) at the University of Miami School of Medicine, Department of Pediatrics. The research being performed at TRI on a variety of pediatric conditions is reported regularly in *Touchpoints, Touch Research Abstracts.*

Building on research done in the 1970s, Field found that preterm neonates who received tactile stimulation during their stay in the transitional care nursery setting experienced greater weight gain, increased motor activity, more alertness, and improved performance on the Brazelton Neonatal Behavioral Assessment Scale. Tactile stimulation was applied by gentle stroking of the head and neck, across the shoulders, from upper back to the waist, from the thighs to the feet, and from the shoulders to the hands. Additional stimulation was provided by passive flexion/extension movements of the arms and legs (Field et al, 1986).

Subsequent research has shown that massage also benefits cocaine-exposed preterm neonates. In addition to better weight gain, massaged infants showed significantly fewer postnatal complications and stress behaviors than the control infants did (Wheeden et al, 1993).

A review of some of the research being done at TRI demonstrates the broad range of situations in which massage is found to be a useful treatment for children. The following list is taken from the Fall and Spring 1995 issues of *Touchpoints:*

- Asthmatic children: 20-minute massages given to asthmatic children by their mothers for one month resulted in decreased anxiety levels and improved mood for both children and parents; the children's cortisol levels decreased;

and they had fewer asthma attacks and were able to breathe better (unpublished data, Field, Henteleff, & Mavunda, 1994).

- Autistic children: After one month of massage therapy, the autistic children were less touch sensitive, less distracted by sounds, more attentive in class, related more to their teachers, and received better scores on the Autism Behavior Checklist and on the Early Social Communications Scales.
- Diabetic children: A pilot study showed that as a result of massage given to diabetic children by their parents, both children and parents showed lower anxiety and less depressed mood levels; the children's insulin and food regulation scores improved, and blood glucose levels decreased to the normal range (unpublished data, Field, Delamater, Shaw, & LaGreca, 1994).
- Depressed adolescent mothers: After 10 massage sessions over a five-week period, depressed adolescent mothers reported lower anxiety; showed behavioral and stress hormone changes, including decreases in anxious behavior and in pulse and salivary cortisol levels; and a decrease in urine cortisol levels, suggesting lower stress levels.
- Infants of depressed adolescent mothers: Full-term infants born to depressed adolescent mothers were given 15 minutes of massage two times a week for six weeks. These infants gained more weight, showed greater improvement on emotionality, sociability, and soothability temperament dimensions and on face-to-face interaction ratings, and had greater decreases in urinary stress catecholamines/hormones (norepinephrine, epinephrine, cortisol) than the controls who were simply rocked.
- Children with posttraumatic stress disorder: Children traumatized by Hurricane Andrew were massaged at their schools two times a week for one month. The massaged children had less depression, lower anxiety levels, and lower cortisol (stress hormone) levels than children in the control group.

Although further research is needed to substantiate much of what has been found to date, massage appears to be a promising adjunct to treatment of children with a variety of disorders.

■ COMPLEMENT TO CHIROPRACTIC

Chiropractic care is gaining increasing recognition as an effective treatment for certain conditions. Massage is often given as a complement to chiropractic care to help prepare the body for chiropractic adjustments, to relieve tension and pain in muscles and related soft tissues, and to prevent future musculoskeletal misalignment.

The term *chiropractic adjustment* is used here to mean a technique in which bones and joints are manipulated to return the body to proper alignment. This often involves a forceful thrusting movement or manipulation. Such adjustments are performed on *subluxations,* a condition of misalignment in a joint, which often results in structural, nervous system, and chemical dysfunctions.

Local massage is sometimes used in preparation for an adjustment. Massage relieves muscle tension and warms up the soft tissues in the area, making joints more pliable and more easily adjusted. Massage may be given along with heat and ultrasound in this preparatory routine.

A general massage (½ to 1 hour long) may also be good preparation for an adjustment. In addition to preparing the immediate area of concern, it helps induce general relaxation and accustoms the recipient to touch. The recipient may be more receptive to other hands-on treatment in such a relaxed state. Massage after an adjustment may help the muscles remain relaxed and prevent a tightening reaction to the treatment. Regular massage may help adjustments last longer by keeping muscles relaxed and lengthened.

Therapeutic massage may also be used to address some of the musculoskeletal problems that bring patients for adjustments. These include nerve constriction due to tight muscles, poor circulation, trigger points, damaged tissues, and the pain–spasm–pain cycle. Massage used with ice can help relieve spasming muscles.

▪ PSYCHOLOGIC ASPECTS OF TREATMENT

Massage is increasingly being used to address the psychologic and emotional problems of patients receiving medical treatment. For example, several of the studies mentioned above found massage to be beneficial in the reduction of the anxiety of patients hospitalized for serious medical conditions.

Massage may also help in the treatment of patients with medical conditions significantly worsened by stress. For example, in a study by Joachim (1983), patients with chronic inflammatory bowel disease, ulcerative colitis, or Crohn's disease (ileitis) who received massage for relaxation had fewer episodes of pain and disability from the disease.

Massage may also help patients hospitalized for psychiatric reasons. In a study by Field et al (1992), hospitalized depressed and adjustment-disorder children and adolescents who received massage were less depressed and anxious and had lower saliva cortisol levels (an indication of less depression) than patients who watched relaxation videotapes.

Psychotherapy patients not hospitalized may also benefit from the effects of massage related to stress and anxiety reduction, improved body awareness, and the ability to receive pleasureable nonsexual touch. For example, some massage therapists work with psychotherapists in the treatment of survivors of sexual and physical abuse. Massage has been found to be beneficial in helping these patients reconnect with their bodies, develop a more compassionate relationship with their bodies, and experience their bodies as a "source of groundedness and eventually of strength and even pleasure—good things instead of a bad thing" (Benjamin, 1995, p. 28).

▪ SUMMARY

Massage has been used to treat medical conditions since ancient times. Massage is indicated when it may contribute directly and measurably to the alleviation of a medical condition, or is sometimes indicated as an adjunct to enhance treatment.

Massage is used in different health care professions within their scopes of practice for a variety of effects.

Massage or manual therapy is used routinely for physical rehabilitation and for the treatment of musculoskeletal problems. It has been used effectively by nurses to relax and reduce the anxiety of patients hospitalized with a variety of conditions. Massage is being used with cancer patients to alleviate some of their symptoms and the side effects from cancer treatment procedures. It has also been used effectively to reduce edema from various causes, and manual lymph drainage is useful in treating lymphedema.

Therapeutic Touch, a form of manual therapy that balances the energy field of the recipient, is used for a wide range of conditions. Considerable research has been done within the nursing profession on the applications of Therapeutic Touch.

Massage is sometimes used as a complement to chiropractic care. Local massage may be used to prepare an area for treatment, or general massage may be used to induce relaxation and promote receptivity to manipulation. Massage after an adjustment may help muscles remain relaxed.

Massage is increasingly used to address psychologic and emotional problems of patients. It is found to be beneficial in reducing the anxiety of patients hospitalized for a variety of reasons and in the treatment of psychiatric patients. It may also help reduce the symptoms of conditions that are made worse by stress. Massage is sometimes used as an adjunct to psychotherapy to help reduce anxiety, improve body awareness, and open patients' receptivity to pleasurable nonsexual touch.

■ REFERENCES

Bauer, W. C., & Dracup, K. A. (1987). Physiological effects of back massage in patients with acute myocardial infarction. *Focus on Critical Care, 14*(6), 42–46.

Benjamin, B. E. (1995). Massage and body work with survivors of abuse: Part I. *Massage Therapy Journal, 34*(3), 23–32.

Chamness, A. (1996). Breast cancer and massage therapy. *Massage Therapy Journal, 35*(1, Winter).

Curties, D. (1994). Could massage therapy promote cancer metastasis. *Journal of Soft Tissue Manipulation,* April–May.

de Bruijn, R. (1984). Deep transverse friction; its analgesic effect. *International Journal of Sports Medicine, 5,* 35–36.

Fakouri, C., & Jones, P. (1987). Relaxation RX: Slow stroke back rub. *Journal of Gerontological Nursing, 13*(2), 32–35.

Ferrell-Torry, A. T., & Glick, O. J. (1993). The use of therapeutic massage as a nursing intervention to modify anxiety and the perception of cancer pain. *Cancer Nursing, 16*(2), 93–101.

Field, T. M., Morrow, C., Valdeon, C., et al. (1992). Massage reduces anxiety in child and adolescent psychiatric patients. *Journal of the American Academy of Child and Adolescent Psychiatry, 31*(1), 125–131.

Field, T. M., Schanberg, S. M., Scafidi, F., et al. (1986). Tactile/kinesthetic stimulation effects on preterm neonates. *Pediatrics, 77*(5), 654–658.

Frazer, J., & Kerr, J. R. (1993). Psychophysiological effects of back massage on elderly institutionalized patients. *Journal of Advanced Nursing, 18,* 238–245.

Heidt, P. (1981). Effect of therapeutic touch on anxiety level of hospitalized patients. *Nursing Research, 30*(1), 32–37.

Joachim, G. (1983). The effects of two stress management techniques on feelings of well-being in patients with inflammatory bowel disease. *Nursing Papers, 15*(5), 18.

Karpen, M. (1995). Dolores Kreiger, Ph.D., R.N.: Tireless teacher of Therapeutic Touch. *Alternative & Complementary Therapies,* April/May, 142–146.

Keller, E., & Bzdek, V. M. (1986). Effects of therapeutic touch on tension headache pain. *Nursing Research, 35*(2), 101–106.

Kramer, N. A. (1990). Comparison of therapeutic touch and casual touch in stress reduction of hospitalized children. *Pediatric Nursing, 16*(5), 483–485.

Kurz, W., Wittlinger, G., Litmanovitch, Y. I., et al. (1978). Effect of manual lymph drainage massage on urinary excretion of neurohormones and minerals in chronic lyphedema. *Angiology, 29,* 64–72.

MacDonald, G. (1995). Massage for cancer patients: A review of nursing research. *Massage Therapy Journal,* Summer, 53–56.

Rattray, F. S. (1994). *Massage therapy: An approach to treatments.* Toronto, Ontario, Canada: Massage Therapy Texts and MAVerick Consultants.

Rhiner, M., Ferrell, B. R., Ferrell, B. A., & Grant, M. M. (1993). A structured non-drug intervention program for cancer pain. *Cancer Practice, 1,* 137–143.

Sims, S. (1986). Slow stroke back massage for cancer patients. *Nursing Times, 82,* 47–50.

Time-Life Books. (1987). *The age of god-kings: Timeframe 3000–1500 B.C.* Alexandria, VA: Time Life Books.

Tope, D. M., Hann, D. M., & Pinkson, B. (1994). Massage therapy: An old intervention comes of age. *Quality of Life—A Nursing Challenge, 3,* 14–18.

Weinrich, S. P., & Weinrich, M. C. (1990). The effect of massage on pain in cancer patients. *Applied Nursing Research, 3,* 140–145.

Wheeden, A., Scafidi, F., Field, T., et al. (1993). Massage effects on cocaine-exposed preterm neonates. *Developmental and Behavioral Pediatrics, 14*(5), 318–322.

Witt, P. L., MacKinnon, J. (1986). Trager psychosocial integration: a method to improve chest mobility of patients with chronic lung disease. *Physical Therapy, 66*(2), 214–217.

Zanolla, R., Monzeglio, C., Balzarini, A., & Martino, G. (1984). Evaluation of the results of three different methods of postmastectomy lymphedema treatment. *Journal of Surgical Oncology, 26,* 210–213.

26

The Art of Healing Touch

Frances M. Tappan

The art of healing touch is a two-way street. A massage that includes the client or patient as a partner will be remarkably more effective than one given as a mere technique of body manipulation. The practitioner who devotes total attention by communicating concern, empathy, and a sincere desire to promote the healing process will spur the receiver of massage to participate more fully in the effort toward regaining health.

The mutual objective of both the practitioner and the recipient is to replace the recipient's dependency with a collaborative effort. To establish this relationship, the client or patient must participate in discussions that include an exchange of ideas, rather than simply receive instructions given by the practitioner. Such an approach will strengthen positive attitudes and minimize feelings of despair.

A pleasant atmosphere, the exchange of laughter, a sense of strength or determination, and feelings of love will strongly encourage the human body toward its own constant search for homeostasis. The body itself will then produce more complicated and comprehensive chemotherapy than is available at any medical center in the world—be it via Eastern or Western medical approaches.

While giving massage, one can encourage the receiver to understand the potential source of healing in his or her own consciousness. The recipient can be encouraged not to be helpless, passive, depressed, or desperate, but rather capable and active in his or her own treatments. According to Bernie Siegle, "The body heals, not the therapy . . . the body can utilize any form of energy for healing . . . even plain water—as long as the patient believes in it" (1986a, p. 129). Everyone wants to love and be loved. Skillful encouragement can stimulate the human body's defense and healing mechanisms

Current research done with plants, animals, and human beings is proving that positive effects are possible through the "laying-on of hands." In an experiment conducted in 1964, Bernard Grad used barley seeds that had been soaked in saline to simulate a "sick" condition. Oskar Estebany worked with Grad as a "healer" and held flasks of water as he would were he doing laying on of hands. An identical saline flask of barley seeds was not treated by the laying-on of hands. The seeds held by Estebany sprouted more quickly, grew taller, and contained more chlorophyll.

In the book *The Secret Life of Plants* (1973), Peter Tompkins and Christopher Bird recorded how Cleve Backster proved without doubt that plants respond if touched with affection. By using lie detector equipment he confirmed Grad's studies that plants respond to loving care and soft music in a positive way. Conversely, they respond negatively to hard rock music and feelings of hate.

In fact, Backster conceived a threat that he would burn an actual leaf of a dracaenia plant to which his lie machine galvanometer was attached. The instant he got the picture of a flame in his mind, and before he could move for a match, there was a dramatic change in the tracing pattern on the graph in the form of a prolonged upward sweep of the recording pen. Backster had not moved either toward the plant or toward the recording machine. Could the plant have been reading his mind?

In fact, there is a lamp on the market, the base of which holds potted plants. When a leaf is touched, a light bulb will go on. A three-way light bulb will cycle through low, medium, and high to off, each time a leaf is touched. During demonstrations, the light refused to go on although the pot had been recently watered. After several people had tried to transfer enough energy to light the bulb and had failed, the demonstrator suggested that the plant must be thirsty and requested a glass of water that was handed to her in a paper cup. Before the plant had even been touched (in fact, the cup of water was at least four inches from the plant), the lamp light turned on. The demonstrator pulled her hand back and the light went off, again before being touched at all. This plant was considered further proof of Backster's theory that plants respond to human thought or mental intent.

In Eastern cultures the transference of attitudes between the healer and the subject is believed to occur via a state of matter for which Western culture has neither a word nor a concept. It is called *prana* in Sanskrit. The nearest translation in English is vitality or vigor. The Chinese call it *chi,* which translates as energy. Regardless of what it is called, however, this phenomenon refers to the balanced functioning of the human body and the vital life force of energy, which keeps people in good physiologic and psychologic health. Think of the world as having a "collective consciousness" and join the "self" to that strength. Lessen thoughts of yourself as "only one."

Advocates of this concept believe that positive energy can be transferred from the healer to the patient through touch (via any medical approach—pulse reading, acupuncture, or more modern medical methods) to return the patient to normal health. They also believe that it is absolutely necessary for the patient to have faith in the healer and to possess a strong will to get well. In an article called *Love Medicine* (1986b), Siegel tells of a woman in the hospital who visualized her X-ray therapy as a "golden beam of sunshine entering her body." He also believes that people set up defenses against sharing their innermost feelings with anyone. If they feel their ability to love shriveling up, they create a vicious cycle that leads to further despair. Anger can really be a cry for help.

Massage and other therapies that are performed with the practitioner's hands are some of the best ways to transfer the strong healing energy from the giver to the receiver. In a controlled study, Kreiger (1976) proved that Therapeutic Touch, or the laying-on of hands, is a uniquely effective human act of healing. Her results showed significant measurable changes in hemoglobin values of patients after receiving Therapeutic Touch. By touching with the intent to help or heal, the patient would feel that heat within the area beneath the hand. Recipients reported feeling profoundly relaxed and having a sense of well-being.

In *Anatomy of an Illness as Perceived by the Patient* (1979), Norman Cousins records how he became, with his doctor, William Hitzig, a participant in the accomplishment of his own recovery. Together they proved that a cheerful atmosphere and an open-minded exchange of ideas related to recovery actually reduced the high sedimentation rate causing his illness. He achieved an almost complete recovery and returned to functional health.

Such attitudes do not develop without concentrated effort on the part of the healer and the one desiring to be healed. All patients are individuals with problems, physical problems that create mental attitudes that may vary all the way from complete rejection of treatment to complete cooperation. Before treating a patient, explain what the treatment will accomplish. Always try to find out what the patient is thinking and feeling by listening more than talking. Work with the patient. Inspire the patient's confidence with a positive attitude that implies that your knowledge and skill are available. This also means that the healer cannot afford to display any personal, negative feelings regardless of anger or rudeness on the part of the patient. A healer's firm, controlled strength of character can guide the patient toward acceptance and belief that the treatment is beneficial.

Sick people become dependent on others in many cases. The health practitioner should strive to replace patient dependency with self-sufficiency; identify important life goals; and eliminate the patient's feelings of despair and loneliness. This can be done by exchanging ideas and sharing knowledge.

Fear can be depressing, if not deadly, so everything possible should be done to strengthen positive attitudes. The atmosphere should always be pleasant. Direct sunlight from windows with a pleasant view is helpful. Tropical fish tanks and tranquil music help the surroundings to be peaceful and interesting. Harmonious relationships should be encouraged.

Illness often follows a crisis that creates a sense of hopelessness and despair. Some theories suggest that each person is ultimately responsible for both illness and the recovery. People from all aspects of health care can help each body in their own special way, but no body is going to heal unless the body itself decides to heal.

The therapist can be most effective by taking careful note of the whole patient at the first moment of contact. Body language can speak louder than words. You can determine how a person feels by the look in her eyes, the way he holds his head, the slump of her shoulders, his tone of voice, or even by noting whether he or she seems to feel happy or depressed.

Above all, the therapist needs to convince the patient that the treatment being given is going to bring relief from pain and recovery from depression. Each patient needs loving support, understanding, a purpose for living, and some sense of satisfaction related to the efforts put forth on his or her behalf.

If massage is to be "healing," both the giver and the receiver will be comfortable with the idea that shared energy and unconditional love provide strong motivation toward healing. Look for the love and light in people. This exchange of healing energy comes in many forms other than massage. It can occur through group concerns with people who share similar problems. People can interact negatively or positively. Never forget, "four hugs a day keep the blues away." People can accept or reject, even subconsciously, the positive energy being extended in their surrounding external environment.

Health practitioners who use touch in their work are in a particularly advantageous position to transfer healing energy by the way in which art, skill, and knowledge are shown during treatment. Each person being treated should be understood by the practitioner as much as possible, relative to the importance of feeling relaxed and at peace, to encourage the caring, loving energy of healing.

There was the case of a dying cancer patient who said to her therapist, "I wish someone would talk to me more about dying! My doctor always changes the subject and my own family refuses to talk about it." The therapist giving massage answered, "You can say anything you want to me." For the remainder of the session they discussed death and the patient's basic beliefs in positive terms.

One person can be terrified under stressful situations, and die of a heart attack. Another person can face the same situation with no terror at all. Those people who are often terrified or angry about situations that occur are less likely to respond to the extension of healing energy.

If you ask seriously ill patients if they would like to live, may of them will say, "No." Nevertheless, ask the same seriously ill people if they would like to live and feel physically well and active, and most of them will say, "Yes!" Do not make the mistake of assuming that all seriously ill people really want to die. An understanding of death at any age is a must for all practitioners, because so many dying people truly need the loving touch of massage.

The human body and mind are ONE. All health practitioners should be aware of their own individual status and know whether they are balanced enough to enhance the healing energy they hope to deliver. They should know how to "center" their own energy toward the well-being of their patients.

In class or group sessions, "energy breaks" may be used to keep the positive energy flowing. One technique is to interrupt the presentation and interject without introduction, "Reach out and touch someone." Responses in the group will vary from those who refuse to touch or to be touched, to those who are not satisfied merely to touch but go beyond, even to a hug. It may take several such breaks in a large group before each member trusts the others enough to transfer any healing energy. These breaks can "sneak in" when people learn to trust, and they may be varied as follows:

- Reach out and touch someone.
- Now reach out, touch someone with a warm, caring touch.

- Find a sensitive, painful spot and touch it gently, projecting healing thoughts, and with warmth.
- Massage the tension away from a painful area.

After asking them to "reach out and touch someone," ask each person to make a fist. Tell the person immediately nearby to open the fist. Reaction will range from those who voluntarily open their own fists to those who strongly resist having anyone try to force their fists open. What does this tell us? People are all different, depending on their internal environment and in how they respond to external stimulation.

The author has witnessed a wide range of reactions. Actually, if one is attempting to get a group of strangers into a peaceful state of mind, it is the responsibility of the leader to use instinct, observation, conversation, and careful notation of the peoples' acceptance or resistance to the idea. From that information the leader may attempt to establish a positive relationship for maximum healing results.

Those in the healing professions should realize that what they see and feel about "what's going on" is not necessarily so. All of us "perform" constantly. For example, when asked, "How do you feel today?" the typical answer is "Fine!" Actually, that person may have a splitting headache or the flu, but is not willing to discuss it at the present time or with that particular person.

The health practitioner needs to find out how a patient really feels most of the time. Loving, caring people do not always find support in their daily family or working routine. People may feel negative, or they may think, "Just do the job! Get it done!" If so, the practitioner will find it difficult to evoke relaxation in that person.

Many a busy executive enjoys a "quick fix" massage. This could help reduce stress; it might even relax an exhausted person right into a peaceful snooze. A good practitioner will realize whether a "quick fix" is enough and advise accordingly.

Many organizations are now hiring massage practitioners to provide "quick fix massage" twice a week at the workplace. This procedure is too new to evaluate its permanent value toward enhanced well-being and productivity. If it contributes to employees' feeling content with and good about themselves and their work benefits, it may revolutionize the profession of massage.

All levels of the desire or need to be touched exist in a normal population. Some folks are just born to love, to be touched, hugged, held, and appreciated. If they get this in living surroundings, they are peaceful people. Others are born, or learn, to reject close contacts. They prefer a more reserved approach to touch. If a massage practitioner who understands these differences can help such people to be less inward oriented and become more outgoing, then massage as a "stress buster" may have positive, even healing, effects.

Anyone could die from a heart attack when not even under stress. However, if one truly has (not pretends to have) a peaceful inner life, chances are better for a strong immune system, and much greater health and healing is possible. Belief systems are powerful enough to cure or kill, often with dramatic effects.

Those people who stop and ask, "Would I choose to live with myself as I am right now?" and answer "Yes," usually have a super immune system that works to keep the body in balance, and these people are the easiest to relax with massage techniques. One should ask of oneself, "If I had only a year to live, what would I do?" A peaceful soul would reply, "Maximize good living without compulsive goals or impossible dreams. Adjust as peacefully as possible to all of life's ups and downs."

If these are not the answers, people could try to change their basic living style toward that goal. Not everyone can do this, and some who do may find it takes more energy than expected. Then the work of the giving of unconditional love to others becomes more readily received. This is the challenge of change. It is said that nothing is sure but death and taxes. Yet there is one more thing we can be sure of, and that is change. Change can be hard to deal with. A person may want to change his or her inner being. That is not, however, as easy as deciding to do so. Everyone looks at his or her own environment and reacts to it depending on his or her DNA (inherited genes). From birth—or even while in fetal development—change that shapes and forms character begins to occur. There are those who feel that one cannot change life patterns. Asking the question "What is your purpose in life?" could start one on the road to positive thinking. An evaluation of one's total belief system could be the beginning of change, and striving to be at peace with yourself could improve one's immune system. Massage practitioners must ask themselves all these questions before they will be able to transfer healing energy to others.

It is, therefore, not how a person perceives the immediate environment, but what this means to the inner environment that strengthens or weakens the immune system. Some people may react to others' actions with anger, then hide that emotion and smile outwardly. Another one may yell and scream over a similar action. In the long run, the inner selves who cannot cope are the ones who deplete the strength of their immune system and eventually kill themselves, because no other course of action seems available. In short, it is not the environment outside the self that is deadly. Rather, it is the way the inner self feels in relation to the outside environment that can be damaging.

Someone once said that people can be divided into three groups: Those who make things happen, those who watch things happen, and those who wonder what happened! It is the practitioner's responsibility to encourage the patient to do all in his or her power to "make things happen."

■ SUMMARY

It should be firmly emphasized that the terms *healing* or *the healer* do not refer to the mystical or occult. It is a proven fact that one is much more likely to achieve the balance of health and happiness with positive attitudes than with negative feelings. The importance of touch, particularly as it relates to massage, can make the difference between healing and the lack of it. Recently more emphasis has been placed on holistic methods of healing, such as control of the autonomic nervous system using imagery, love, touching, and stressing the importance of attitude.

▪ REFERENCES

Cousins, N. (1979). *Anatomy of an illness as perceived by the patient: Reflections on healing and regeneration.* New York: Norton.

Grad, B. et al. (1964). A telekinetic effort on plant growth, part 2. Experiments involving treatment with saline in stoppered bottles. *International Journal of Parapsychology, 6,* 473.

Krieger, D. (1976). Nursing research for a new age. *Nursing Times, 72* (April), 1.

Siegel, B. S. (1986a). *Love, medicine & miracles.* New York: Harper & Row.

Siegel, B. S. (1986b). Love medicine. *New Age Journal, 50* (April), 512.

Tompkins, P., & Bird, C. (1973). *The secret life of plants.* New York: Avon.

VI

Supplemental Learning Materials

Summary Charts
of Comparative Techniques

The following summary chart shows the results of a survey done by Frances Tappan in 1948 comparing the massage techniques of three of the pioneers of physical therapy in the early twentieth century with practitioners in the late 1940s. The three pioneers were Albert Hoffa of Germany, James Mennell of England, and Mary McMillan of the United States. The 25 graduate operators interviewed were from 15 different schools. These schools were: D.T. Watson School of Physical Therapy (Leetsdale, PA); Children's Hospital (Los Angeles); Harvard University, Medical School, Courses for Graduates (Boston); University of Southern California (Los Angeles); Mayo Clinic (Rochester, MN); University of Minnesota (Minneapolis); Northwestern University, Medical School (Chicago); New York University, School of Education (New York City); Stanford University (Stanford, CA); University of Wisconsin, Medical School (Madison, WI); Reed College (Army training school, Portland, OR); Fitzsimmons General Hospital (Army training school, Denver); O'Reilly General Hospital (Army training school, Springfield, MO); Walter Reed General Hospital (Army training school, Washington DC); and The Institute of Southern Sweden (Stockholm).

To prevent any one school from influencing the results, not more than three from each school were interviewed. In some instances, when the operator was teaching in one school but a graduate of another, the information gathered was considered representative of the school in which that person was currently teaching.

SUMMARY CHART OF COMPARATIVE TECHNIQUES

TABLE A–1

Question	Hoffa	McMillan	Mennell	Conclusions from Questionnaire Results
1. Are there any exceptions to following the venous flow?	The only exception is in the massage of the back, where the stroke may go in either direction	No exceptions are made	Exceptions include superficial stroking and following the principle of beginning away from the injured area	The trend seems to be progressively toward making exceptions to following the venous flow as Mennell does
2. What do you consider adequate treatment time for the back, a limb, and total body?	6 to 10 min is used for back or limb and 15 min for whole body	10 to 15 min is recommended for beginners to use for the back or limb and not more than 50 min for a general massage	Treatment time must depend on the pathology and reaction of the patient. No time can be suggested	Treatment time must be adjustable to the pathology and reactions of the patient, but average between 10 to 20 min for back or limb and up to 45 for the whole body, which is more than Hoffa recommends and similar to McMillan's suggested time
3. What do you prefer as a medium?	Anything to make the part pliable can be used	Dry rubbing is preferred but for certain pathologies oil, cocoa butter, or lanolin is suggested	Mennell's prescription combines oil of Bergamot and French chalk	Except in cases where pathology demands one or the other, choice of medium is up to the therapist, as Hoffa suggests
4. Do you massage by muscle groups or is massage done by other anatomic divisions of the body?	All massage is done by dividing the body into various muscle groups	Some areas are divided by muscle groups and others, such as the back, are divided using other anatomic landmarks	Only the fact that one begins away from the injured part and works toward it, is mentioned as to how the area is covered	The majority of operators still divide the body into specific muscle groups for massage as Hoffa does
5. Is the most proximal part of the limb massaged before the distal?	Every description of a part to be massaged progresses from the distal aspect of the limb to the proximal	Descriptions progress from the distal aspect of the limb to the proximal	The proximal aspect of a limb should always be massaged before the more distal	The practice of massaging the most proximal aspect of a limb before the distal as Mennell recommends is now being widely used
6. Is the whole extremity or back effleuraged before petrissage is begun?	Each muscle or muscle group is given effleurage and petrissage before the next group is begun	Massage of the leg is done by giving effleurage to the whole lower leg and then petrissage	No definite routine in this respect is stated	Most operators are still following the technique of massaging each muscle or muscle group with effleurage and petrissage before going to the next group as Hoffa does, rather than effleuraging a whole part and then giving it petrissage

7. Is the patient always placed in a recumbent position?	The only time that the patient is in a recumbent position is in massage of the back, and even here the patient may be in a seated position	The patient is always in a recumbent position unless pathology is such that this position cannot be held comfortably	The patient is preferred in a recumbent position, but each patient must be considered individually. Thus sitting, or even standing, positions may be used if necessary	Most massage to the upper extremity is done with the patient in a seated position. The tendency seems to be that of making exceptions to the recumbent position as Mennell does
8. Which parts are usually supported, (1) in a back-lying position; and (2) in a face-lying position?	(1) No back-lying position is described; (2) no mention of support is made with reference to the face-lying position	(1) A rolled towel is placed under the knee; (2) a small pillow is placed under the abdomen	(1) Support is placed under the knee; (2) the body is supported in slight hyperextension for back massage, with one pillow under the legs and another under the chest	(1) Knees are supported in the back-lying position as by McMillan and Mennell; (2) most people follow the technique of McMillan and support the abdomen, and all but three support the ankles or have them over the edge of the plinth (table)
9. What arm position is preferred when the patient is face-lying?	The arms are "out horizontally"	Arms are shown in T position and also down at the sides	Arms are folded over the head (chest is supported by a pillow which relieves weight on the arms)	McMillan's two positions are the ones used the most (T and at the sides), but the patient's comfort and ability to relax is the primary guide for selection of arm position
10. In massage of the lower extremity is the patient usually turned from back-lying to face-lying?	The patient is turned to make the posterior thigh more accessible and is placed on the side to massage the tensor fascia lata	The patient is not usually turned, but may be if pathologic conditions are such that it seems best to do so	The patient is turned to make the posterior thigh more accessible	McMillan's policy of not turning the patient unless pathology indicates its necessity seems to be followed
11. Must the part being massaged always be in elevation?	Hoffa seems to prefer a neutral position	All illustrations show the part in a neutral position	Elevation is preferred whenever possible	Following Hoffa and McMillan, the trend is still that of elevating the part for pathologic conditions and treating it otherwise in a neutral position
12. Is emphasis placed on stance of the therapist?	No reference is made to stance	No reference is made to stance	Mennell mentions the operator should stand at the side of the table and not at the end. One should be comfortable, with no strain on the back or knees	Little emphasis other than good body mechanics is placed on stance by everyone

Question	Hoffa	McMillan	Mennell	Conclusions from Questionnaire Results
13. Do you alternate sides of the table during massage of the back?	The operator is instructed to move to the opposite side of the back when doing the other side	No reference is made as to alternating sides of the table in massage of the back	Mennell does alternate sides of the table during a back massage	McMillan and the majority of the operators do not alternate sides of the table during massage of the back
14. Do you always massage in a standing position?	Most of the massage is done with the operator or seated, even in giving a massage to the back	All illustrations show the operator in a standing position	It is advised that all massage be done in a standing position	Whereas people do not remain seated to the extent that Hoffa did, neither do they stand without exception. Hands and forearms are usually done with the operator seated
15. Do you usually repeat a given stroke any particular number of times before progressing to a different stroke?	Hoffa refers to repeating a stroke "three or four" times but sets up no definite routine	Suggestions for "three or four" strokes are included in descriptions. The number of strokes vary up to six and no set number is recommended	Mennell makes no reference to number of strokes to be given	The trend seems to be moving away from grouping strokes by numbers as indicated by the lack of mention of such in Mennell's text, and the fact that the majority of the people interviewed do not do so, except as a guide for beginners, which may have been all the basic texts meant it for
16. Does return stroke always maintain contact?	Hoffa seems not to maintain contact with his return stroke	The hand should return to its original position without pressure but without losing contact with the part being massaged	The return stroke does not always maintain contact with the body, particularly with superficial stroking	McMillan's technique of maintaining contact on the return stroke is being used by most operators
17. Do you ever "stroke off" a whole area, such as the back, the upper extremity, or the lower extremity?	No description of such a technique can be found in Hoffa's text	The back is stroked off when each division has been effleuraged and on the forearm as a final stroke	Mennell's "superficial stroking" is similar but of a superficial nature only	McMillan's influence has been felt in that the majority use this technique

USE OF THE VARIOUS STROKES

Question	Hoffa	McMillan	Mennell	Conclusions from Questionnaire Results
1. Which of the effleurage strokes are used?	Hoffa describes the use of light and deep stroking; knuckling; circular effleurage; thumb stroking; alternate-thumb stroking; simultaneous stroking	McMillan describes the use of light and deep stroking; simultaneous stroking; alternate-hand stroking	Mennell describes the use of superficial stroking; deep effleurage; simultaneous stroking	The majority of the operators use an effleurage that is predominantly the same, light and deep stroking, and simultaneous stroking. Alternate-hand stroking, which was mentioned by McMillan, is widely used as well as one-hand-over-the-other for deeper pressure. Also of note is the tendency for the operator to pick up Mennell's idea of superficial stroking, although they do not do it in the prescribed manner
2. Which of the petrissage strokes are used?	Hoffa describes the use of petrissage which is one-handed; two-handed (with flat hand for large flat surfaces and pickup where possible); two-fingered	McMillan describes the use of petrissage, which is one-handed; two-handed; with alternate hands; finger and thumb; for small areas; flat-handed on the back	Mennell describes use of kneading (circular movements in opposite directions); petrissage (raising muscle mass away from subjacent tissues); one-handed	Hoffa's techniques for petrissage are predominantly in use; McMillan's two-hand petrissage and Mennell's are very similiar and this stroke is used by some
3. Which of the friction strokes are used?	Hoffa describes the use of friction that uses the thumb; the index finger; both thumb and index finger	McMillan describes the use of friction that uses the thumb; two or three fingers; the thenar eminence	Mennell describes friction that uses any part of the hand, but especially the tips of the fingers or the balls of the thumbs	Use of the heel of the hand and one-over-the-other for pressure are not described by any of the basic texts, but are being used widely. Other techniques concerning friction are predominantly the same, except for the few people who combine friction and petrissage into a stroke that resembles both strokes

Table A–2 (Continued)

Question	Hoffa	McMillan	Mennell	Conclusions from Questionnaire Results
4A. Is tapotement used routinely? B. Which of the tapotement strokes are used?	A. Tapotement is used routinely B. Hacking is the only tapotement stroke that is described	A. McMillan describes the use of tapotement routinely for a general massage B. Tapotement strokes described are hacking, clapping, tapping, beating	A. Mennell describes the use of tapotement but does not use it routinely B. He describes the use of hacking, clapping, beating	A. Whereas Hoffa used tapotement routinely and McMillan described its use in a general massage, Mennell states that he does not use it routinely and the majority of the people surveyed use it for certain pathologic conditions only. B. Use of the various strokes is fairly uniform
5. How is vibration used?	Hoffa does vibration either with the points of the fingers or with a flat hand but advises the use of a mechanical vibrator	McMillan describes vibration as being done with one finger or several and also with the flat hand	Mennell believes that the hand is a poor substitute for a mechanical vibrator	Although described by all three of the basic texts, it is used very little
6. Which other strokes are used?	None	The five fundamental procedures can form the basis for a large variety of manipulations	Mennell describes "shaking" in which the hand grasps the part giving quick firm vibrations that shake it from side to side. He also mentions a stroke that is similar to friction, but it is applied in a transverse plane to the muscle fibers	Horizontal stroking for the low back is rather widely used although very few have a name for this stroke. Mennell's frictionlike stroke, which is done in a transverse plane, is used by some. Although used by only a few, Storms's technique for nodules has made some impression in this country

Organizations and Publications

■ ORGANIZATIONS

American Massage Therapy Association
820 Davis Street Suite 100
Evanston, IL 60201-4444
(847) 864–0123

AMTA Foundation
744 Thayer Avenue
Silver Spring, MD 20910
(301) 585–7240 or (301) 589–0123

American Oriental Bodywork Association
(AOBTA)
Suite 510, Glendale Executive Park
1000 White Horse Road
Voorhees, NJ 08043
(609) 782–1616

American Polarity Therapy Association
2888 Bluff Street Suite 149
Boulder, CO 80301
(303) 545–2080

Amma Institute of Traditional Japanese
Massage
1881 Post Street
San Francisco, CA 94115
(415) 564–1103

Associated Bodywork & Massage
Professionals
28677 Buffalo Park Road
Evergreen, CO 80439-7347
(800) 458–2267 or (303) 674–8478

Commission on Massage Training
Accreditation/Approval (COMTAA)
820 Davis Street Suite 100
Evanston, IL 60201-4444
(847) 864–0123

Dr. Vodder School—North America
P.O. Box 5701
Victoria, British Columbia, Canada, V8R 6S8
(604) 598–9862

International Institute of Reflexology
P.O. Box 12642
St. Petersburg, FL 33733-2642
(813) 343–4811

Jin Shin Do® Foundation for Bodymind
Acupressure™
1084G San Miguel Canyon Road
Watsonville, CA 95076
(408) 763–7702

MFR Treatment Center & Seminars
  (Myofascial Release)
Routes 30 & 252
10 South Leopard Road, Suite 1
Paoli, PA 19301
(610) 644–0136

NANMT (National Association of Nurse
  Massage Therapists)
P.O. Box 67
Tuckahow, NY 10707
(914) 961–3251

National Certification Board for Therapeutic
  Massage and Bodywork (NCBTMB)
8201 Greensboro Drive, Suite 300
McLean, VA 22102
(800) 296–0664 or (703) 610–9015
http:\\www.NCBTMB.com

North American Vodder Association
  of Lymphatic Therapy (NAVALT)
P.O. Box 861
Chesterfield, OH 44026
(216) 729–3258

Nurse Healers–Professional Associates, Inc.
P.O. Box 444
Allison Park, PA 15101
(412) 355–8476

Skilled Touch Institute of Chair Massage
584 Castro Street #555
San Francisco, CA 94114–2578
(415) 621–6817
70411,335@Compuserve.Com

Touch Research Institute
University of Miami School of Medicine
Department of Pediatrics
P.O. Box 016820
Miami, FL 33101

▪ PUBLICATIONS

Massage & Bodywork Quarterly
(Publication of Associated Bodywork
  & Massage Professionals, ABMP)
28677 Buffalo Park Road
Evergreen, CO 80439-7347
(800) 458–2267 or (303) 674–8478

Massage Therapy Journal
(Publication of the American Massage Therapy
  Association, AMTA)
820 Davis Street Suite 100
Evanston, IL 60201-4444
(847) 864–0123

MASSAGE Magazine
1315 W. Mallon
Spokane, WA 99201
(800) 872–1282

Boards Administering
Massage Practice Laws*

ALABAMA
(*note: at press time, Alabama's Board information was not available. Please contact the member of the Alabama Massage Therapy Board below for an update*)
Ron Pate
One Independence Plaza,
Suite 305
Birmingham, AL 35209
(205) 879–3949

ARKANSAS
Arkansas State Board of
  Massage Therapy
PO Box 34163
Little Rock, AR
72203-4163
(501) 682–9170

CONNECTICUT
Connecticut Massage
  Therapy Inquiries

Department of Public Health
150 Washington St.
Hartford, CT 06106
(860) 509–7566

DELAWARE
Committee on
  Massage/Bodywork
  Practitioners
Cannon Bldg., Ste. 203
PO Box 1401
Dover, DE 19903
(302) 739–4522

DISTRICT OF COLUMBIA
Department of Consumer
  and Regulatory Affairs
Occupational and Professional
  Licensing Administration
Room 910
614 H St., NW
Washington, DC 20001
(202) 727–7823

FLORIDA
Florida Department of
  Professional Regulation
Board of Massage
Northwood Center
1940 N. Monroe St.
Tallahassee, FL
32399-0774
(904) 488–6021

HAWAII
State of Hawaii Professional &
  Vocational Licensing Division
Department of Commerce
  & Consumer Affairs
PO Box 3469
Honolulu, HI 96801
(808) 586–3000
  or (808) 586–2699

IOWA
Board of Massage Therapy
  Examiners

*From: The American Massage Therapy Association 1996–97 Membership Registry (printed with permission).

Iowa Department of Public
Health
Lucas State Office Bldg. 4th Fl.
Des Moines, IA 50319-0075
(515) 242–5937

LOUISIANA
Louisiana Board of Massage
Therapists
P.O. Box 1279
Zachary, LA 70791
(504) 658–8941

MAINE
Department of Professional
& Financial Regulation
Licensing & Enforcement
Division
35 State House Station
Augusta, ME 04333-0035
(207) 624–8603

MARYLAND
Maryland Board of Chiropractic
Examiners
4201 Patterson Ave.
Baltimore, MD 21215-2299
(410) 764–4726

NEBRASKA
State of Nebraska
Department of Health
Bureau of Examining Boards
301 Centennial Mall South,
3rd Floor
PO Box 95007
Lincoln, NE 68509-5007
(402) 471–2115

NEW HAMPSHIRE
Bureau of Health Facilities
Administration
Division of Public Health
Services
Health and Welfare Bldg.
6 Hazen Dr.
Concord, NH 03301-6527
(603) 271–4592

NEW MEXICO
Board of Massage Therapy

Regulation and Licensing
Department
PO Box 25101
Santa Fe, New Mexico 87504
(505) 827–7013

NEW YORK
New York State Educational
Department
Division of Professional
Licensing Services
Cultural Education Ctr.
Albany, NY 12230
(518) 473–1417
or (518) 474–3866
for handbook: (518) 474–3800

NORTH DAKOTA
North Dakota Massage Board
Albert Dahlgren RMT
22 Fremont Dr.
Fargo, ND 58103
(701) 235–9208
or (701) 237–4036

OHIO
State Medical Board
77 South High St.
17th Fl.
Columbus, OH 43215
(614) 466–3934

OREGON
Oregon Board of Massage
Technicians
407B State Office Bldg.
800 NE Oregon St., #21
Portland, OR 97232
(503) 731–4064

RHODE ISLAND
Rhode Island Department
of Health
Division of Professional
Regulation, Room 104
Cannon Bldg.
3 Capitol Hill
Providence, RI 02908
(401) 277–2827

SOUTH CAROLINA
South Carolina Department
of Labor
Licensing and Regulation
3600 Forest Drive
PO Box 11329
Columbia, SC 29211
(803) 734–4294

TENNESSEE
Health Related Boards
Attn: Massage Therapy
283 Plus Park Blvd.
Nashville, TN
32747-1010
(615) 367–6393

TEXAS
Texas Department of Health
Massage Therapy Program
1100 West 49th St.
Austin, TX 78756-3138
(512) 834–6616

UTAH
State of Utah Department
of Commerce
Division of Occupational and
Professional Licensing
Heber M. Wells Bldg.
160 E. 300 South
PO Box 45805
Salt Lake City, Utah 84145-0805
(801) 530–6628

VIRGINIA
Virginia Board of Nursing
6606 West Broad St.
Richmond, VA 23230
(804) 662–9909

WASHINGTON
State of Washington Department
of Health
HPQA Division
Health Professions
Section One
PO Box 1099
Olympia, WA 98507-1099
(360) 586–6351

Please note: *The above listings reflect information available at the time of publication. Please contact each board directly to obtain the most current information.*

For the states not listed above, refer to local or county government.

There are some 3,100 counties and 7,200 cities, towns, townships, and villages in the United States, as listed in *County Executive Directory* and *Municipal Executive Directory* (Caroll Publishing Co., Washington, DC, updated several times a year). Your local public library should have these or similar directories. You can easily and quickly obtain contact addresses and phone numbers for any local or county official, sometimes just by telephoning your library. Usually the city attorney, mayor, or county commissioner's office is the contact that will provide direct information about the regulation of massage practice.

For additional information, contact the AMTA chapter in the state. It may also be helpful to contact an AMTA massage therapist practicing in the locality.

Local laws may apply even in states with statewide licensing. In addition to massage ordinances and statutes, local business and zoning laws must be checked before setting up a massage practice.

If you experience difficulty in contacting any of the above state boards, please call AMTA for assistance at (847) 864–0123.

Performance Evaluation Forms

The performance evaluation, or practical testing, of massage techniques and their applications is important in the educational setting. Students benefit from receiving feedback about their performance as they are learning how to give safe and effective massage. Teachers need to determine if students have achieved a minimum level of competency.

The following forms are offered as examples of a format that can be used in giving performance evaluations to students of massage. The general format takes into consideration the need for giving a numerical value or grade to what is in many ways a subjective evaluation. It also honors the teachers' more intuitive sense of how students are grasping the material to be learned, while encouraging them to be specific about what they are seeing.

One of the most important elements in developing an evaluation instrument is determining which items will receive evaluation. These are based generally on the learning outcomes stated for the course of study. The following instruments have been developed for evaluating performance of the classic massage techniques described in Chapter 6; the application of skills in giving a full-body massage session as described in Chapter 8; and the application of skills in giving treatment to a specific part of the body, for a specific medical condition, or to a special population as described throughout the text.

The rating scale used is from 0 to 5. Zero indicates total incompetence; 1 = very poor; 2 = poor; 3 = adequate; 4 = good; 5 = excellent. A simple way for evaluators to use the rating scale is to first determine whether students are adequate (rating = 3) using their experience and judgment in observing performance, and taking into consideration all relevant factors. If students are not at least "adequate," evaluators can identify specific factors that are detracting from the performance and determine if the rating is 2, 1, or 0. If students appear more than adequate, evaluators can identify specific factors that make the performance good or excellent and choose a rating of 4 or 5. Reasons for the rating given and ways to improve performance may be noted in the "comments" section. The more specific evaluators can be about what they are looking for, the more objective and consistent evaluations will be.

The comments section of the form provides a place for evaluators to identify the factors they observed that had an impact on the rating. For example, an observation that the student forgot to put a bolster under the knees of a recipient who was supine might help account for the rating given for "positioning." Students receive specific feedback about their performance from the comments. In this sense, an evaluation may also be a learning tool.

In the school setting, translating a rating into a grade is a matter of determining the level of competence desired in students who pass a course or section of a course. In some situations, an average rating of 3 or adequate may be deemed satisfactory or passing. Other situations may call for more than adequate for a passing grade. Traditional schools may need to translate numerical evaluations into A, B, C, D, or F grades. These performance evaluation forms provide a basis for assigning grades, but do not dictate what a passing grade is. The particular school or teacher needs to take that next step in assigning grades.

■ PERFORMANCE EVALUATION OF INDIVIDUAL MASSAGE TECHNIQUES: CLASSIC WESTERN MASSAGE

Student's Name: Date of Evaluation:
Evaluator's Name: Class:

0 = incompetent; 1 = very poor; 2 = poor; 3 = adequate; 4 = good; 5 = excellent

Effleurage techniques slide or glide over the skin with a smooth continuous motion.

Technique/Rating   **Comments**

1. Basic sliding effleurage

    0   1   2   3   4   5

2. Bilateral tree stroking

    0   1   2   3   4   5

3. Three-count stroking of the trapezius

    0   1   2   3   4   5

4. Horizontal stroking

    0   1   2   3   4   5

5. Mennell's superficial stroking

    0   1   2   3   4   5

6. Nerve strokes

    0   1   2   3   4   5

7. Knuckling

    0   1   2   3   4   5

8. Sedating effleurage of the back

    0   1   2   3   4   5

Petrissage techniques lift, wring, or squeeze soft tissues in a kneading motion; or press or roll the tissues under or between the hands.

9. Basic two-handed kneading

    0   1   2   3   4   5

10. One-handed kneading

   0 1 2 3 4 5

11. Alternating one-handed kneading

   0 1 2 3 4 5

12. Circular two-handed petrissage

   0 1 2 3 4 5

13. Alternating fingers-to-thumb petrissage

   0 1 2 3 4 5

14. Skin rolling

   0 1 2 3 4 5

15. Compression

   0 1 2 3 4 5

Friction is performed by rubbing one surface over another repeatedly.

16. Superficial warming friction

   0 1 2 3 4 5

17. Sawing friction

   0 1 2 3 4 5

18. Superficial friction using knuckles

   0 1 2 3 4 5

19. Deep cross-fiber friction

   0 1 2 3 4 5

20. Circular deep friction

   0 1 2 3 4 5

Tapotement consists of a series of brisk percussive movements following each other in rapid, alternating fashion.

21. Hacking

   0 1 2 3 4 5

22. Cupping

0   1   2   3   4   5

23. Clapping

0   1   2   3   4   5

24. Slapping

0   1   2   3   4   5

25. Tapping

0   1   2   3   4   5

26. Pincement

0   1   2   3   4   5

27. Quacking

0   1   2   3   4   5

Vibration may be described as an oscillating, quivering, or trembling motion; or movement back and forth, or up and down, performed quickly and repeatedly.

28. Fine vibration with fingertips

0   1   2   3   4   5

29. Light effleurage with vibration

0   1   2   3   4   5

30. Shaking—coarse vibration

0   1   2   3   4   5

31. Jostling—coarse vibration

0   1   2   3   4   5

Touch without movement

32. Passive touch

0   1   2   3   4   5

33. Direct static pressure

0   1   2   3   4   5

Total Points _____/33 = _____ Average Rating   Student's Name:

▪ PERFORMANCE EVALUATION OF FULL-BODY MASSAGE

Student's Name: Date of Evaluation:
Evaluator's Name: Class:

0 = incompetent; 1 = very poor; 2 = poor; 3 = adequate; 4 = good; 5 = excellent

Items	Comments

1. Professional demeanor

    0   1   2   3   4   5

2. Environment

    0   1   2   3   4   5

3. Draping

    0   1   2   3   4   5

4. Positioning the receiver

    0   1   2   3   4   5

5. Body mechanics

    0   1   2   3   4   5

6. Use of lubricant

    0   1   2   3   4   5

7. Organization of session

    0   1   2   3   4   5

8. Application of techniques

    0   1   2   3   4   5

9. Pressure

    0   1   2   3   4   5

10. Rhythm and pacing

    0   1   2   3   4   5

11. Safety considerations

    0   1   2   3   4   5

12. Overall effectiveness

    0   1   2   3   4   5

Total points _____ /12 = _____ Average Rating   Student's Name:

▪ PERFORMANCE EVALUATION OF MASSAGE TREATMENT

Student's Name: Date of Evaluation:
Evaluator's Name: Class:

Special condition/assessment/diagnosis: _____ .

Part of body treated: _____ .

Treatment goals: _____ .

0 = incompetent; 1 = very poor; 2 = poor; 3 = adequate; 4 = good; 5 = excellent

Items for Evaluation	**Comments**

1. Professional demeanor

    0   1   2   3   4   5

2. Environment

    0   1   2   3   4   5

3. Draping

    0   1   2   3   4   5

4. Positioning the receiver

    0   1   2   3   4   5

5. Body mechanics

    0   1   2   3   4   5

6. Choice of techniques (appropriateness)

    0   1   2   3   4   5

7. Skill in application of techniques

    0   1   2   3   4   5

8. Adjunct modalities used

    0   1   2   3   4   5

9. Organizations of session

    0   1   2   3   4   5

10. Safety precautions observed

    0   1   2   3   4   5

11. Effectiveness of treatment

    0   1   2   3   4   5

Total points _____/11 = _____**Average Rating**   **Student's Name:**

Health History Forms
for Massage Therapy

Health history information is essential for planning safe and effective massage sessions. In the wellness model, health information is used to plan massage sessions that help the receiver progress further along the path to high-level wellness. In the treatment model, information about medical conditions, diagnoses from health care providers, and treatment goals help the therapist apply massage to alleviate the condition for which massage is indicated.

An important purpose of health history information is to alert the practitioner to situations for which massage is contraindicated, or for which special cautions apply. The receiver may not be aware that massage can be harmful under certain limited conditions, and so it is the practitioner's responsibility to gather enough information to make such a judgment. Certain areas of the body may be avoided, certain techniques omitted, or applications modified based on information from health history.

The following two examples of health history forms may serve as models for developing a written form that fits your practice and your potential clients or patients. One form may be used to gather information for a general wellness session, and the other asks for more detailed medical information.

■ HEALTH HISTORY FOR MASSAGE THERAPY—GENERAL WELLNESS

Name _____ Date of initial visit ——————————

Address _____ Phone _____

Occupation _____ Date of birth _____

Sports/physical activities/hobbies _____

The following information will be used to help plan safe and effective massage sessions. Please answer to the best of your knowledge.

1. Have you had professional massage before?　Yes　No

2. Do you have any difficulty lying on your front, back, or side?　Yes　No

   If yes, please explain _____

3. Do you have allergic reactions to oils, lotions, ointments, liniments, or other substances put on your skin?　Yes　No

   If yes, please explain _____

4. Do you wear contact lenses (　) dentures (　) a hearing aid (　)?

5. Do you sit for long hours at a workstation, computer, or driving?　Yes　No

   If yes, please describe _____

6. Do you perform any repetitive movement in your work, sports, or hobby?　Yes　No

   If yes, please describe _____

7. Do you experience stress in your work, family, or other aspect of your life?　Yes　No

   If yes, how do you think it has affected your health? muscle tension (　) anxiety (　) insomnia (　) irritability (　) other _____

8. Is there a particular area of the body where you are experiencing tension, stiffness, or other discomfort?　Yes　No

   If yes, please identify _____

9. Do you have any particular goals in mind for this massage session?　Yes　No

   If yes, please explain _____

In order to plan a massage session that is safe and effective, we need some general information about your medical history.

10. Are you currently under medical supervision?   Yes   No

    If yes, please explain _____

11. Are you currently taking any medication?   Yes   No

    If yes, please list _____

12. Please check any condition listed below that applies to you:

_____ contagious skin condition	_____ joint disorder
_____ open sores or wounds	rheumatoid arthritis
_____ easy bruising	_____ osteoporosis
_____ recent accident or injury	_____ epilepsy
_____ current fever	_____ headaches
_____ swollen glands	_____ cancer
_____ allergies	_____ epilepsy
_____ heart condition	_____ diabetes
_____ high or low blood pressure	_____ decreased sensation
_____ circulatory disorder	_____ recent surgery
_____ contagious skin condition	_____ joint disorder
varicose veins	_____ artificial joint
atherosclerosis	
phlebitis	

Comments:

_____

_____

_____

13. For women: Are you pregnant?   Yes   No   If yes, how many months?_____

14. Is there anything else about your health history that you think would be useful for your massage practitioner to know to plan a safe and effective massage session for you?

    _____

    _____

    _____

I understand that these massage sessions are for general wellness purposes and that I should see a doctor or other appropriate health care provider for diagnosis and treatment of any suspected medical problem. Also, that it is my responsibility to keep my massage practitioner informed of any changes in my health, and any medications that I may begin to take in the future.

Signature _____ Date _____

■ HEALTH HISTORY FOR MASSAGE THERAPY TREATMENT

Name _____ Date of initial visit _____

Address _____ Phone _____

Occupation _____ Date of birth _____

Name of physician _____ Phone _____

Other health care provider_____

Referred by _____

1. Have you had massage therapy before?   Yes   No

2. For women: Are you pregnant?   Yes   No   If yes, how many months?_____

3. Do you have any difficulty lying on your front, back, or side?   Yes   No

   If yes, please explain _____

4. Do you have allergic reactions to oils, lotions, ointments, liniments, or other substances put on your skin?   Yes   No

   If yes, please explain _____

5. Do you wear contact lenses ( ) dentures ( ) a hearing aid ( )?

6. Do you sit for long hours at a workstation, computer, or driving?   Yes   No

   If yes, please describe _____

7. Do you perform any repetitive movement in your work, sports, or hobby?   Yes   No

   If yes, please describe _____

8. Do you experience stress in your work, family, or other aspect of your life?   Yes   No

   How would you describe your stress level?   Low   Medium   High   Very high

   If high, how do you think stress has effected your health? muscle tension ( ) anxiety ( ) insomnia ( ) irritability ( ) other _____

9. Is there a particular area of the body where you are experiencing tension, stiffness, or other discomfort?   Yes   No

    If yes, please identify _____

In order to plan a massage session that is safe and effective, we need some general information about your medical history.

10. Are you currently under medical supervision?   Yes   No

    If yes, please explain _____

11. Are you currently taking any medication?   Yes   No

    If yes, please list _____

12. Please check any condition listed below that applies to you:

    _____ Skin condition (eg, acne, rash, skin cancer, allergy, easy bruising, contagious condition)

    _____ Allergies

    _____ Recent accident, injury, or surgery (eg, whiplash, sprain, broken bone, deep bruise)

    _____ Muscular problems (eg, tension, cramping, chronic soreness)

    _____ Joint problems (eg, osteoarthritis, rheumatoid arthritis, gout, hypermobile joints, recent dislocation)

    _____ Lymphatic condition (eg, swollen glands, nodes removed, lymphoma, lymphedema)

    _____ Circulatory or blood conditions (eg, atherosclerosis, varicose veins, phlebitis, arrhythmias, high or low blood pressure, heart disease, recent heart attack or stroke, anemia)

    _____ Neurologic condition (eg, numbness or tingling in any area of the body, sciatica, damage from stroke, epilepsy, multiple sclerosis, cerebral palsy)

    _____ Digestive conditions (eg, ulcers)

    _____ Immune system conditions (eg, chronic fatigue, HIV/AIDS)

    _____ Skeletal conditions (eg, osteoporosis, bone cancer, spinal injury)

    _____ Headaches (eg, tension, PMS, migraines)

    _____ Cancer

    _____ Emotional difficulties (eg, depression, anxiety, panic attacks, eating disorder, psychotic episodes). Are you currently seeing a psychotherapist for this condition?   Yes   No

    _____ Previous surgery, disease, or other medical condition that may be affecting you now (eg, polio, previous heart attack or stroke, previously broken bones)

Comments:

_____

_____

_____

13. Is there anything else about your health history that you think would be useful for your massage practitioner to know to plan a safe and effective massage session for you?

_____

_____

_____

14. Has your physician or other health care provider recommended massage for any of the conditions listed above?   Yes   No

If yes, please explain _____

15. Do you have any particular goals in mind for this massage session related to any of the conditions mentioned above?   Yes   No

If yes, please explain _____

I understand that I should see a doctor or other appropriate health care provider for diagnosis and treatment of any suspected medical problem. It may be beneficial for my massage practitioner to speak to my doctor about my medical condition to determine how massage may help the healing process, and to avoid worsening the condition. I will be asked for permission to contact my doctor, if the massage practitioner thinks that it might be useful. I also understand that it is my responsibility to keep my massage practitioner informed of any changes in my health, and any medications that I may begin to take in the future.

Signature _____ Date _____

Glossary

Active movements are performed voluntarily by a person with no or some assistance from a practitioner. Types of active movements are free, assistive, and resistive.

Acupressure is a Western term for a form of bodywork based in traditional Chinese meridian theory in which acupuncture points are pressed to stimulate the flow of energy or *chi*.

Amma is a form of traditional Japanese massage.

Assistive movements are a type of active movement in which the recipient initiates the movement, and the practitioner helps perform the movement.

Benefits are positive outcomes. The benefits of massage are experienced by recipients when the effects of massage support their general health and well-being.

Body mechanics refers to the posture of the practitioner when performing massage. Good body mechanics is the use of the body in a structurally and mechanically sound way to maximize the effectiveness and safety of performing massage techniques.

Bodywork is a general term for practices involving touch and movement in which the practitioner uses manual techniques to promote health and healing in the recipient. The healing massage techniques described in this text are considered forms of bodywork.

Chair massage refers to massage given with the recipient seated in an ordinary or a special massage chair. Receivers remain clothed in chair massage. It has been called "on-site massage" when the chair is taken to a public place such as an office or commercial establishment.

Classic full-body massage refers to a massage session lasting from 30 minutes to 1½ hours, in which traditional Western massage techniques are combined into a routine to address the whole body. These sessions are generally wellness oriented and aim to improve circulation, relax the muscles, improve joint mobility, induce general relaxation, promote healthy skin, and create a general sense of well-being.

Classic massage techniques are those techniques that have been refined over time and remain in use today. The term *classic* suggests simplicity, style, excellence, and enduring value.

Classic Western massage refers to those techniques used traditionally in Europe and the United States since the late nineteenth century, when the word *massage* itself came into general use. The five technique categories commonly used to describe classic Western massage are effleurage, petrissage, tapotement, friction, and vibration.

Contraindications are conditions or situations that make receiving massage inadvisable because of the harm that it might do.

Deep friction is a type of friction in which the practitioner's fingers do not move over the skin, but instead, move the skin over tissues underneath. Cross-fiber and circular friction are the most common types of deep friction.

Deep transverse friction is a specific type of deep friction used in rehabilitation to break adhesions, facilitate healthy scar formation, and treat muscle and tendon lesions. It is performed across the tissues, causing broadening and separation of fibers. Deep transverse friction was popularized by James Cyriax.

Direct pressure, or **direct static pressure,** is the application of force to compress tissues in a specific spot; it is usually applied with a thumb, finger or fingers, elbow, or knuckles. It can be considered a form of compression without movement and has also been called **static friction.**

Draping refers to the use of sheets, towels, or other materials to cover recipients of massage to preserve their privacy and modesty, to maintain professional boundaries, and for warmth.

Effects of massage refers to the basic physiologic and psychologic changes that occur to the recipient during a massage session.

Overall effectiveness of a massage performance refers to the degree to which intended goals are achieved and to which the recipient is satisfied.

Effleurage is a classic Western massage technique category that includes movements that slide or glide over the body with a smooth continuous motion.

Endangerment sites are areas of the body where delicate body structures are less protected and, therefore, may be more easily damaged when receiving massage.

Environment for massage includes the room, air quality, lighting, sound, dressing arrangements, equipment, and overall cleanliness and neatness of the space in which a session is given.

Esalen massage is a genre of bodywork based on a simplified form of classic Western massage, whose main purpose is to enhance non-verbal connection with the inner self and with others. It emphasizes the sensual aspectes of massage. It was developed at the Esalen Institute in Big Sur, California in the 1970's as part of the Human Potential Movement.

Free active movements or **free exercises** are performed entirely by a person with no assistance from a practitioner.

Friction is a classic Western massage technique category that includes movements that rub one surface over another repeatedly and includes superficial and deep friction.

General contraindications are conditions or situations that make receiving *any* massage inadvisable because of the harm that it might do.

Healing means enhancing health and well-being and the process of regaining health or optimal functioning after an injury, disease, or other debilitating condition. "To heal" means to make healthy, whole, or sound; restore to health; or free from ailment.

Holistic massage refers to those forms of massage that take into account the wholeness of human beings, ie, body, mind, emotions, and spirit.

Indication is used in the treatment model to mean that when a specific medical condition is present, a particular modality is indicated or advised to alleviate the condition. Massage is indicated as a treatment for a number of medical conditions.

Jin Shin Do® is a modern synthesis of traditional Chinese acupressure/acupuncture theory and techniques, breathing exercises, Taoist philosophy, and modern psychology. It was developed by Iona Marsaa Teeguarden in the 1970s in the United States.

Joint manipulations, sometimes called adjustments or chiropractic adjustments, refer to techniques that take a joint beyond its normal range of motion and that are specific attempts to realign a misaligned joint, usually using a thrusting movement. Joint manipulations are not part of classic Western massage and are not within the scope of this text.

Joint movements, or mobilizations, are passive movements performed within the normal pattern and range of joint motion. Joint movements cause motion in the soft tissues surrounding joints, stimulate circulation and the production of synovial fluid, aid muscle relaxation, and increase kinesthetic awareness.

Local contraindications are conditions or situations that make receiving massage on a particular part of the body inadvisable because of the harm that it might do; also called **regional contraindications.**

Lubricants are topical substances used in some massage sessions to enhance the effects of techniques and to minimize skin friction. Common lubricants include liniments, vegetable and mineral oils, jojoba, lotions, and combinations of these substances.

Manual lymph drainage is a form of massage designed to assist the function of the lymphatic system by the application of slow, light, and repetitive strokes that help move lymph fluid through the system of vessels and nodes.

Massage is the intentional and systematic manipulation of the soft tissues of the body to enhance health and healing. Joint movements and stretching are commonly performed as part of massage. The primary characteristics of massage are touch and movement.

Massage therapy is a general term for health and healing practices involving touch and movement, which are based in massage and related manual techniques. It is sometimes used synonymously with the term **bodywork**. The term *massage therapy* has been adopted by some massage practitioners to define their profession, which is a licensed profession in many states.

Modality is a method of treating a medical condition. Massage is considered a modality in the tradition of physiotherapy, along with other modalities such as ice packs, hot packs, ultrasound, or whirlpool baths.

Myofascial massage is a general term for techniques aimed at restoring mobility in the body's fascia and softening connective tissue that has become rigid. It is sometimes called myofascial release, or myofascial unwinding.

Pacing refers to the speed of performing techniques, which may vary from very slow to very fast for different effects.

Passive movements are body movements initiated and controlled by the practitioner, while the recipient remains totally relaxed and passive.

Passive touch is simply laying the fingers, one hand, or both hands lightly on the body. Passive touch may impart heat to an area, have a calming influence, or help balance energy.

Petrissage is a classic Western massage technique category that includes movements that lift, wring, or squeeze soft tissues in a kneading motion; or press or roll the soft tissues under or between the hands.

Polarity therapy is a form of bodywork that uses simple touch and gentle rocking movements with the intention to balance life energy by affecting general and muscular relaxation. It was developed by Randolph Stone in the mid-twentieth century.

Positioning the receiver refers to placing the recipient of massage in a position (eg, supine, prone, side-lying, seated) to maximize his or her comfort and safety. Bolsters and other props may be used to support specific body areas.

Practitioner refers to someone trained in massage techniques and who uses massage in the practice of his or her profession.

Pressure is related to the force used in applying techniques and to the degree of compaction of tissues as techniques are applied. The amount of pressure used in massage will depend on the intended effect and the tolerance or desires of the recipient.

Professional demeanor refers to the appearance, language, and behavior of practitioners, which meets professional standards and inspires trust and respect.

Organization of a session refers to the overall structure of a massage session into beginning, middle, and end; the progression from one section of the body to another; and the ordering of techniques into sequences. Organization includes the use of opening techniques, transitions, and finishing techniques.

Reflexology is a form of bodywork based on the theory of zone therapy, in which specific spots of the body are pressed to stimulate corresponding areas in other parts of the body. **Foot reflexology,** in which pressure techniques are applied only to the feet, is the most common form of reflexology.

Resistive movements are a type of active movement in which the practitioner offers resistance to the movement, thereby challenging the muscles used.

Rhythm refers to a recurring pattern of movement with a specific cadence, beat, or accent and may be described as smooth, flowing, or uneven.

Scope of practice describes the legally allowed, or professionally accepted, methods used by practitioners, as well as the intention in performing them. Different professions have different scopes of practice as defined by law or by the profession. Massage techniques fall within the scope of practice of several professions.

Session refers to a period of time in which massage is given to a recipient by a practitioner. Sessions have logical organization, have a wellness or a treatment purpose, and generally vary from 10 minutes to two hours.

Shiatsu is a general term for Japanese bodywork based in traditional Chinese meridian theory and Western science, in which *tsubo* (ie, acupoints) are pressed to balance the flow of energy or *ki*.

Sports massage is the science and art of applying massage and related techniques to ensure the health and well-being of the athlete and to enhance athletic performance. The major applications of sports massage are recovery, remedial, rehabilitation, maintenance, and event (ie, pre-, inter-, and post-event).

Stretching is a passive movement performed to the limit of the range of motion of a joint. Stretching increases flexibility at the joint, lengthens the muscles and connective tissues that cross the joint, and helps relax muscles involved.

Superficial friction is a type of friction in which the hand rubs briskly back and forth over the skin to improve circulation in superficial tissues and to create heat.

Swedish massage is a genre of bodywork that includes classic Western massage, Swedish movements, various forms of hydrotherapy, heat lamps, and other modalities. Swedish massage is a popular form of massage found in health clubs, spas, and resorts. The hey day of Swedish massage was from about 1920 to 1950 in the United States.

Tapotement is a classic Western massage technique category consisting of brisk percussive movements that are performed in rapid rhythmic fashion. The most common classic forms of tapotement are hacking, rapping, cupping, clapping, slapping, tapping, and pincement.

Technique refers to the technical aspects of the application of massage, or how the body moves while performing massage. The broader concept of the term technique also includes the intent.

Touch means "to come into contact with." Massage practitioners touch their clients or patients in many ways, but primarily with their hands. Touch may happen on a physical or an energetic level.

Touch without movement is a type of classic massage technique in which the practitioner comes in contact with the recipient either physically or energetically, but no perceptible movement occurs that fits into the five traditional classic Western massage categories. Two common types of touch without movement are passive touch and direct static pressure.

Treatment refers to interventions aimed at alleviating a specific medical condition.

Treatment model is a concept that explains the intention of using specific interventions or modalities to alleviate medical conditions.

Trigger points are small hyperirritable spots in muscle or related connective tissue that may cause local pain or pain in a distant referral zone. Trigger points may be relieved manually with ischemic compression techniques, deep friction, deep stripping, and stretching.

Vibration is a classic Western massage technique category that includes oscillating, quivering, or trembling movements; or movement of soft tissues back and forth, or up and down, performed quickly and repeatedly. Vibration may be described as fine or coarse (eg, shaking, jostling).

Wellness refers to a condition of optimal physical, emotional, intellectual, spiritual, social, and vocational well-being.

Wellness massage is massage performed with the intention of promoting the receiver's general well-being. It goes beyond the treatment of specific conditions to help the receiver achieve high-level wellness.

Wellness model is a concept that explains the intention of behaviors aimed at living a healthy and vibrant, meaningful life. It goes beyond the idea of the absence of disease and emphasizes personal responsibility.

Bibliography

Academy of Traditional Chinese Medicine. (1975). *An outline of Chinese acupuncture.* Peking: Foreign Language Press.

Alternative medicine: Expanding medical horizons: A report to the National Institutes of Health on alternative medicine systems and practices in the United States. (1994). Available from the Office of Alternative Medicine, National Institutes of Health, 6120 Executive Blvd #450, Rockville, MD 20892-9904.

Arano, L. C. (1976). *The medieval health handbook: Tacuinum sanitatis.* New York: George Braziller.

Armstrong, D., & Armstrong, E. M. (1991). *The great American medicine show: Being an illustrated history of hucksters, healers, health evangelists, and heroes from Plymouth Rock to the present.* New York: Prentice Hall.

Armstrong, M. E. (1972). Acupuncture. *American Journal of Nursing,* September.

Barnes, J. F. (1987). Myofascial release. *Physical Therapy Forum,* September 16.

Bauer, W. C., & Dracup, K. A. (1987). Physiological effects of back massage in patients with acute myocardial infarction. *Focus on Critical Care, 14*(6), 42–46.

Baumgartner, A. J. (1947). *Massage in athletics.* Minneapolis, MN: Burgess.

Beals, K. R. (1978). Clubfoot in the Maori: A genetic study of 50 kindreds. *New Zealand Medical Journal, 88,* 144–146.

Beard, G., & Wood, E. C. (1964). *Massage principles and techniques.* Philadelphia: W. B. Saunders.

Bell, A. J. (1964). Massage and the physiotherapist. *Physiotherapy,* 50, 406–408.

Benjamin, B. E. (1995). Massage and bodywork with survivors of abuse: Part I. *Massage Therapy Journal, 34*(3), 23–32.

Benjamin, P. J. (1989). Eunice D. Ingham and the development of foot reflexology in the United States. Part one: The early years—to 1946. *Message Therapy Journal,* Spring, 38–44.

Benjamin, P. J. (1989). Eunice D. Ingham and the development of foot reflexology in the United States. Part two: On the road 1946–1974. *Message Therapy Journal,* Winter, 49–55.

Benjamin, P. J. (1993). Massage therapy in the 1940's and the College of Swedish Massage in Chicago. *Massage Therapy Journal, 32*(4), 56–62.

Benjamin, P. J. (1994). *On-site therapeutic massage: Investment for a healthy business.* Information brochure. Rockford, IL: Hemingway Publications.

Benjamin, P. J. (1996). The California revival: Massage therapy in the 1970–80's. Presentation at the AMTA National Education Conference in Los Angeles, CA, June.

Benjamin, P. J., & Lamp, S. P. (1996). *Understanding sports massage.* Champaign, IL: Human Kinetics.

Bilz, F. E. (1898). *The natural method of healing: A new and complete guide to health.* Translated from the latest German edition. Leipiz: F. E. Biltz.

Bohm, M. (1913). *Massage: Its principles and techniques.* Translated by Elizabeth Gould. Philadelphia: Lippincott.

Brown, C. C. (ed.). (1984). *The many facets of touch.* Skillman, NJ: Johnson & Johnson Baby Products Company.

Byers, D. C. (1991). *Better health with foot reflexology.* St. Petersburg, FL: Ingham Publishing.

Cailliet, R. (1981). *Shoulder pain,* 2nd ed. Philadelphia: F. A. Davis.

Cailliet, R. (1988). *Soft tissue pain and disability,* 2nd ed. Philadelphia: F. A. Davis.

Cantu, R. I., & Grodin, A. J. (1992). *Myofascial manipulation: Theory and clinical application.* Gaithersburg, MD: Aspen Publishers.

Chaitow, L. (1996) *Modern neuromuscular techniques.* London: Churchill Livingston.

Chamness, A. (1996). Breast cancer and massage therapy. *Massage Therapy Journal, 35*(1) Winter.

Chopra, D. (1991). *Perfect health: The complete mind/body guide.* New York: Harmony Books.

Claire, T. (1995). *Bodywork: What type of massage to get, and how to make the most of it.* New York: William Morrow.

Collinge, W. (1996). *The American Holistic Health Association complete guide to alternative medicine.* New York: Warner Books.

Crosman, L. J., Chateauvert, S. R., & Weisburg, J. (1985). The effects of massage to the hamstring muscle group on range of motion. *Massage Journal,* 59–62.

Cunliffe, B. (1978). *The Roman baths: A guide to the baths and Roman museum.* City of Bath: Bath Archeological Trust.

Curties, D. (1994). Could massage therapy promote cancer metastasis? *Journal of Soft Tissue Manipulation,* April–May.

Cyriax, J. H., & Cyriax, P. J. (1993). *Illustrated manual of orthopedic medicine,* 2nd ed. Boston: Butterworth & Heinemann.

de Bruijn, R. (1984). Deep transverse friction: Its analgesic effect. *International Journal of Sports Medicine, 5*(suppl), 35–36.

Downing, G. (1972). *The massage book.* New York: Random House.

Dychtwald, K. (1977). *Body-mind.* New York: Jove Publications.

Eisenberg, D. M., Kessler, R. C., Foster, C., Norlock, F. E., Calkins, D. R., & Delblanco, T. L. (1993). Unconventional medicine in the United States. *The New England Journal of Medicine, 328*(4), 246–252.

Fakouri, C., & Jones, P. (199) Relaxation RX: Slow stroke back rub. *Journal of Gerontological Nursing, 13*(2), 32–35.

Fay, H. J. (1916). *Scientific massage for athletes.* London: Ewart, Seymour & Co.

Ferrell-Torry, A. T., & Glick, O. J. (1993). The use of therapeutic massage as a nursing intervention to modify anxiety and the perception of cancer pain. *Cancer Nursing, 16*(2), 93–101.

Field, T. M., Fox, N., Pickens, J., Ironsong, G., & Scafidi, F. (1993). Job stress survey. Unpublished manuscript, Touch Research Institute, University of Miami School of Medicine. Reported in *Touchpoints: Touch Research Abstracts, 1*(1).

Field, T. M., Morrow, C., Valdeon, C., et al. (1992). Massage reduces anxiety in child and adolescent psychiatric patients. *Journal of the American Academy of Child and Adolescent Psychiatry, 31*(1), 125–131.

Field, T. M., Schanberg, S. M., Scafidi, F., et al. (1986). Tactile/kinesthetic stimulation effects on preterm neonates. *Pediatrics, 77*(5), 654–658.

Fitzgerald, W. H., & Bowers, E. F. (1917). *Zone therapy.* Columbus, OH: I. W. Long.

Ford, C. W. (1993). *Compassionate touch: The role of human touch in healing and recovery.* New York: Simon & Schuster.

Fraser, J., & Kerr, J. R. (1993). Psychophysiological effects of back massage on elderly institutionalized patients. *Journal of Advanced Nursing, 18,* 238–245.

Frierwood, H. T. (1953). The place of the health service in the total YMCA program. *Journal of Physical Education, 21.*

Gach, M. R. (1990). *Acupressure's potent points: A guide to self-care for common ailments.* New York: Bantam Books.

Georgii, A. (1880). *Kinetic jottings.* London: Henry Renshaw.

Gordon, R. (1979). *Your healing hands. The polarity experience.* Santa Cruz, CA. Unity Press.

Grafstrom, A. (1904). *A text-book of mechano-therapy (massage and medical gymnastics), prepared for the use of medical students, trained nurses, and medical gymnasts.* Philadelphia: W. B. Saunders.

Graham, D. (1884). *Practical treatise on massage.* New York: Wm. Wood and Co.

Graham, D. (1902). *A treatise on massage, its history, mode of application and effects.* Philadelphia: Lippincott.

Heidt, P. (1981). Effect of therapeutic touch on anxiety level of hospitalized patients. *Nursing Research, 30*(1), 32–37.

Hoffa, A. (1978). *Technik der massage,* 13th ed. Stuttgart, Germany: Ferdinand Enke.

Ingham, E. D. (1938). *Stories the feet can tell: Stepping to better health.* Rochester, NY: author.

Issel, C. (1993). *Reflexology: Art, science, & history.* Sacramento, CA: New Frontier Publishing.

Joachim, G. (1983). The effects of two stress management techniques on feelings of well-being in patients with inflammatory bowel disease. *Nursing Papers, 15*(5), 18.

Johnson, W. (1866). *The anatriptic art.* London: Simpkin, Marshall & Co.

Jordan, K., & Osborne-Sheets, C. (1995). *Maternity massage.* Somatic Learning Associates.

Juhan, D. (1987). *Job's body: A handbook for bodywork.* Barrytown, NY: Station Hill Press.

Kaard, B., & Tostinbo, O. (1989). Increase of plasma beta endorphins in a connective tissue massage. *General Pharmacology, 20*(4), 487–489.

Keller, E., & Bzdek, V. M. (1986). Effects of therapeutic touch on tension headache pain. *Nursing Research, 35*(2), 101–106.

Kellogg, J. H. (1923). *The art of massage.* Battle Creek, MI: Modern Medicine Publishing Co.

Kellogg, J. H. (1929) *The art of massage: A practical manual for the nurse, the student and the practitioner.* Battle Creek, MI: Modern Medicine Publishing Co.

King, R. K. (1996). *Myofascial massage therapy: Towards postural balance.* Self-published training manual by Bobkat Productions, Chicago.

King, R. K. (1993) *Performance massage.* Champaign, IL: Human Kinetics.

Knaster, M. (1996). *Discovering the body's wisdom.* New York: Bantam.

Kramer, N. A. (1990). Comparison of therapeutic touch and casual touch in stress reduction of hospitalized children. *Pediatric Nursing, 16*(5), 483–485.

Kresge, C. A. (1983). Massage and sports. In O. Appenzeller & R. Atkinson (eds.), *Sports medicine: Fitness, training, injuries* (pp. 367–380). Baltimore: Urban & Schwarzenberg.

Kunz, K., & Kunz, B. (1982). *The complete guide to foot reflexology.* Englewood Cliffs, NJ: Prentice-Hall.

Kurz, W., Wittlinger, G., Litmanovitch, Y. I., et al. (1978). Effect of manual lymph drainage massage on urinary excretion of neurohormones and minerals in chronic lymphedema. *Angiology, 29,* 64–72.

Kurz, I. (1986). *Introduction to Dr. Vodder's manual lymphatic drainage.* Vol. 2, therapy 1. Heidelberg: Haug Publishers.

Kurz, I. (1990). *Introduction to Dr. Vodder's manual lymphatic drainage.* Vol. 3, therapy 2. Heidelberg: Haug Publishers.

Leboyer, F. (1982). *Loving hands: The traditional art of baby massage.* New York: Alfred A. Knopf.

Ling, P. H. (1840). The general principles of gymnastics. In *The collected works of P. H. Ling.* (1866). Stockholm, Sweden. Translated by Lars Agren and Patricia J. Benjamin. Unpublished.

Ling, P. H. (1840). Notations to the general principles. In *The collected works of P. H. Ling.* (1866). Stockholm, Sweden. Translated by Lars Agren and Patricia J. Benjamin and published in *Massage Therapy Journal,* Winter 1987.

Ling, P. H. (1840). The means or vehicle of gymnastics. Translated by R. J. Cyriax. *American Physical Education Review, 19*(4), April 1914.

MacDonald, G. (1995). Massage for cancer patients: A review of nursing research. *Massage Therapy Journal,* Summer, 53–56.

MacKenzie, J. (1923). *Angina pectoris.* London: Henry Frowde and Hodder and Stoughton.

Masunaga, S. (1983). *Keiraku to shiatsu.* Yokosuka: Ido-No-Nihonsha.

Masunaga, S., & Ohashi, W. (1977). *Zen shiatsu.* Tokyo: Japan Publications.

McGarey, W. A. (1974). *Acupuncture and body energies.* Phoenix: Gabriel Press.

McKenzie, R. T. (1915). *Exercise in education and medicine,* 2nd ed. Philadelphia: W. B. Saunders.

McMillan, M. (1921). *Massage and therapeutic exercise.* Philadelphia: W. B. Saunders.

McMillan, M. (1925). *Massage and therapeutic exercise,* 2nd ed. Philadelphia: W. B. Saunders.

Mennell, J. B. (1945). *Physical treatment,* 5th ed. Philadelphia: Blakiston.

Miesler, D. W. (1990). *Geriatric massage techniques: Topics for bodyworkers no. 2.* Guerneville, CA: Day-Break Productions.

Montagu, A. (1978). *Touching: The human significance of the skin,* 2nd ed. New York: Harper & Row.

Monte, T., & the Editors of EastWest Natural Health. (1993). *World medicine: The EastWest guide to healing your body.* New York: Putnam.

Murrell, W. (1890). *Massotherapeutics or massage as a mode of treatment.* Philadelphia: Blakiston.

Namikoshi, T. (1969). *Japanese finger-pressure, shiatsu.* Tokyo: Japan Publications.

Namikoshi, T. (1969). *Shiatsu.* San Francisco: Japan Publications.

Namikoshi, T. (1981). *The complete book of shiatsu therapy.* Tokyo: Japan Publications.

Nelson, D. (1994). *Compassionate touch: Hands-on caregiving for the elderly, the ill, and the dying.* Barrytown, NY: Station Hill Press.

Nissen, H. (1889). *A manual of instruction for giving Swedish movement and massage treatment.* Philadelphia: F. A. Davis.

Nissen, H. (1920). *Practical massage and corrective exercises with applied anatomy.* Philadelphia: F. A. Davis.

Norman, L., & Cowan, T. (1988) *Feet first: A guide to foot reflexology.* New York: Simon & Schuster.

Ohashi, W. (1976). *Do-it-yourself shiatsu.* New York: E. P. Dutton.

Omura, Y. (1982). *Acupuncture medicine.* Tokyo: Japan Publications.

Ostom, K. W. (1905). *Massage and the original Swedish movements.* Philadelphia: Blakiston's.

Palmer, D. (1995). What is kata? *TouchPro Massage Manual.* San Francisco: Skilled Touch Institute of Chair Massage.

Palmer, D. (1995). The death of on-site massage? *Massage Therapy Journal, 34*(3), 119–120.

Perrone, B., Stockel, H. H., & Krueger, V. (1989). *Medicine women, curanderas, and women doctors.* Norman, OK: University of Oklahoma Press.

Pollard, D. W. (1902). Massage in training. An unpublished thesis, International Young Men's Christian Association Training School, Springfield, MA.

Posse, N. (1895). *The special kinesiology of educational gymnastics.* Boston: Lothrop, Lee & Shepard.

Prudden, B. (1980). *Pain erasure: The Bonnie Prudden way.* New York: M. Evans.

Prudden, B. (1984). *Myotherapy: Bonnie Prudden's complete guide to pain-free living.* New York: Ballantine Books.

Rattray, F. S. (1994). *Massage therapy: An approach to treatments.* Toronto, Ontario: Massage Therapy Texts and MAVerick Consultants.

Rhiner, M., Ferrel, B. R., Ferrel, B. A., & Grant, M. M. (1993). A structured non-drug intervention program for cancer pain. *Cancer Practice, 1,* 137–143.

Robbins, G., Powers, D., & Burgess, S. (1994) *A wellness way of life,* 2nd ed. Madison, WI: Brown & Benchmark.

Roth, M. (1851). *The prevention and cure of many chronic diseases by movements.* London: Churchill.

Sampson, C. W. (1926). *A practice of physiotherapy.* St. Louis: C. V. Mosby.

Schneider, Vimala. (1982). *Infant massage: A handbook for loving parents.* New York: Bantam Books.

Serizawa, K. (1972). *Massage, the oriental method.* Tokyo: Japan Publications.

Serizawa, K. (1984). *Effective tsubo therapy.* Tokyo: Japan Publications.

Serizawa, K. (1984). *Tsubo, vital points for oriental therapy.* Tokyo: Japan Publications.

Siedman, M. (1982). *Like a hollow flute: A guide to polarity therapy.* Santa Cruz, CA: Elan Press.

Siegel, A. (1986). *Live energy: The power that heals.* Bridgeport, Dorset, England: Prism Press/Colin Spooner.

Seiger, L., Vanderpool, K., & Barnes, D. (1995). *Fitness and wellness strategies.* Madison, WI: Brown & Benchmark.

Sims, S. (1986). Slow stroke back massage for cancer patients. *Nursing Times, 82,* 47–50.

Stillerman, E. (1992). *Mother-massage: A handbook for relieving the discomforts of pregnancy.* New York: Dell Publishing.

Teeguarden, I. M. (1978). *Acupressure way of health: Jin Shin Do®.* New York/Tokyo:Japan Publications (distributed by Putnam).

Teeguarden, I. M. (1981). *Jin Shin Do® handbook,* 2nd ed. Felton, CA: Jin Shin Do® Foundation.

Teeguarden, I. M. (1987). *Joy of feeling: Bodymind acupressure™*. New York/Tokyo: Japan Publications (distributed by Putnam).

Teeguarden, I. M. (1996). *A complete guide to acupressure.* New York/Tokyo: Japan Publications (distributed by Putnam).

Tope, D. M., Hann, D. M., & Pinkson, B. (1994). Massage therapy: An old intervention comes of age. *Quality of Life—A Nursing Challenge, 3,*14–18.

Torres, (no date). *The folk healer: The Mexican-American tradition of curanderismo.* Kingsville, TX: Nieves Press.

Tsay, R. C. (1974). *Textbook of Chinese acupuncture medicine, general introduction to acupuncture.* Vol. 1. Wappinger Falls, NY: Association of Chinese Medicine and East-West Medical Center.

Travell, J. G., & Rinzler, S. H. (1952). The myofascial genesis of pain. *Postgrad Med, 11,* 425–434.

Travell, J. G., & Simons, D. G. (1983). *Myofascial pain and dysfunction: The trigger point manual.* Baltimore: Williams & Wilkins.

Travell, J. G., & Simons, D. G. (1992). *Myofascial pain and dysfunction: The lower extremeties.* Vol. 2. Baltimore: Williams & Wilkins.

Travis, J. W., & Callander, M. G. (1990). *Wellness for helping professionals.* Mill Valley, CA: Wellness Associates Publications.

Weinrich, S. P., & Weinrich, M. C. (1990). The effect of massage on pain in cancer patients. *Applied Nursing Research, 3,* 140–145.

Wheeden, A., Scafidi, F., Field, T., et al. (1993). Massage effects on cocaine-exposed preterm neonates. *Developmental and Behavioral Pediatrics, 14*(5), 318–322.

Whitt, P. L., & MacKinnon, J. (1986). Trager psychosocial integration: A method to improve chest mobility of patients with chronic lung disease. *Physical Therapy, 66*(2), 214–217.

Wittinger, H., & Wittinger, G. (1986). *Introduction to Dr. Vodder's manual lymphatic drainage.* Vol. 1. (3rd rev. ed.). Heidelberg: Haug Publishers.

Wood, E. C., & Becker, P. D. (1981). *Beard's massage,* 3rd ed. Philadelphia: W. B. Saunders.

Yamamoto, S., & McCarty, P. *The shiatsu handbook.* Eureka, CA: Turning Point Publications.

Yates, J. (1990). *A physicians guide to therapeutic massage: Its physiological effects and their application to treatment.* Vancouver BC, Canada: Massage Therapists Association of British Columbia.

Zanolla, R., Monzeglio, C., Balzarini, A., & Martino, G. (1984). Evaluation of the results of three different methods of postmastectomy lymphedema treatment. *Journal of Surgical Oncology, 26,* 210–213.

Index

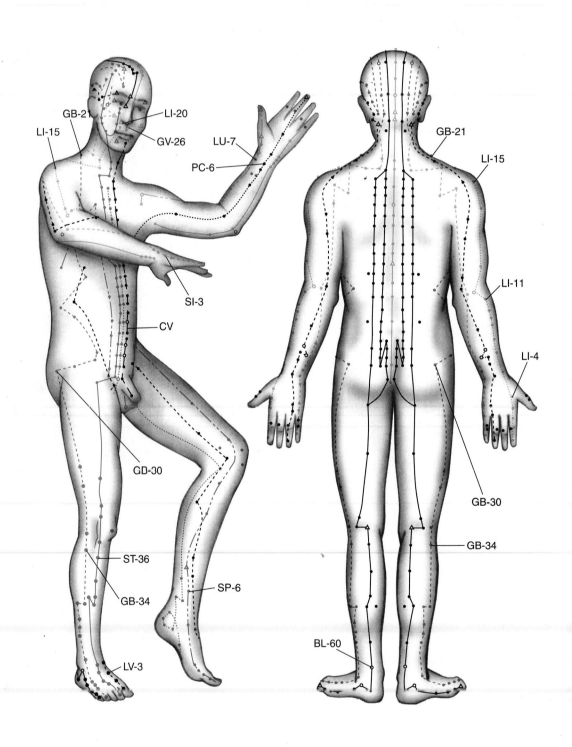